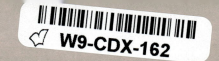

SAFE DELIVERY:
PROTECTING YOUR BABY DURING HIGH RISK PREGNANCY

DEDICATION

To *Angie*,
my wife, for her support,
encouragement and love

ROGER K. FREEMAN, M.D.

To *Ruby Langley West*,
my grandmother, for always
believing in "her Susie"

SUSAN C. PESCAR

SAFE DELIVERY:
PROTECTING YOUR BABY DURING HIGH RISK PREGNANCY

Roger K. Freeman, M.D.
Susan C. Pescar

Facts On File, Inc.
460 Park Avenue South, New York, N.Y. 10016

Safe Delivery:
Protecting Your Baby
During High Risk Pregnancy

by
Roger K. Freeman, M.D. and Susan C. Pescar

Library of Congress Cataloging in Publication Data

Freeman, Roger K.
   Safe delivery.

   Bibliography: p.
   Includes index.
   1. Pregnancy, Complications of. I. Pescar, Susan C.
II. Title.
RG571.F73   618.3   82-1523
ISBN 0-87196-666-2   AACR2

Printed in the United States of America
10 9 8 7 6 5 4 3 2 1

ACKNOWLEDGMENTS

The authors gratefully acknowledge the contributions of and wish to especially thank the following people—who deserve special credit—for their help, suggestions and many hours of work in the development and completion of this book: CHRISTINE A. NELSON, M.D., Associate Adjunct Professor of Pediatrics, University of California, Irvine, and Pediatric Education Coordinator, Miller Children's Hospital, Long Beach, CA; ELEANORA SCHOENEBAUM, Editorial Director, Facts on File, Inc., New York; SUSAN COHAN, copy editor; GLENN COWLEY, our Literary Agent; and ELIZABETH MENZE, research assistant.

We would also like to thank the following people who graciously provided information, art work or photography for the book: (in alphabetical order) *Carol E. Anderson, M.D.*, Assistant Professor of Pediatrics, University of California, Irvine, and Medical Geneticist, Memorial Hospital Medical Center, Long Beach, CA; *Anita Barnette, R.D.M.S.*, Chief Technologist, Department of Diagnostic Ultrasound, Memorial Hospital Medical Center, Long Beach, CA; *Darlene Bullock, R.N., A.C.C.E.*, Labor and Delivery, Women's Hospital, Long Beach, CA; *Christine Friese*, B.S., Executive Secretary, Women's Hospital, Long Beach, CA; *Thomas J. Garite, M.D.*, Assistant Professor of Obstetrics and Gynecology, University of California, Irvine, and Associate Medical Director for Perinatology, Women's Hospital, Long Beach, CA; *Kathy Keiser, M.A.*, Genetics Associate, Long Beach, CA; *Dennis McQuown, M.D.*, Director of Diagnostic Ultrasound, Memorial Hospital Medical Center, Long Beach, CA; *John Melnyk, Ph.D.*, Director of Cytogenetics Laboratories, Memorial Hospital Medical Center, Long Beach, CA; *Ruth E. Redmann, R.N., M.A.*, Coordinator, Perinatal Outreach Education Program, Women's Hospital and Miller Children's Hospital, Long Beach, CA; and *Catherine Rommal, R.N.C.*, Perinatal Nurse Coordinator, Women's Hospital, Long Beach, CA.

CONTENTS

Introduction 1
Section I.   Thinking of Getting Pregnant 5
  1. The Could I Be High-Risk Checklist 7
  2. Some High Risk Problems 10
  3. Risks After 35 48
  4. Teratogens 54
  5. What Everyone Should Know About Birth Defects 81
  6. Problems Many Women May Experience
     During Pregnancy 114
  7. Sex, Exercise and Diet During Pregnancy 124
  8. Competent Obstetrical Care 134
  9. Psychological Effects of A High Risk Pregnancy 141
Section II.   What Advanced Medical Care Can Do 153
  10. A Bird's-Eye View: Ultrasound 158
  11. Diagnosing the Unborn Baby 168
  12. Identifying Problems Early 179
  13. Tests to Determine Fetal Fitness 190
  14. What You Should Know About Labor
      and Delivery 201
  15. Drugs Used to Stop Premature Labor 225
  16. Cesarean Birth 235
Section III.   Perinatal Care 261
  17. The Special Role of the Health Care Team 264
  18. Regionalized Perinatal Care 274
  19. Infant Special Care Units 283
  20. A Glimpse into the Future 294
Glossary 306
Works Consulted 310
Index 311

INTRODUCTION:

ASSISTING THE MIRACLE
OF BIRTH

Thirty years ago this book could not have been written. Comparatively little could then be said or done about problems during pregnancy, labor or delivery—or about caring for the newborn after delivery.

Today—it is an entirely different story—and one well worth telling.

The process of pregnancy and birth is truly miraculous, not only because it results in the production of a new life, but also because, despite the almost infinite chances for disaster, the new person usually enters the world perfectly formed and ready for a life destined to last over 70 years. Nevertheless, more often than most people realize, things can go wrong. This book will attempt to familiarize prospective parents with the risks for less than optimal outcome and the many medical solutions that are now available.

Because of extraordinary advances in what is now called "high-risk obstetrics" (maternal-fetal medicine or perinatology) and specialized care for the sick newborn (neonatology), there is every reason for those who are high-risk to be optimistic about having a safer pregnancy with better results. The fact is—there is a great deal to be excited about and much more progress to look forward to in the near future.

This is where the value and importance of this book come in. Its role is to bridge the gap in parents' knowledge by reporting the results of more than 30 years of medical progress in "giving birth."

We don't have all the answers, because all the answers are not known—nor can all the problems be remedied. But we have tried to put all the pieces together by discussing what medical science does know about high-risk pregnancy and its management, and what can be done to help make a pregnancy safer and optimize its results.

We will look at the issues—the facts—as they are now known and explain them in detail. We hope to give some insight to those who may be high-risk, by discussing the real problems and the real results. We intend to sort out fact from fiction, answer questions and address your concerns. Our purpose is to provide you with an excellent, honest and straightforward reference guide if you're thinking of getting pregnant or are now pregnant.

The book is also an invaluable resource for fathers-to-be, grandparents and others who may not understand what you are talking about or what the doctor meant by a certain test or procedure.

Let's go back. Three decades ago it was much more difficult to identify those at risk for a problem pregnancy—and little could have been done to manage many potential problems even if they had been identified.

No one had yet found a safe and accurate way to evaluate a fetus inside his or her mother's womb; there were no drugs to stop premature labor; a great deal less was known about genetics and the identification of hereditary problems; and if a woman had heart disease, diabetes, hypertension, Rh disease, a kidney disorder, or any other chronic or potentially troublesome medical problem, she was simply discouraged from having children. Such women were told that pregnancy for them would be dangerous—if not disastrous—and it often was.

And for those women over 35 years of age who were having children, little was known about the possible risk of birth defects and congenital disorders. Little was known about being "fit" for pregnancy, or about the importance of prenatal care, following a recommended diet and eliminating the risk of problems due to alcohol use, smoking and certain medications and drugs.

Suddenly a revolution in knowledge occurred after years and years of dedicated, diligent medical research and study. From this new information came exciting and important diagnostic and treatment capabilities. The long, hard work was finally beginning to pay off: Doctors could identify those at risk for many problems, and various genetic disorders could be singled out. When a problem occurred during pregnancy, labor or delivery—many more steps could be taken to either alleviate or lessen it.

The results were promising and have become more so every year. New knowledge and advanced technology have turned the odds in favor of the mother and baby in most instances.

But with all the progress has come some confusion. Much has been reported in the news media about progress in the management of pregnancy and high-risk problems. Along with the praise have come many criticisms, some of which have been well-founded, while others have not. But with so many people saying so many conflicting things—fact and fiction have somehow been jumbled together. With new advances occurring so rapidly, no wonder false or inaccurate information has spread swiftly.

It is important for those who may be or have been identified as high-risk to have the maze unscrambled. What is a high-risk pregnancy? What does it mean for me and my baby? Should my husband and I first have genetic counseling? What is perinatal care? If I am high-risk, what do I do? Whom do I see? What should I expect? What are all these tests everyone is always talking about? Is fetal monitoring a help or a hindrance? Will I need a cesarean section? What role do I play in all this, anyway?

For many women today's advances have allowed them to play a new and exciting role in giving birth. For many who would have been told 30 years ago that they should not try to have children or that they could not have children, the new technology has given them a special lease on life. For many women, having the pregnancy carefully managed by highly skilled, specially trained professionals experienced in high-risk obstetrics means a safer pregnancy and better results.

One thing is certain—the new obstetrics, perinatology and neonatology are exciting areas that represent new hope, more promise and greater dimensions of care when it comes to giving birth.

Birth will always be a very special miracle. But today medicine can do so much more to assist that miracle. Greater knowledge and technological advances have allowed us to take a giant step toward better assuring a safer and healthier pregnancy, labor and delivery.

We would like to emphasize that this book should in no way replace your personal physician. Especially with high-risk pregnancy, your doctor is vital to your care and will always be the best source of information when it comes to your own personal situation. Your doctor knows you, your medical history, what risks might be involved for you, what problems you and your husband or mate might face, and what tests and treatment would best be recommended for your particular needs. Whenever you have a question or concern, always ask your doctor.

ONE

THINKING OF GETTING PREGNANT OR ALREADY PREGNANT?

More growth occurs and more patterns are set that will affect a human being for the rest of his or her life in those first nine months preceding birth than during any other period. From the time of conception and its resultant single cell, cells begin dividing and multiplying rapidly. Even before the newly fertilized egg drops down into the uterus, cell division has begun. As early as the third week of gestation, the embryo develops a rounded head and trunk—with an umbilical cord attached. Certainly this tiny embryo does not yet look anything like a baby, but the form is taking shape as cells furiously multiply in their orderly fashion.

By the fourth week the embryo is only about one-eighth of an inch long but has a transparent-looking spot where his or her eyes are forming; a column-like structure that will develop into a spine; and primitive structures that will develop into the heart, mouth, aorta, bladder, rectum and blood vessels. Still it does not look like a human baby.

But by sometime near the 30th day of gestation, it has become more clearly human. At this point the embryo begins growing a quarter of an inch each week, and blood is pumped by the almost microscopic heart. At the sixth week stubby little protuberances seem to punch out: The extremities—arms and legs—are beginning to develop. The face and body, although still very tiny, begin to look more and more human, as light areas in the hands show where bone is forming.

Only around one-half inch long now, this tiny embryo—a forming human being—is miraculously well developed and human, even though only six weeks have passed since conception. And it is possible that the expectant mother still doesn't even know this tiny being exists!

Intrauterine photographs show a network of little blood vessels through the entire fetus—and show that all major physical structures are in place at 10 weeks of gestation. The embryonic stage is over—and this tiny fetus must start the long task of further enlarging and developing its existing body systems. Muscles are beginning to flex and stretch, while little eyes seem half-closed.

Imagine—only two and one-half months have passed since the woman's last menstrual cycle—and even now no one may know for sure that this new and growing human being exists. At three months this two-inch phenomenon will continue to grow rapidly.

At four and one-half months, the fetus may already be sucking its thumb, exercising and moving about—all within its protective environment. The mother may begin to sense the baby's movement, a truly marvelous phenomenon. As time goes on, the fetus's muscles grow stronger, and the bones and spine grow harder. The expectant mother may even get a swift kick now and then. At times the baby sleeps, and much of the time he or she seems to be rousting around in there—testing and stretching new muscles.

The point is, the first three months of life for the baby are paramount in his or her growth and development, and the months after that are also vitally significant. As we will discuss throughout Section 1, things that at any other time might be insignificant may have grave consequences to the developing little organism during these all-important first nine months.

Because so much more is known and such a great deal can be done for women "at risk" for problems during pregnancy, more women in this group are having children than ever before.

Section 1 (Chapters 1 through 9) details important information about high-risk or at risk pregnancy. The information is useful for those already pregnant who have been identified as high-risk, and for others who are thinking of getting pregnant and know they would be or might be at risk.

ONE

THE "COULD I BE HIGH-RISK?" CHECKLIST

The term "high-risk pregnancy" means something different to everyone. The fact is—most people really don't know what the term means—and many women don't know if they would be considered high-risk if pregnant. The term itself is rather deceiving—or in some cases misleading. The confusion has allowed the phrases "high-risk pregnancy," "at risk pregnancy" or "complicated pregnancy" (used synonymously) to be thrown around a great deal in newspapers, magazines, on radio and television, and among the general public.

In many situations being high-risk simply means the need for the pregnancy to be carefully followed to ensure that a *potential* problem doesn't occur or to recognize it quickly if it does. This allows necessary steps to be taken promptly to lessen the problem's impact or eliminate it altogether. In still other cases more intense medical intervention is necessary throughout the pregnancy to manage *known* problems.

You would be considered high-risk if you had a condition *before pregnancy* that would make you or your unborn child have an increased potential for developing problems. *During pregnancy* you or your unborn baby might develop a problem or condition that would then put one or both in the high-risk category. Again, whether the problem is present before or develops during the pregnancy, the high-risk designation simply means that a woman and her unborn child will benefit from careful and specialized evaluation, management and, where indicated, treatment throughout pregnancy.

High risk involves a large group of different known or potential problems. A woman may have one or more of these problems or be "at risk" to develop one. A "high-risk pregnancy," or at risk pregnancy then, means that either a specific, identifiable problem or a potential problem exists for mother, baby or both—and that the pregnancy requires optimal prenatal/perinatal management for the best possible outcome.

You would be considered high-risk if you have:

- Diabetes
- Hypertension
- Heart disease
- Rh incompatibility
- Kidney disease
- Liver disease
- Some thyroid disorders
- Severe asthma
- Incompetent cervix and uterine malformation
- A sexually transmitted (venereal) disease
- Cancer
- Some other disease state that could affect the pregnancy's outcome

You could also be considered at increased risk for potential problems if you have a history of:

- Miscarriage
- Premature birth
- Stillbirth
- Bleeding problems
- A previous abnormal child

Your risk would be increased if you had been exposed to:
- Rubella and you are not immune
- Certain toxins
- Extensive radiation
- Certain chemicals
- Specific drugs

Other special risk factors include:
- A family history (on either the mother's or father's side) of hereditary disease or genetic disorder
- Smoking cigarettes
- Chronic alcohol consumption
- Taking unnecessary or potentially damaging drugs

• Being seriously overweight or underweight

Women over age 35 may make up a special category in the high-risk group (Chapter 3) because many tend to have age-related illnesses (such as hypertension, heart disease, diabetes) that may affect their safety or that of the unborn baby. There is also a higher incidence of chromosomal abnormalities in the offspring of older women.

As you can see, the high-risk status includes a greater number of pregnancies than most people realize. Generally, it appears that more than 3 millions births a year in the United States, 20 percent to 25 percent are probably in the high-risk group. And that number is rising yearly because, for one, more women over 35 years of age are having children.

Because so much more can be done today than ever before, and since, in most cases, there is every reason to be optimistic, it is very important to know if you are or would be high-risk.

If you know you have an existing medical problem and want to raise a family, (if possible before pregnancy) you should learn all you can about the increased risks for you, discuss the pros and cons of a pregnancy with your husband or mate, learn what role each of you would play in the management of the pregnancy—and see your doctor for a complete evaluation and consultation. Your doctor should be an invaluable source of information and help in explaining specific and potential problems for you in this pregnancy, as well as the various diagnostic and treatment procedures that might be necessary.

If you are not sure you would be at increased risk for problems during pregnancy—see your doctor for a pre-pregnancy evaluation and consultation. He or she will be the best judge of your health status and be able to give you his or her best recommendation. In some cases your doctor may want you to see a specialist in high-risk obstetrics for consultation and possible management. Your own doctor will be the best judge as to the need for specialized intervention, if he or she is not an obstetrician who specializes in high-risk obstetrics (a maternal-fetal specialist or sometimes called a perinatologist).

CHAPTER 2:

SOME HIGH RISK PROBLEMS, THEIR POTENTIAL IMPACT AND MANAGEMENT

Because great strides have been made in the identification, management and treatment of certain problems or medical conditions that put an expectant mother and/or her unborn/newborn baby "at risk" for a complicated pregnancy, it is important for you to know more about some of them and what can be done to vastly improve the outcome for both mother and baby. Therefore, this chapter is a basic discussion about some high risk problems and what can be done about them.

Hypertension (Toxemia, Pre-Eclampsia and Eclampsia)

Hypertension, toxemia, pre-eclampsia and eclampsia are terms which confuse most people. The fact is—the terms *are* confusing and the problems difficult to understand. Things become even more complicated when other terms such as "primary hypertension," "secondary hypertension," "essential hypertension," "hypertensive vascular disease" or "hypertensive cardiovascular disease" are tossed around. Here are the terms you need to know:

- *Chronic hypertension* is due to increased pressure in the arteries and often associated with atherosclerosis (collections of fatty substances on the inside of the arteries). It is not caused by pregnancy but may cause problems if a woman with chronic hypertension becomes pregnant. In about 85 percent of people with identified hypertension, the cause is unknown and the disease is called "essential" or "primary" hypertension. In the remaining 15 percent of patients an underlying cause is identified. We will refer to both primary and essential hypertension as "chronic hypertension."

- *Toxemia* is a term most often used to refer to the hypertensive disorders of pregnancy. "Toxemia," however, is a rather misleading term, since there is no known toxin (poison) associated with hypertension, but the use of the word has endured over the years. You will more than likely hear the phrase "toxemia of pregnancy," which means hypertensive disorders of pregnancy.
- *Pre-eclampsia* and *Eclampsia* are hypertensive disorders unique to pregnancy that occur in the last three months (trimester). There is usually edema (swelling and fluid retention) and often protein is found in the urine. Toxemia of pregnancy (pre-eclampsia and eclampsia) are most commonly seen in a woman's first pregnancy. The woman with pure pre-eclampsia does not have chronic hypertension but becomes hypertensive in late pregnancy, and her blood pressure returns to normal after delivery. With pre-eclampsia the woman does not experience convulsions or coma. In rare instances, pre-eclampsia worsens and the woman experiences convulsions or goes into a coma. When this occurs, it is called eclampsia. Women with chronic hypertension who become pregnant often develop superimposed pre-eclampsia. We will discuss chronic hypertension, chronic hypertension with superimposed eclampsia, pre-eclampsia and eclampsia in more detail.

Chronic Hypertension

Chronic hypertension, as we noted earlier, has an unknown cause 85 percent of the time. Therefore, 15 percent of the time chronic hypertension is secondary to a primary problem—that is, a renal disorder, heart disease, endocrine disorder or some other condition is the cause of the hypertensive disease. In some cases the primary problem can be corrected, and in others they can be carefully managed.

Chronic hypertension usually first affects men and women between the ages of 25 and 55, and often there is a family history of the problem. Hypertensive disease is seen more often in women than in men and more frequently in blacks than in other races. Predisposing factors also include advanced age, obesity, diabetes (and other endocrine disorders), heart disease or renal disorders. Therefore, those who should be evaluated on a reasonably routine basis so that early detection can occur are women over 25, blacks and those with a family history of hypertensive disease. If chronic hypertension is not carefully managed and treated, it can become uncontrolled and affect almost every organ of the body (in particular the heart, brain, kidneys, eyes and pregnant uterus).

With mild to moderate chronic hypertension, a person is usually asymptomatic (has no symptoms). Headaches, dizziness and chest pain are warning signs that should indicate the need for prompt medical attention. If left unchecked, the disorder can lead to heart disease, brain hemorrhage, visual disturbances resulting in blindness and renal (kidney) damage. If hypertensive disorders are not treated or damage is permanent, then heart failure, cerebral thrombosis (blockage of an artery within the brain) or cerebral hemorrhage (bleeding from a blood vessel of the brain), renal failure and blindness may all occur.

You can see why it is important for both men and women to be evaluated for hypertensive disease at routine intervals. Most often if high blood pressure is identified in its early stages, it can be successfully managed by diet, exercise, and where necessary the use of diuretics and other anti-hypertensive drugs. Hypertensive individuals would be wise to stop smoking if they smoke, because nicotine causes further narrowing of the arteries. In fact, hypertension is one of those problems in medicine where careful management makes a very major difference. The vast majority of hypertensive people can live happy and healthy lives with careful management.

However, when the woman with chronic hypertension becomes pregnant—the pregnancy is truly high risk. Because of arterial narrowing, the blood supply to the uterus is compromised and the growth and oxygenation of the fetus are jeopardized. Pre-eclampsia and eclampsia are also likely to develop, with characteristic tissue swelling and proteinuria (protein in the urine). In the extreme, full blown eclampsia (convulsions or coma) may also occur. Women with chronic hypertension are at higher risk for fetal growth retardation, stillbirth and a 4 to 5 times greater risk for placental abruption (discussed later in this chapter) as well.

Hypertension with superimposed pre-eclampsia means that a woman has already been diagnosed (before pregnancy) as having chronic hypertension. Then she is diagnosed as having pre-eclampsia when her blood pressure rises above its already abnormally high level after the 26th week of pregnancy (and she has proteinuria, edema and sometimes visual changes).

The greatest problem with superimposed pre-eclampsia or eclampsia is that it intensifies the already existing hypertension. Therefore, women with chronic hypertension need to be carefully evaluated routinely throughout pregnancy—and especially in the last few months—to identify superimposed pre-eclampsia immediately. About 15 percent of women with chronic hypertension will experience pre-eclampsia in addition to their usual chronic hypertension.

Pre-Eclampsia

As noted earlier, pre-eclampsia (high blood pressure) is a complication of pregnancy that occurs in the *last* trimester. (If elevation of blood pressure occurs *before* the 26th week, it is likely to be due to chronic hypertension that has not been diagnosed.) Also, pre-eclampsia is very much a disease of a woman in her first pregnancy (called a primagravida). If the problem is seen in a second, third or later pregnancy, it is probably not pure pre-eclampsia but more likely due to underlying chronic hypertension.

So that your doctor will have a means of comparison, it is always best to know what your blood pressure was before pregnancy occurred. This is particularly important if you are seeing a different doctor during pregnancy or have recently moved and must find a new doctor. It is always wise to have your medical records forwarded to your new doctor, particularly if you have a chronic medical problem.

The first sign of pre-eclampsia may be high blood pressure and/ or swelling with rapid weight gain. Headaches, nervousness, intermittent blurred vision and undue fatigue may also occur. The reason your blood pressure is taken, your weight recorded and a urinanalysis performed at each prenatal visit is to make sure pre-eclampsia is not developing.

Many of these symptoms and signs are normal during pregnancy, so you should not over-react if you have one or more of them occasionally. The real test will be your blood pressure and the absence or presence of protein in the urine. If, however, these symptoms become uncomfortable during your pregnancy and your next visit is not scheduled for several weeks, it's always a good idea to call your doctor or schedule an earlier appointment to be evaluated. This is particularly important if these symptoms occur after the 26th week.

Many women don't realize that pre-eclampsia can also begin during labor or *after* delivery. (One-third of pre-eclampsia is manifested before labor, one-third of cases occur during labor and another one-third take place after delivery.) In most women this is readily managed. Early detection is important and is one of the reasons for the continual "harassment" by nurses who keep taking your blood pressure during labor and following delivery. It is done to detect not only low blood pressure (from excessive blood loss, for example) but also pre-eclampsia, so prompt management can occur.

If pre-eclampsia is not carefully managed, the fetus can be affected. The disorder can cause inadequate oxygenation of the fetus resulting in fetal distress (discussed in Chapters 12 and 13). Fetal distress can lead to brain damage or even death if it is severe or long-lasting enough. To put this into perspective, until 1966 around 25,000 stillbirths and neonatal deaths (due to prematurity) in the United States each year were directly attributed to hypertensive disorders. Because of early detection and management of pre-eclampsia today, as well as advances in neonatology for the care of the premature infant—this number has declined significantly.

Eclampsia

Although the majority of women who experience pre-eclampsia never get eclampsia—if the blood pressure gets out of hand suddenly, the disease may progress to eclampsia. Eclampsia is pre-eclampsia that has progressed to the point of convulsions and possible coma. Everything possible is done to prevent convulsions if they have not occurred or to prevent further seizures if the woman is already eclamptic. As with pre-eclampsia, eclampsia can affect every organ and body system, causing either permanent damage or death of the mother and baby if not vigorously managed and its progression halted.

Management and Treatment of Hypertensive Disorders

Women with hypertensive disorders are managed by rest, diet, and medications to control blood pressure and to prevent convulsions.

Both mild and moderate chronic hypertension and pre-eclampsia require frequent evaluation by your doctor. If at any point your doctor feels the problem is worsening and needs more intense management, hospitalization will be recommended.

If you are hospitalized, you would be kept at bed rest. Your blood pressure as well as other bodily functions would be checked frequently, and your baby's well-being would also be monitored. The type of medication recommended will very much depend on the extent of your problem and is determined by a careful evaluation of your individual needs. You would most likely stay in the hospital until the baby was delivered and the hypertensive problem was resolved or brought under control.

Because hypertensive disorders can cause fetal damage or death due to uteroplacental insufficiency (UPI)—which means inadequate supply of oxygen or nutrients to the fetus—fetal surveillance testing is necessary. The type and frequency of testing are dependent on the severity of the problem. Tests to determine fetal well-being include the contraction stress test (CST), non-stress test (NST) and determination of estriol levels in the mother's blood. These are described in detail in Chapter 13. Ultrasound (discussed in Chapter 10) is often recommended to determine or verify fetal growth retardation, which may result from severe or prolonged hypertension. Fetal lung maturity is evaluated by what is called the L/S ratio or PG level in the amniotic fluid (discussed in Chapter 13). Your doctor may use one or more of these tests to determine whether premature delivery is required, based on your fetus's needs and condition.

For the woman with mild pre-eclampsia who is at term—the best treatment is delivery, since this will cure the pre-eclampsia. If the expectant mother is not at term and the disease is mild, bed rest, careful observation of the mother and fetal fitness testing will most likely be recommended. If the mother is pre-term and delivery is indicated, amniocentesis (to determine the L/S ratio for fetal lung maturity) may be recommended. Delivery would be recommended if the fetus's lungs were mature, but if the L/S ratio were not optimal, further monitoring and treatment of the pre-eclampsia could be continued until the baby was mature, as long as both mother and fetus continue to do well. If, however, the pre-eclampsia is not controllable or convulsions occur, the only option may be to deliver the baby—even if it is premature.

With today's management and treatment, maternal death and disability due to hypertensive disorders are very, very rare. Fetal and newborn death and disability have also markedly decreased because of new methods of fetal evaluation, prompt intervention and the enormous improvements in the care of premature infants. However, it is vital for women to seek prenatal care early in pregnancy and follow the doctor's recommended schedule of visits.

Endocrine/Glandular Problems: Diabetes and Thyroid Disease

Although there are quite a number of endocrine diseases (those of the ductless glands), the two most significant in pregnancy involve the pancreas (diabetes) and the thyroid gland.

Diabetes

One of the most impressive examples of the impact of technology and medical advances on pregnancy is seen in the care of the diabetic mother and her unborn baby. Diabetes complicates about 1 percent to 2 percent of all pregnancies. Usually a chronic disease, diabetes mellitus (generally called "diabetes") is thought to be inherited but may also involve some environmental factors.

A deficiency in insulin production (or inefficient insulin action) results in the body's inability to break down and use the blood sugar for energy; body fat is then broken down for energy use. However, fat breakdown and buildup of the blood sugar may produce real problems. The result is the production of ketones, which are products of fat metabolism. This is called "ketosis" and leads to a buildup of acid in the body—acidosis. In ketoacidosis this buildup of abnormal products poisons the cells of the body. Symptoms of diabetes include excessive thirst, abnormally frequent urination, and weight loss despite increased food intake due to an increased appetite.

Two kinds of diabetes are seen in pregnancy: pre-existing diabetes (which involves both insulin-dependent and non-insulin-dependent women who have had the disease before pregnancy) and what is called gestational diabetes (which involves women not known to be diabetic before pregnancy who suddenly manifest the disease for the first time during pregnancy).

Gestational diabetes tends to confuse people. Pregnancy itself is a diabetogenic state—that is, it increases the potential for diabetes. The fact is, some of the hormones present in pregnancy, in particular HPL (human placental lactogen), cause insulin resistance in some pregnant women. Increased insulin production is needed to keep up with the body's metabolic needs. Generally, most women while pregnant will increase their insulin production to meet this requirement. Women who have this same increased insulin resistance but cannot meet this challenge with increased insulin production by the pancreas become diabetic during pregnancy.

The disease may or may not be severe or troublesome in pregnancy. Most gestational diabetics will either revert to a non-diabetic state after pregnancy, or the severity of the diabetes will lessen. At times a woman who has a history of diabetes in her family (but who does not have the disease herself) becomes diabetic during pregnancy. She may or may not return to a non-diabetic state after pregnancy.

The severity of *diabetes* has a great deal to do with the possible problems for mother and baby. Basically, as the severity of the diabetes increases, the risks increase for the mother and most particularly for the baby. It also determines the extent of medical testing, management and intervention.

It is important to put the problem of diabetes and pregnancy into perspective. Until 60 years ago women of childbearing age with moderate to severe diabetes simply did not have children. Without the availability of insulin (developed in 1922), these women were simply too sick, and many died when the disease became totally out-of-control. With the development of insulin came a better, healthier life for all diabetics and new hope for diabetic women and their husbands to have the children they may have always wanted.

But with this new hope came a major unforeseen problem. The initial perinatal mortality rate was 50 percent or more. Often those babies who did survive had serious congenital abnormalities. They were abnormally large and often sustained serious birth injuries. Of those fetuses who died before birth, death most often occurred one to two months before the end of the pregnancy. It therefore seemed logical to prematurely deliver the babies of moderate to severe (insulin-dependent) diabetic mothers. This procedure reduced perinatal mortality from 50 percent to 25 percent in the late 1950s and 1960s. But with this came new, significant problems for the premature baby (in particular, serious breathing problems, which made it difficult for many to survive). The worse the diabetes, the earlier the baby was delivered, often by cesarean birth—and consequently, the more premature the baby.

Part of the answer came in 1969–70 with the availability of the contraction stress test (CST), the later non-stress test (NST) and estriol measurements which allowed doctors to better determine fetal well-being. (These tests are discussed in detail in Chapters 11, 12 and 13.) Other tests, such as determining the L/S ratio and PG level (described in Chapters 11 and 13), allowed doctors to determine fetal lung maturity or the lack of it.

In this way *a fetus who was doing fine* but whose lungs were not yet mature would not be delivered, and the problems of prematurity would be avoided. *Those at risk* could be identified as early as possible so intervention could take place. It was the availability of these diagnostic methods—*surveillance of fetal well-being* and *determining fetal lung maturity*—that have made progress. With the careful management of the diabetes and the utilization of these special tests, fetal mortality rates have been *dramatically* reduced to 3 percent to 4 percent—and nearly all these deaths are due to serious congenital malformations incompatible with survival.

New, innovative programs may prove to lower the fetal and neonatal mortality rate even further and reduce the number of severe congenital malformations. At our institution (Women's Hospital in Long Beach, California), there is a special program for diabetic mothers—and the results have been encouraging. In this program, women and their partners are put through an educational program, and the mother's diabetes is put under tight control before the couple tries to conceive. Because careful controls for the mother's blood sugar appear to improve pregnancy outcome, traditionally diabetics required several weeks of hospitalization to achieve the frequent measurement of blood sugar levels along with frequent changes in insulin dosage. Recently, most centers have begun having patients monitor their own blood sugar levels with special instruments that need only a drop of blood from a fingerstick. This has allowed of excellent control with a minimum of hospitalization.

These mosthers are monitored by an evaluation of hemoglobin A_{1C} (found in the blood) long before pregnancy. Hemoglobin A_{1C} appears to be a "marker" of the control of the diabetes during the preceding 60 days to 90 days. It has recently been shown that when the hemoglobin A_{1C} is high (greater than 9 percent in early pregnancy), the diabetes was not under good control prior to or around the time of conception and during the first three months of fetal development. The babies of women with high hemoglobin A_{1C} have a greater incidence of congenital malformations than those with a normal level of this blood substance. Therefore, in our special program the diabetes can be and is put under tight control long before pregnancy and hemoglobin A_{1c} is evaluated to verify excellent control of the diabetes.

Once the woman becomes pregnant, she is carefully managed throughout the pregnancy and the diabetes tightly controlled. Fetal testing is performed based on the severity of the mother's disease and an evaluation of the overall clinical picture.

At the present time then, diabetes and its effects on pregnancy are approached in a multifaceted manner:

- *Congenital malformations* are attacked by establishing tight control of diabetes long before and during early pregnancy.
- *Stillbirth* is attacked by careful fetal surveillance—contraction stress testing (CST), non-stress testing (NST) and measurement of estriol levels.
- *Prematurity* is attacked by determining the L/S ratio in the amniotic fluid (and/or the PG level may be used in the future) as a measure of fetal lung maturity and by postponing delivery if at all possible until the fetus's lungs can mature.
- *Birth injury* is attacked by measuring the fetus's size with ultrasound and recommending cesarean delivery if the baby is so large that vaginal delivery would be risky.

A non-insulin-dependent diabetic mother whose fetus is doing well will usually be delivered (labor induced) at 40 weeks if spontaneous labor and delivery have not already taken place. If delivery is not recommended, then fetal surveillance (contraction stress testing and measurement of estriol levels) would begin at 40 weeks gestation. Ultrasound may be performed to determine fetal size. If the baby is too big and cannot pass through the birth canal, then cesarean delivery would be recommended to avoid birth injury or death.

If the insulin-dependent expectant mother does not have vascular complications and the baby is growing well, fetal fitness testing (the contraction test) will be performed once a week and estriol levels determined daily—beginning at about the 32nd or 34th week of pregnancy if the L/S ratio in the amniotic fluid verifies fetal lung maturity.

For those diabetic women with vascular complications or hypertension, or those in whom the baby is not growing well, fetal surveillance testing may begin as early as the 26th to 28th week of pregnancy (the time when it is possible for the fetus to survive outside the womb if delivery were mandatory). Delivery of the baby will depend on the test results. If the baby is not doing well— he or she may be delivered early—if the chance for fetal survival is better outside the womb than if the fetus were left unattended inside the womb.

Babies of diabetic mothers may have hypoglycemia (low blood sugar) in the newborn stage. Essentially, the baby has been existing in a "sugar-syrup environment" and controlling its own blood sugar with increased insulin production. (Insulin does not cross the placenta, whereas *glucose does*.) To balance this, the fetus produces a lot of insulin to control the blood sugar. Once born, the baby is no longer getting this barrage of glucose from the mother but keeps producing insulin at the same rate. Therefore, the baby's blood sugar goes way down during the first few hours to days of the newborn period. He or she is usually carefully monitored and may be treated in a newborn intensive care unit until the blood sugar level is under control.

The point is—when it comes to diabetes and pregnancy there is every reason for greater optimism today than ever before and for new hope for the future as more becomes known and even more can be accomplished. Although there are still some risks for congenital malformation (3 to 4 times greater than for the general population of women having babies) and stillbirth—with new programs becoming available and careful management, it is hoped that in the near future the risks for these complications in the diabetic mother will be no greater than those for the low risk mother. It is an area of care where progress has been phenomenal, representing a turnaround in statistics and outcomes in favor of both mother and baby.

Thyroid Disease

No one really knows why, but thyroid disease is more common among pregnant women. The thyroid gland, located in the neck, is responsible for controlling the body's metabolism, and has an effect on all vital body processes.

When it is mild, hyperthyroidism (overactivity of the thyroid gland) has symptoms that are difficult to distinguish from some of the normal symptoms of pregnancy. All pregnant women experience a faster heartbeat, an increase in appetite, heat intolerance and a flushed feeling off and on. But expectant mothers with hyperthyroidism also lost weight or fail to gain enough weight—which is obviously not characteristic during pregnancy. If hyperthyroidism is not treated, the expectant mother can lose an excessive amount of weight—enough to be unsafe for her developing fetus.

Uncontrolled hyperthyroidism may ultimately lead to "thyroid storm," in which the thyroid gland suddenly produces an excessive amount of thyroid hormone and releases it into the bloodstream. With this, all symptoms intensify to the dangerous level—severe tachycardia (rapid heart rate), dehydration, delirium, diarrhea, vomiting and often an extremely high fever—all culminating in heart failure. Therefore, it is imperative for both mother and fetus that hyperthyroidism be recognized and controlled as early as possible.

Hyperthyroidism can usually be easily managed by what are called "anti-thyroid drugs"—which control the amount of thyroid hormone produced by the overactive gland. These drugs, however, cross the placenta and may also potentially affect the fetus's thyroid gland. But when the drugs are carefully chosen and their dose regulated, the mother's disease can usually be controlled without adversely affecting her baby. Radioactive iodine treatment, often used to control this disease in other situations, *should not* be given during pregnancy. In some situations in which drug control is not possible, surgical removal of the thyroid may be needed.

The newborn infant of a hyperthyroid mother may also have symptoms of hyperthyroidism in some cases, because the mother's naturally produced hormone overstimulates both mother and fetus. This is usually temporary, but treatment must be started if the signs of overactivity do not resolve themselves.

Conversely, if the mother is being treated with anti-thyroid drugs that affect the fetus, the baby may show *hypothyroidism* (underactivity of the thyroid gland) at birth. If hypothyroidism in the newborn is not recognized promptly and treated, it can result in severe mental retardation—a condition called "cretinism." However, if hypothyroidism is treated immediately, it appears that these infants do extremely well.

Untreated *hypothyroidism* in expectant mothers is rarely seen, since most often women with this problem are infertile—a situation that can be reversed by treatment with thyroid hormone. Women who are being treated for hypothyroidism should be monitored carefully during pregnancy to assure that the amount of thyroid they are taking is correct.

Another thyroid problem seen in pregnancy is when the mother has a lump or lumps in her thyroid gland. Although the vast majority of these lumps are benign, in some situations they can be cancerous. (Thyroid cancer has a very high curability rate.) However, pregnant women should not be given the radioactive iodine uptake test (a test in which radioactive iodine is taken orally, followed by a special scan of the thyroid gland) to diagnose potential cancer or other potential thyroid problems. Radioactive iodine can lead to fetal malformation so the test must be avoided. A biopsy of the nodule (surgical removal of the lump, followed by careful microscopic examination) may be recommended as an alternative method of making a diagnosis. If thyroid cancer is diagnosed, the thyroid gland is removed and a synthetic thyroid hormone is taken orally to meet the body's needs. Additional anti-cancer therapy may or may not be necessary.

Those women who have had a subtotal to total *thyroidectomy* (surgical removal of part or all of the thyroid gland) and others who are taking synthetic thyroid hormone should see their doctors for a pre-pregnancy visit to have their thyroid function checked (by blood test) and the dosage of their thyroid drug adjusted if necessary.

Heart Disease

Heart disease in pregnant women is relatively uncommon today when compared to years ago. This is due to a reduction in rheumatic heart disease, which used to be responsible for the majority of heart disease seen in these women. Basically, when there was no cure for strep throat, it frequently progressed into rheumatic fever, which in turn caused varying degrees of damage—to the heart valves, in particular. With the advent of antibiotics to combat strep infections, rheumatic heart disease was dramatically reduced.

Today five types of heart disease are seen in pregnant women: congenital heart disease, which is the most common; rheumatic heart disease due to rheumatic fever; arteriosclerotic heart disease, which is more often seen with hypertension and diabetes; cardiomyopathy, which is a rare abnormality of the cardiac muscles causing them to become dysfunctional; and hypertensive cardiac decompensation, which is hypertension and diabetes; cardiomyopathy, which is a rare abnormality of the cardiac muscles causing them to become dysfunctional; and hypertensive cardiac decompensation, which is hypertension that progresses to the point of cardiac involvement and damage.

Because heart disease is such a technically complex area, and each woman is managed so individually, it is virtually impossible to make valid generalizations. However, we can say that maternal heart disease does not appear to affect the growth and development of the fetus unless: the mother is in chronic heart failure (the heart muscle is not as efficient in pumping blood as it should be); she has very advanced heart disease; or she is cyanotic (has a type of heart disease in which she is blue because her blood cannot receive enough oxygen).

Pregnancy itself though can markedly affect a woman's heart disease. Unfortunately, the demands pregnancy puts on the heart may result in decompensation or worsening of the mother's condition during pregnancy. Decompensation (also called "congestive heart failure") is most likely to occur at three times during the pregnancy:

- Between the 28th and 32nd weeks, when the work demand of the heart is reaching a peak
- During labor and delivery, because of the increased cardiovascular demands
- During the postpartum period, when the mother has many fluid shifts, which can result in congestive heart failure

Management will differ depending on the type of heart disease and the severity of the problem. The expectant mother with no cardiac insufficiency and no limitations on physical activity due to heart disease is usually restricted to moderate activity when pregnant, and is frequently checked to evaluate her heart disease in order to be on guard for signs of decompensation. For others who have trouble breathing, experience fatigue, palpitations and angina pains, or even more severe symptoms with marked minimal or no physical activity in the non-pregnant state, the recommended treatment is maximum rest, which is usually quite beneficial because it decreases the demands on the heart. Because of the three periods in the pregnancy that seem to make greater demands on the heart, women with heart disease are more closely watched and monitored during these specific times. A woman with heart disease will usually be managed by both her internist or cardiologist and her obstetrician (or the maternal-fetal specialist to whom she was referred).

Depending on the extent of the cardiac problem and each woman's needs, management (besides bed rest) may also include avoiding excessive weight gain through special diet, control of abnormal fluid retention by salt restriction and at times fluid restriction as well. Doctors also do everything possible to prevent anemia and hypertension, both of which increase the demands on the heart.

If the heart disease worsens during pregnancy, most often the woman will be hospitalized and restricted to complete bed rest. Care may also include a sodium (salt) restricted diet and drugs such as diuretics (to eliminate excess water) and digitalis (a drug that helps the heart to beat more efficiently) where necessary. During labor and delivery and the postpartum period, these women will be monitored carefully—including pulse, blood pressure and respiratory rate.

Women with artificial valves have a special problem, because they take anticoagulant drugs, which prevent blood from clotting on the artificial valve. This can be a problem because warfarin (Coumadin[R]—the drug most often used) crosses the placenta and can affect the fetus adversely (causing fetal malformations and bleeding in the fetus). However, heparin (another anticoagulant) does not cross the placenta. Heparin has to be given by injection or by continuous infusion for a long time. One problem: most women with heart disease who are on warfarin become pregnant first—and see their doctors after pregnancy has occurred—which is too late to stop the potential effects of the warfarin. Therefore, all women who have valve replacements and others taking an anticoagulant drug such as warfarin/Coumadin[R] for another reason should see their doctors long before pregnancy to discuss the risks of the drug and the possibility and safety of using heparin instead. Often anticoagulant drugs will be stopped before labor and delivery to avoid excessive bleeding.

So much progress has been made to this point that women have successfully had open heart surgery and bypass surgery while pregnant or experienced a heart attack and survived. The overall outcome has improved—in particular, for those with mild to moderate heart problems.

Women with *very severe cardiac problems*, however, are significantly risking their own health and well-being if they become pregnant—due to the heart problem(s) and the increased demands pregnancy places on cardiac function. In this case, the woman could be told that pregnancy is not recommended and that—for her own safety—a very effective method of birth control should be used. Although this can be very difficult for the woman who really wants a child—her well-being is vitally important, too. On most cases, if the mother would be in great jeopardy—her baby would be equally at risk, since she would not be able to meet the baby's requirements for adequate oxygenation.

As a safety precaution—all women with cardiac problems should see their internist or cardiologist if they are considering getting pregnant. A complete evaluation should be performed, and the doctor should discuss the potential and real risks if pregnancy were to occur.

Urinary Tract and Kidney (Renal) Disease

Acute and chronic urinary tract and kidney (renal) problems range from those easily managed and treated to those that are more rare, serious and potentially fatal. Women with chronic kidney disease or those with a history of acute episodes of urinary tract or kidney infections need to be carefully evaluated prior to conception to determine the potential risks if pregnancy occurred.

Urinary tract infections are problems common for women in general and are the most frequently seen urinary tract problems seen in pregnancy. During pregnancy the urinary tract dilates, causing less rapid flow of urine down the system, leading to stasis (pooling and collection of stagnant urine in certain areas). This then predisposes expectant mothers to urinary tract infections (UTIs), which may start in the bladder but may later extend upward and develop into kidney infection.

Symptoms of a lower urinary tract infection are burning and irritation upon urination, frequency of urination, urgency (the feeling of needing to urinate often), lower abdominal pain and possibly a low-grade fever. (The doctor may call this *cystitis*—which is an inflammation of the bladder.) When the kidneys are involved (called "pyelonephritis," or kidney infection), the woman usually experiences low back pain and higher fever and generally feels poorly.

When a woman develops a urinary tract or kidney infection during pregnancy: her risk for premature labor may increase; if she has a very high fever, particularly during early pregnancy, there is an increased risk for developmental abnormalities in the fetus; and, since drugs must be used to eradicate the problem, there is a slight risk of their adversely affecting the fetus (therefore, the drug used must be wisely chosen).

If a urinary tract or kidney infection is not carefully diagnosed and treated, the potential for chronic kidney infection develops. Chronic infection—called chronic pyelonephritis—can ultimately damage the kidneys themselves which may eventually lead to kidney failure and can be fatal if not treated.

Both *temporary and chronic kidney disease* are seen in pregnancy.

Temporary kidney problems may be due to urinary tract infection (as we discussed) or can be associated with hypertension (either chronic hypertension or pre-eclampsia and eclampsia). When these conditions include kidney involvement, they are characterized by protein in the urine (proteinuria), decreased kidney function (buildup of waste products in the blood and often swelling because of water retention) and, in some rare situations, even kidney failure. With true pre-eclampsia or eclampsia, these symptoms will usually cease soon after the baby's delivery. With chronic hypertension the extent of the kidney involvement will depend on how well the hypertension can be managed and kept under control.

Chronic kidney problems that predate pregnancy are very complex and for the most part fairly rare in the majority of pregnant women. But these problems can have a serious effect on the fetus and mother if not carefully managed.

Chronic pyelonephritis is a long-term, smoldering kidney infection that damages the collecting system. The extent of damage will determine the degree of renal (kidney) insufficiency and the amount of kidney deterioration. Chronic pyelonephritis can lead to chronic hypertension as kidney damage progresses.

Chronic glomerulonephritis is not an infection but a kidney disease that progressively destroys the working part of the organ which filters waste products from the blood. With this, renal insufficiency can occur, and the woman may develop hypertensive cardiovascular disease as well. (Confusing as it may sound, kidney disease can lead to hypertension, and hypertension can cause kidney damage.) If superimposed pre-eclampsia takes place along with these other problems—both kidney failure and heart failure may occur. When the disease reaches this point, it can also have devastating effects on the fetus—resulting in fetal hypoxia and even fetal death—without successful intervention.

With chronic glomerulonephritis where there is no hypertension and where renal function is fairly normal—the mother and baby usually do well. If the problem is progressing or the expectant mother experiences an acute episode of inflammation—she is usually hospitalized at bed rest and carefully monitored. Drugs are given to reduce her high blood pressure, great care is taken to maintain a balance in fluids, and salt (sodium) intake is restricted.

Although pregnancy does not appear to worsen chronic glomerulonephritis, women with this disease have a higher incidence of spontaneous abortion (miscarriage), stillbirth, premature labor, placental abruption and even infertility. The main problem with the chronic kidney diseases seen during pregnancy is that women with them will more often have secondary hypertension and be at greater risk of developing toxemia of pregnancy or superimposed pre-eclampsia or eclampsia. These women also have an increased risk of having growth retarded babies and all the problems associated with growth retardation—fetal distress, decreased oxygen supply, and a higher perinatal mortality and morbidity rate (because of the damage to the placenta from the hypertension).

However, since the extent of the problems experienced in pregnancy is directly related to the severity of the kidney disease and the degree of damage it has caused, it is vital that *any woman with a chronic renal disease* see her doctor for a complete evaluation *before* trying to get pregnant. In this way, an evaluation can be made to determine if pregnancy would constitute a significant risk for both mother and a potential baby.

Women who have had a *kidney transplant* are now getting pregnant and have done remarkably well—even though they are on strong drugs to protect them from rejection of the transplant. The outcome for these women and their babies is not 100 percent positive, and there is an increased risk for fetal malformation—but they have done much, much better than anyone had expected.

Also, pregnant women with *one normal kidney* (if the other was surgically removed) often do well when carefully managed and followed. There is, however, some significant risk-taking with this—in that if the remaining kidney develops a problem, the woman has no backup kidney to support her or the baby. Again consultation with the doctor is highly recommended *before* pregnancy.

The point is—progress has been made in the management of urinary tract and kidney infections and in chronic renal disease during pregnancy. However, women with chronic renal disease with moderate to severe damage must seriously consider the risks pregnancy might bring and carefully weigh the recommendations of their doctors in planning a pregnancy.

Liver Disease

Actually, it is rare to find primary liver disease in women who are pregnant. *Hepatitis* is the most common primary liver disease seen in pregnancy. Hepatitis A and B are viruses that cause acute inflammation and swelling of the liver. The infected woman initially has symptoms of a low grade fever, loss of appetite, muscle aches and sometimes vomiting. As the disease progresses the expectant mother turns yellow (jaundiced) and may experience some pain in the upper right side of her abdomen. Her urine turns dark brown and she has abnormal enzymes as well as bilirubin in her blood (detected by blood test).

Once the disease has been diagnosed, adequate rest and a well-balanced nutritional plan are recommended. Absolute avoidance of alcohol, and all drugs and medications is required, so as not to stress the liver. Remember, liver function is responsible for detox-ification of many substances, so anything that would require the liver to work harder must be avoided to allow it to recover. Hepatitis can last several weeks to several months. Usually if the doctor's recommendations are carefully followed, the woman recovers, and the fetus is not affected.

However, if the hepatitis (either A or B) does not improve after several months, it is then considered *chronic hepatitis*. With chronic hepatitis there is a continual low-grade progression of the disease and eventual scarring of the liver. This can ultimately result in cirrhosis and liver failure, which can be fatal. The pregnant woman with chronic hepatitis faces greater problems than if she were not pregnant—because of the baby's demands on the mother's liver for his or her detoxification needs. Also, all women show some slug-gishness of liver function during pregnancy, so the degree of de-toxification normally decreases to some extent.

The fetus, too, would be at greater risk for problems. There is a risk that the fetus can get chronic hepatitis from the mother—which could have very serious consequences. And, if the mother's liver cells are damaged, they cannot manufacture protein, vitamin K and other nutrients that the fetus needs for growth and devel-opment.

You may also have heard about a problem called *cholestasis*, in which the products of the liver don't drain properly and instead build up in the blood and are then deposited in the skin. Certain chemicals called "bile acids" cause intense itching. Women of Scan-dinavian and Chilean origin (in particular) get exaggerated choles-tasis, however, the problem can reoccur in subsequent is usually gone within hours after the baby is born. Although cholestasis usually doesn't affect fetal well-being it can be very irritating for the woman. The problem can reoccur in subsequent pregnancies and if these women use oral contraceptives.

Severe Asthma

Bronchial asthma is a chronic disease causing off and on mild to severe difficulties in breathing. Emotional stress seems to make its symptoms worse. Those who experience recurrent asthma attacks know they cause difficulty in breathing, wheezing, and cough—first a dry cough, then one in which mucus can be coughed out. Some attacks may be resolved without treatment, but most require treatment with bronchodilator drugs (drugs that relax the muscles in the bronchi and cause the airways to reopen), as well as rest and avoidance of stress and of whatever triggered the attack (allergy, infection, irritating substances, cold air, exercise, etc.).

Most women with mild to moderate asthma tolerate pregnancy very well. The drugs most often used to treat them are quite safe and do not seem to significantly increase the risk for fetal problems.

However, the fetus of a mother with severe asthma (or any other severe lung disease) is at increased risk of potentially serious problems if the asthma is not kept under control. With severe asthma, as with other lung diseases, the mother's blood oxygen content may decrease significantly. Because of this, these babies tend to be smaller and have a higher incidence of fetal distress (a problem that results from inadequate oxygenation). If severe asthma is not treated, it may lead to fetal/neonatal damage or death.

When asthma is very severe, cortisone-like drugs may be necessary. These drugs cause some anomalies in rats, but are not clearly related to problems in the human fetus. The questionable risk associated with using the appropriate drugs is less than the risk of chronic hypoxia (low blood oxygen content), which can significantly affect both mother and fetus. Therefore, it is vitally important that severe asthma be kept under control throughout pregnancy, both for the well-being of the fetus and that of the mother.

If the asthma becomes a problem, or your doctor(s) are concerned about the effects of the disease on your fetus, then tests to determine fetal fitness may be recommended as early as the 26th week of pregnancy or anytime thereafter. (Fetal distress is discussed in Chapter 12 and tests to determine fetal fitness in Chapter 13.)

Blood Incompatibility (Rh Disease and ABO Incompatibility)

Each of us inherits certain characteristics in our blood—called "blood groups." These are determined by certain unique materials called red blood cell *antigens*, which are found on the surface of the red blood cells. These antigens make it possible for the body to recognize its own blood (or blood of the same type) as "self" and other blood antigens as "foreign." Each antigen is part of a blood group system. The blood plasma (the liquid portion of the blood) contains other substances called *antibodies*, which guard against "foreign antigens." Part of the body's immune (protection) system, antibodies destroy anything recognized as foreign to the body. Foreign antigens are seen as invaders and a threat to the body's well-being.

Therefore, the immune system produces antibodies to foreign blood cells and continues to make more and more antibodies to destroy the invaders if the blood is exposed to more foreign antigens. This action and reaction when two different blood groups mix together is the principle that forms the basis for the problems that may result from blood group incompatibility between mother and baby.

While there are actually many different blood antigens that can be identified in the laboratory, two major blood group systems—the ABO *blood type* system and the Rh system—are most important in pregnancy (or if blood transfusion is necessary). These systems often confuse expectant mothers (and most people in general) because if they are told they are Rh positive (Rh+) or that they have the Rh factor (meaning Rh+), they think their blood type is Rh+.

This is not the case, however. Rh+ simply means that the red blood cells have the Rh antigen (usually called the "Rh factor") on them.

In reality, then, blood type and Rh are two separate considerations (that is, they involve two different blood group systems), as follows:

- In the *ABO blood type system*, you will have one of four blood types—*A, B, AB* or *O*. These letters refer to the antigens on the red blood cells. If you have type A blood, *A* antigens are found on the surfaces of your red blood cells; with type B, there are *B* antigens; type AB blood has both *A* and *B*

surface antigens; and type O blood has *neither* A nor B antigens on the red blood cells.
- In the *Rh system*, you will be Rh positive (Rh+, meaning
that the Rh factor is present on your red blood cells), or you
will be Rh negative (Rh−, meaning that the Rh factor is not
present).

Hence, your blood type is determined by the ABO system, and
in addition you are Rh+ or Rh−.

A system has been developed to make it simpler to discuss these
two groups of blood antigens. For example, instead of saying you
have type A blood with an Rh+ factor—this would shorten to
A+. Those with type A blood with no Rh factor would be A−.
In other words, the letter (A, B, AB or O) represents the blood
type, and the + or − represents the presence (+) or absence
(−) of the Rh factor. Each of us, then, will be one of the following:
A+, A−, B+, B−, AB+, AB−, O+ or O−.

We will now discuss two types of problems due to blood antigen
incompatibility. The first—and by far the most significant—is Rh
disease (which may result from incompatibility between the
mother's and the fetus's Rh factors), and the second is ABO incompatibility (which may result from incompatibility between the
mother's blood type and that of the baby).

Rh Disease

Rh disease used to be responsible for the deaths of around 10,000
babies every year in the United States, but that has changed because
of a better understanding of how the immune system works, genetics and blood typing. Not only was it a common cause of perinatal mortality, but it was responsible for mild to severe brain
damage and cerebral palsy before the early 1970s. At that time a
serum (Rhogam®) was developed to prevent the disease in many
situations. This, along with better tools for fetal surveillance and
treatment and technological improvements in caring for the very
sick newborn, has improved the outlook for those mothers and
infants at risk for this disease. Death of a fetus or newborn from
Rh disease is increasingly rare, and brain damage and cerebral palsy
due to the disease continue to decrease. Nonetheless, Rh disease
is still a potential threat in 10 percent to 15 percent of expectant

mothers who are Rh negative if they are carrying an Rh positive fetus.

The most common set of circumstances is as follows: the mother is Rh− (has no Rh factor), and the father is Rh+ (has the Rh factor). With this combination, each baby has at least a 50 percent chance of being Rh+, since this factor is inherited. Rh sensitization occurs during an Rh− an *Rh− woman's pregnancy with an Rh+ fetus*. During the pregnancy—most often during the process of labor and delivery—minor "leaks" between the baby's bloodstream and the mother's (via the placenta) are fairly common. If Rh+ blood cells from the baby enter the mother's bloodstream, her immune system will begin to make antibodies to destroy the foreign invaders. Usually antibody production takes about a week or so, and once it has occurred, the mother's blood will be sensitized (Rh sensitization) to Rh positive blood. Antibodies would now be formed rather rapidly if there were any later exposures to the Rh factor (Rh+ blood)—for example, in a later pregnancy.

Therefore, it is *usually* a prior pregnancy that sensitizes the mother—and a subsequent pregnancy with an Rh+ fetus (where a leak occurs) in which the mother's immune system responds immediately and progressively destroys the baby's blood. With each exposure to the Rh+ cells (due to leaks), the mother's antibody response strengthens, and the resulting Rh disease in the fetus worsens. That means once the mother has been sensitized, Rh disease potentially worsens with each subsequent pregnancy in which the fetus is Rh+. Because Rh sensitization of Rh− mothers most commonly occurs late in the first sensitized pregnancy—this baby tends not to be seriously affected or shows no effect at all.

There are, however, other sets of circumstances in which *Rh disease can occur in a first pregnancy*:

- An Rh− woman had received an Rh+ blood transfusion or blood products prior to pregnancy. Because antibodies are already present, the potential exists for the first Rh+ fetus of an Rh− mother to have significant Rh disease.
- A leak between the mother and baby occurs, and Rh sensitization develops *early* in the first pregnancy of an Rh− mother and Rh+ fetus (which means antibody production can progress throughout the pregnancy).
- A previous pregnancy of an Rh− mother and Rh+ fetus resulted in a spontaneous or therapeutic abortion.
- An Rh− daughter (now the expectant mother) was sensi-

tized by being exposed to *her Rh+ mother's* blood (basically the opposite circumstances as would happen in her own pregnancy). This has been called the "grandmother theory."

The effects of Rh disease on the fetus are the result of the breakdown (called "hemolysis") of the fetus's blood cells by the mother's Rh antibodies. As the cells are destroyed, the fetus gets progressively more anemic. This ultimately leads to heart failure, because the heart overworks to make up for the lack of oxygen the fetus is experiencing. When the heart fails (that is, when it does not pump efficiently), fluids back up, and the baby becomes swollen.

In addition to the anemia and all of its side effects, destruction of the blood cells leads to an overproduction of bilirubin (a yellow substance that forms when the blood cells are broken down). Before delivery, the placenta can carry away enough of this material so that the fetus is not jeopardized by its presence. However, after delivery the affected baby usually becomes very jaundiced (yellow), because he or she cannot get rid of the excess bilirubin. Accumulation of bilirubin in the baby's brain beyond a critical level—called "kernicterus"—leads to brain damage, usually a form of cerebral palsy.

With mild Rh disease, the baby may reach term safely and can usually be treated for the anemia and excessive bilirubin production. With more severe disease (usually in later pregnancies), babies may have very serious problems earlier in pregnancy, and stillbirth might result if either premature delivery or vigorous intrauterine treatment does not occur.

Today the control of Rh disease is based on two principles: (1) *prevention* of sensitization of Rh negative mothers (when possible) and (2) *early detection* of fetal disease, careful fetal surveillance and aggressive treatment of affected unborn/newborn babies. This entire process starts at the first prenatal visit, when all pregnant women have their lbood groups determined—both ABO blood type (which we will discuss in detail in the next section) and Rh. If you are Rh−, your blood will also be checked for Rh antibodies to determine if you are already sensitized to the Rh factor.

If you have no Rh antibodies, your blood will be tested again for Rh antibodies around the 30th week of pregnancy and again every four to six weeks until delivery. If you still have no antibodies, a final test would be done right after the baby is delivered, and Rhogam® would be given if no antibodies were detected. Rhogam® is a special gamma globulin that can destroy Rh positive cells that may have leaked into your blood—before your body has produced its own antibodies. It therefore prevents you from being sensitized to the Rh factor. The administration of Rhogam® *to Rh negative mothers who do not have Rh antibodies* is recommended in the following situations:

- Within 72 hours of delivery of an Rh+ baby
- After a spontaneous abortion (miscarriage), therapeutic abortion, or ectopic pregnancy
- In some situations, after diagnostic amniocentesis

While Rhogam® is not 100 percent effective in preventing Rh sensitization—it is nearly so and has led to a major reduction in the incidence of Rh disease and perinatal death and damage.

If you have Rh antibodies or develop them during pregnancy, your antibody titer (the amount of antibody production, determined by a special blood test) would be monitored in early pregnancy—as often as every four to six weeks. If the titer is above a critical level, amniocentesis would be recommended to help monitor the severity of the Rh disease in the fetus. The level of bilirubin (the yellow pigment) in the amniotic fluid, along with an evaluation of fetal lung maturity can help doctors determine the best method(s) of management—simply careful watchfulness, intrauterine blood transfusion to delay the necessity for early delivery, or premature delivery of the baby if sufficient fetal maturity is documented.

Intrauterine blood transfusion is performed when the fetus is so anemic that it would likely die if the pregnancy continued but would not be expected to survive if delivered so prematurely. The intrauterine transfusion is done in a way similar to amniocentesis. Ultrasound and/or X-ray is used to carefully locate the fetus's position, and a needle is inserted through the amniotic fluid around the baby into the baby's abdominal cavity. Blood that will not be destroyed (Rh negative blood without antibodies) is injected. The baby's body is able to use this transfused blood temporarily, while its own Rh+ blood is being destroyed. A fetus may need several intrauterine transfusions before it can be safely delivered. While there is some risk of bleeding or damage to the fetus with the procedure, the outcome without it is almost certain death.

At the time of birth, babies with Rh disease are immediately evaluated for severe anemia, and their bilirubin level is checked. They are monitored carefully and frequently for any rapid rise in the bilirubin level, as well as any worsening of the anemia. Treatment today is quite successful in the vast majority of cases and includes the use of blood transfusions to combat anemia and elevated bilirubin levels and often the use of phototherapy (ultraviolet light therapy that helps reduce the level of bilirubin) as well. Exchange transfusions are frequently necessary for babies with Rh disease and involve the systematic withdrawal of the baby's blood (a small amount at a time), followed by replacement with new blood that will not be destroyed by the maternal Rh antibodies. As the blood is progressively removed, some of the antibodies that have been causing the problem are also removed, as is the bilirubin.

The point is—with the availability of Rhogam®, early detection of Rh disease, the use of diagnostic amniocentesis (discussed in detail in Chapter 11) and blood transfusions, where indicated, as well as early delivery of the baby, when necessary, and sophisticated care of newborns with the disease—the great majority of babies never get Rh disease and those that do have satisfactory outcomes, in most cases. Although the problem has not been totally eliminated—progress in preventing and fighting the disease has been remarkable over the years.

ABO Incompatibility

ABO incompatibility is often confused with Rh disease and misunderstood. Because of the confusion, it is important that we discuss it—even though the problem is seen *after birth* rather than during the pregnancy. As we discussed earlier, a number of different blood antigens are found on the surface of each person's red blood cells. The groups of antigens (blood group systems) that are most important in pregnancy are the Rh system, discussed above, and the ABO blood type system.

People are born with *antibodies* to those ABO antigens that their blood does not have. That means most adults with type O blood have antibodies to A and B antigens (called "anti-A" and "anti-B"). Those with type A have anti-B antibodies, and those with type B blood have anti-A antibodies. People with type AB blood do not develop antibodies against either A or B blood (and have therefore been called the "universal recipients" in terms of blood transfusions).

If a mother has one ABO blood type and her baby another—there is a potential risk that ABO incompatibility may develop. Again, ABO incompatibility differs significantly from Rh disease, because there is not an increased risk of a problem *during* pregnancy. ABO incompatibility is not detected until *after* the baby is born, and it generally produces mild to moderate problems (if any) in a newborn. The mother's antibodies can attack the baby's blood because it sees it as "foreign." The baby's red blood cells are broken down (hemolyzed), and the baby may become slightly to moderately anemic. However, the most common problem seen in these babies is jaundice (due to a buildup of bilirubin).

Some facts about ABO disease are well worth mentioning:

- ABO incompatibility can occur in *any* pregnancy, including the first one. One cannot predict whether or not it will occur, or if it does occur, how serious it will be. However, it is usually of much less concern than Rh disease.
- ABO problems are seen in infants after birth probably because the degree of fetal red blood destruction is low grade, bilirubin is cleared by the mother and there is minimal anemia produced in the fetus.
- Mothers with type O blood who have babies with either type A or type B blood are most commonly involved with ABO incompatibility, because they have antibodies against these other blood types. Type O babies, on the other hand, or babies whose ABO blood type is the same as their mothers' do not get this disease. Because of the increased risk for this disease in infants of type O mothers, many hospitals routinely determine the blood types of infants of type O mothers at the time of birth and do other special tests on the blood of those babies who do not have type O blood.
- Babies with ABO incompatibility usually do not experience serious problems. In fact, some will show no disease (jaundice or anemia) at all. If, however, the degree of anemia and/or the elevation of the bilirubin level are more severe, treatment may be necessary. Phototherapy alone is usually quite successful in managing the jaundice. However, on rare occasions, exchange transfusion may be needed to treat the anemia, the jaundice or both.

On the whole, identification and treatment of ABO incompatibility is extremely successful, and parents have little to worry about in most cases.

Post-date Pregnancy (beyond Term)

Thirty-eight to 42 weeks is considered "Term" pregnancy. Anywhere from 10 percent to 15 percent of expectant mothers will be past 42 weeks gestation (by available dates). This is called *post-date pregnancy*. One of the most common causes for extended pregnancy is that the due date is wrong. Often women on birth control pills have delayed ovulation which makes it difficult to determine the time of conception and others have not kept accurate records of their menstrual cycle. Still other women are uncertain because their menstrual cycles are quite irregular normally. All of these situations make "dating" a pregnancy a real guessing game.

Studies have shown that of these 10 percent to 15 percent of post-date pregnancies—around 3 percent to 4 percent of women will experience a prolonged pregnancy. *Prolonged pregnancy* means that the "dates" were correct, and the pregnancy is *actually* extended. The concern about prolonged pregnancy involves a problem called postmaturity syndrome. *Postmaturity syndrome* is a problem of decreased placental function that may accompany prolonged pregnancy—but it doesn't develop in all prolonged pregnancies.

"Postmaturity syndrome" is characterized by a lack of appropriate fetal growth or even loss of fetal weight. Essentially, the fetus stops growing because the placenta is not providing adequate nutrition. Other noted symptoms of postmaturity syndrome include a decrease in amniotic volume, the presence of meconium (the intestinal waste products of the fetus, expelled into the amniotic fluid with fetal distress), and a decrease in the respiratory function of the placenta (oxygenation of the fetus—fetal distress). When the baby is born, he or she has a very characteristic look—small, with very little subcutaneous fat (in fact, looking very much like a wrinkled old man or woman), peeling, yellow-stained skin and often long fingernails.

Chronic fetal distress may lead to serious damage to the brain and other organs and even death, if appropriate intervention does not occur at a critical time. With particularly severe, long-term placental insufficiency, the fetus may be so damaged by lack of oxygenation that stillbirth may occur.

Serious problems are also associated with the presence of meconium in the amniotic fluid, either before delivery or right at the time of delivery. If inhaled (aspirated) into the baby's lungs, either by breathing movements before birth or most often by breaths taken after birth, this sticky greenish-black material can plug up the baby's airways and cause various breathing disturbances—including pneumonia and pneumothorax (collapse of the lung caused by air leak). Meconium aspiration and its resultant problems can often be prevented if the baby's mouth and windpipe are suctioned carefully before he or she takes a deep breath. This is a time when the doctor would prefer that the baby *not* breathe or cry until suctioning is completed. (The reason we mention this is that parents often panic if they see rather quick work on the baby, and they have not heard the baby cry or make any noise. They tend not to understand what is happening and think the worst, when what the doctor and his or her associates are doing is trying to suction the baby immediately—before that first breath or cry.)

A third problem with postmaturity syndrome results from the lack of nutrition provided by the failing placenta. The baby may show temporary hypoglycemia (low blood sugar) for several hours or days after delivery, because it does not have the usual reserve of a normally nourished baby. Because of this risk, the baby will be carefully monitored for this complication (by simple, quick blood tests) and will often need to be fed earlier and more often than other babies. Postmaturity babies are smaller than their potential but not below normal in most cases.

The basic problem then, in post-date pregnancy is in distinguishing between those women whose dates are wrong—and those with true prolonged pregnancy and therefore at risk for postmaturity syndrome. Since postmaturity can be a very serious problem, a specific approach to post-date pregnancy has been developed. Fetal fitness testing is begun at 42 weeks gestation (or 294 days from the last menstrual period) and continued once a week until delivery. (Fetal fitness testing is described in detail in Chapter 13.) As long as testing is normal (indicating normal uteroplacental oxygen transfer) intervention is not necessary, since it is well-known that many post-date pregnancies are not truly prolonged—but rather the dates are wrong. In this way we can identify those fetuses at risk for damage or death who require intervention—and also recognize those not presently at risk.

If the fetal fitness testing is clearly abnormal at any point—then the baby must be delivered by the most expeditious means—often cesarean birth, since the stress of labor may put the fetus at increased risk for further fetal distress and hypoxia. However, in some situations labor may be induced with careful monitoring of the fetus, in hopes of allowing a safe vaginal delivery. Although it is impossible for doctors to know for sure if a woman is really overdue or not—fetal fitness testing has given us a reasonable and reliable means of evaluation for identifying those fetuses who require intervention. This ability has saved countless lives and increased the quality of life for many other babies.

Multiple Births

One in 89 births will result in twins and 1 in 7,900 births in triplets. The chance for quadruplets is 1 in 1 million. Because of the fertility drugs available today, we are seeing more multiple births (even quintuplets) than ever before.

"Identical" (monozygotic) twins come from a single ovum, are always the same sex and remarkably resemble each other the vast majority of the time because they are genetically identical. "Fraternal" (dizygotic) twins come from two ova and often don't look alike and can be of the opposite sex. Having fraternal twins is inherited on the mother's side of the family, and there appears to be a correlation between increased maternal age and the incidence of twins.

If a woman is carrying twins (or more) her uterus is larger than would be expected for the time of gestation. If twins are suspected, ultrasound is performed to verify the diagnosis. Because multiple births are more likely to be premature (15 percent, compared to 5 percent for single babies), and since the mother is essentially supporting two or more fetuses—once the diagnosis of a multiple pregnancy is made, it is important for the mother to get as much rest as possible. As a safety precaution mothers are told to get off their feet and into bed as much as possible after the 20th week of pregnancy. This constant rest may be helpful in prolonging the pregnancy.

Besides the potential for premature delivery—carrying multiple fetuses increases the risk for pre-eclampsia and eclampsia, breech presentation of one or more of the babies, anemia (so supplemental iron is prescribed), differential growth of the fetuses (one fetus gets more from the placenta than the other), prolapsed cord or some other cord accident, and partial placental separation between the deliveries of the fetuses (which may result in decreased oxygenation of the fetus not yet delivered).

When mothers are carefully managed and follow the prescribed program of rest, diet, office visits and other measures, the majority of twins (and other multiple births) do well today—which is a vast improvement over the outcome years ago.

Incompetent Cervix and Uterine Malformation

Repeated spontaneous abortion (miscarriage) or premature delivery may result from abnormalities of the cervix or uterus. There are preventive measures that may be helpful once the problem is recognized, but unfortunately recognition usually only occurs after a pregnancy loss.

Incompetent cervix refers to a situation in which the cervix dilates very early in pregnancy, resulting in spontaneous abortion or premature delivery. It may be due to deformities of the lower part of the uterus and conditions that result in scarring or deformity of the cervix itself—previous tears of the cervix (sometimes related to induced abortions), and scars that have resulted from cervical surgery (surgical biopsy, or a procedure called "conization," in which a segment of the cervix is removed). Conization may be done in order to diagnose suspicious lesions of the cervix (for example, in women with abnormal Pap smears). It is also used to treat carcinoma *in situ* of the cervix (the earliest form of cervical cancer).

While the cause of cervical incompetence can't be identified in the majority of women who have it, it can be successfully treated in an increasingly large number of women. The problem is suspected if a woman has a known cervical problem and/or has experienced repeated spontaneous midtrimester abortion or prematurity. Treatment consists of suturing (sewing) the cervix closed after the 14th week of pregnancy. Using a method called either the McDonald or Shirodkar procedure, a large stitch is placed around the cervix while the pregnant mother is under anesthesia. The stitch must be removed when labor starts in order to allow vaginal delivery. The success rate varies depending on what caused the incompetent cervix in the first place.

Uterine malformation can either be congenital (such as double-horned uterus) or a result of later events in a woman's life (such as the formation of fibroid tumors or uterine surgery). Depending on the type and extent, these malformations can cause one or more of the following problems: abnormal or faulty implantation of the placenta; repeated miscarriage or premature delivery; dystocia—failure of labor to progress (discussed in Chapter 14); or various fetal malformation due to abnormal pressure on the developing fetus (discussed in Chapter 2).

Some of the problems can be treated through surgery allowing for a subsequent successful pregnancy. Your doctor may wish to evaluate you in detail for a uterine problem if you have had previous miscarriages, premature infants or infants with certain characteristic deformities.

History of Vaginal Bleeding and Placental Problems

We know that 15 percent to 30 percent of women will experience some vaginal bleeding during pregnancy. If the bleeding occurs in the first three months of pregnancy, there is risk of miscarriage— called a *threatened abortion*. Little can be done about this since in the majority of cases this means that the "conceptus" (the word for the fetus very early in pregnancy) has a significant abnormality that would make survival impossible. Therefore, threatened abortion (in the first trimester of pregnancy) many times ends in spontaneous abortion (miscarriage). Later in pregnancy—after the 20th week— bleeding is usually due to a placental problem: either placental abruption or placenta previa.

Placental abruption is characterized by painful bleeding associated with either uterine contractions or cramping, or just constant, very severe pain in the uterus. In this situation, part of the placenta "abruptly separates" from the wall of the uterus before delivery has occurred. The pain is usually caused by the accumulation of blood between the placenta and the uterine wall. The uterus can go into constant, very painful contraction, which markedly decreases the blood flow to the baby. Blood loss is usually from the mother's side of the placenta, so she can develop shock (low blood pressure because of inadequate blood to circulate), which also decreases the oxygen supply to the baby. With massive abruption, fetal death can occur rapidly, even with prompt intervention. Fortunately, placental abruption is usually partial rather than complete, and successful intervention can occur.

When a significant placental abruption occurs (unless it happens very early in pregnancy), the recommended treatment is most often prompt delivery, before the fetus dies and the mother experiences a serious loss of blood. Rapid vaginal delivery or emergency cesarean delivery is performed, and blood transfusion is often necessary to manage shock from blood loss and to avoid serious maternal complications. Fetal death (stillbirth) and newborn death usually result from sudden uteroplacental insufficiency (lack of oxygen through the placenta because of partial or complete abruption) or the problems associated with prematurity (respiratory distress syndrome, organ system immaturity, etc.).

Women who are older, those with chronic hypertension and those who have had many other children are at greater risk for premature separation of the placenta than other expectant mothers. Trauma to the mother's abdomen may also cause placental abruption, although this is uncommon. These at-risk women and those who have a history of previous placental abruption should be carefully evaluated and followed throughout pregnancy. Those with hypertension may improve their odds of avoiding placental abruption by getting the condition under control.

It is very important to remember that if bleeding of any kind occurs during pregnancy—you should call your doctor immediately. Significant bleeding requires that you go immediately to a hospital for evaluation. If the problem is placental abruption and the placenta has only partially separated, immediate delivery of the baby may save his or her life. Therefore, a very rapid response to bleeding on your part is paramount.

Placental abruption can occur during labor and can be detected by electronic fetal monitoring (see Chapter 12). Prompt cesarean delivery is usually necessary, and such intervention can be life-saving.

Placenta previa is a distinctly different problem from placental abruption and occurs in about 1 in every 200 pregnancies. Placenta previa is most often recognized when it causes painless bleeding. Characteristically, the expectant mother wakes up after a nap or a night's sleep and first thinks she has ruptured her membranes (her "water" has broken) or fears she has urinated. However, she discovers that the liquid is blood. Her amazement comes from the lack of any pain to signal that something was wrong. (Although a small number of women experience minor cramping or contractions with bleeding from placenta previa, this problem is painless in most cases.)

With placenta previa, a portion or all of the placenta is lying in the lower part of the uterus near or directly over the cervix. Bleeding usually occurs when blood vessels are disrupted from minor tears in the placental attachment to the uterus or partial detachment of the placenta. Some dilatation of the cervix is often involved. Most bleeding from placenta previa is not massive. However, if severe, uncontrollable bleeding occurs, shock can result, and immediate cesarean delivery is necessary.

If a woman experiences spotting or painless bleeding in later pregnancy, the bleeding is first managed by bed rest. Ultrasound (see Chapter 10) is performed to locate the placenta and verify or rule out the diagnosis of placenta previa. If the diagnosis is verified, complete bed rest is recommended—most often in the hospital—until delivery. In some very specific situations, women are allowed to go home after the bleeding has stopped, provided they are absolutely committed to complete bed rest at home except for bathroom privileges. If any bleeding begins again, the woman is again hospitalized, for her well-being and that of her fetus. Complete bed rest may be recommended in later pregnancy, even without bleeding, in order to turn the odds in favor of the woman *who has experienced the previous loss of a baby because of placenta previa.* The time in pregnancy that bed rest would be recommended is based on each individual woman—her previous pregnancy history and whether or not there has been bleeding from the low-lying placenta.

Cesarean birth is required when placenta previa is found, since vaginal delivery would not only be dangerous to both mother and baby because of bleeding but also virtually impossible, because the cervix is obstructed by the placenta.

The goal in managing placenta previa is to stop the bleeding, carefully monitor the mother and baby (as necessary) and keep both in shape until approximately the 37th week. At this tiem, fetal lung maturity is determined, and if the fetus is mature, cesarean birth is performed. This mode of management is important, since there is a significant risk of serious bleeding if labor occurs (see Chapter 14).

At times blood loss from the mother may be serious enough that she will need one or more blood transfusions. Placenta previa increases the risk for prematurity and its many associated problems, as well as perinatal death. With today's technology and knowledge, however, the outlook is vastly improved for the baby and maternal death due to placenta previa has become increasingly rare.

History of Premature Birth

In humans "term pregnancy" (which means the baby has reached full gestation—full maturity) is 280 days on the average. To simplify this, the time of pregnancy is expressed in weeks or months

(40 weeks or 9 months). There are, however, built-in variations on this average gestational time period. Pregnancies that go to "term" (also called "term delivery") are those in which delivery occurs between the 38th and 42nd weeks of pregnancy.

Premature birth is generally defined as delivery after the 20th week of pregnancy but before the 38th week. Statistically, 7 percent of babies will be premature. The basic problem of prematurity is that the baby's organs—in particular the lungs—are not fully developed and therefore may have minor to serious difficulty functioning efficiently. While in the uterus, the baby's respiratory, nutritional and detoxification functions are provided by the mother through the placenta. After birth the baby must be able to perform these functions (and several others) on his or her own. The lungs present the most significant problem, because they mature in the last few weeks of pregnancy. If the baby is born prematurely—then the lungs have usually not had time to reach the level of maturity required to totally support the baby without difficulty. Some premature babies require only supplemental oxygen. Others need the support of a respirator (a mechanical device that either completely breathes for the infant or assists in this vital function), as well as other rather dramatic life-support measures.

The more premature the baby—the less developed his or her organs will be and the less capable (for the most part) he or she will be of functioning well or without medical assistance. Because of this, babies born before the 36th week of pregnancy usually require special care—some level of intensive care in a special nursery (which is discussed in detail in Chapter 19). Because prematurity is still the major cause of neonatal death, doctors try to stop premature labor if it occurs. (Discussed in detail in Chapter 15.)

Although many of the reason(s) for premature delivery still represent a major unanswered question, we do know that certain problems or conditions increase the risk. These include chronic hypertension, pre-eclampsia, eclampsia, placental abruption, placenta previa, premature rupture of the membranes, umbilical cord prolapse, uterine abnormalities, uterine infections, cigarette smoking, multiple births, teratogens, congenital and genetic abnormalities, Rh disease and uteroplacental insufficiency (inadequate oxygen and nutrient supply to the fetus for a variety of reasons).

Advances in obstetrics and neonatology have markedly decreased neonatal death and disability over the years—when the pregnancy is carefully managed medically, and the woman diligently follows the doctor's recommendations. Although prematurity can prove to be a serious problem, much progress has been made, and more is expected in the near future.

History of Spontaneous Abortion (Miscarriage)

Statistically, 15 to 20 percent of pregnancies end in spontaneous abortion (also called "miscarriage"). The first sign of a threatened abortion is vaginal bleeding, and the second sign is usually pain (a result of the cervix opening). Any time bleeding occurs, you should contact your doctor immediately for advice. If bleeding is severe and accompanied by pain—it may be best to go to the nearest emergency room. At times "spotting" or "episodic minor bleeding" may mean little and may have no effect on the fetus. However, depending on the time in the pregnancy—bleeding can signify spontaneous abortion, placenta previa, placental abruption or another minor to serious problem. Therefore, it is important for the doctor to evaluate the situation and determine the cause of the bleeding.

The vast majority (75 percent) of spontaneous abortions occur before the 16th week of pregnancy, and the majority of these are due to serious structural malformations in the "conceptus" (the term for the fetus very early in pregnancy). This, then, appears to be nature's way of terminating the gestation of a conceptus who could not survive. Loss of the conceptus before the 20th week of pregnancy is considered a spontaneous abortion, because before that time the survival of the fetus is virtually impossible.

However, there are other possible causes of spontaneous abortion, such as severe chronic hypertension, hypertensive vascular disease, hyperthyroidism, abnormal uterus, serious infection, maternal trauma, incompetent cervix, uncontrolled diabetes, hormonal deficiencies and the effects of teratogens (factors that can induce malformation in the developing conceptus). If you have a history of spontaneous abortion, then you would want to see your doctor *before* pregnancy or very early in pregnancy (at worst) for a complete evaluation. In this way, any underlying problem and/or cause that is preventable, treatable or manageable may be identified so appropriate care can be given.

Although tragedies such as miscarriage and stillbirth (discussed in the next section) are very difficult for parents—there is a great deal of hope. We know that a couple have a 70 percent to 80 percent chance of maintaining a pregnancy to the time of fetal viability (when survival is possible) even if they have already experienced three miscarriages. Those who have experienced even four or five spontaneous abortions still have a 65 percent to 70 percent chance of maintaining a pregnancy until the fetus is capable of surviving. Also, even though little can be done about the loss of the conceptus with a serious structural malformation (since survival is impossible), much more can be done today than ever before when it comes to maternal conditions or other potential problems associated with spontaneous abortion.

History of Stillbirth

Stillbirth means that a fetus died in the uterus or during labor and was born dead. This term is used for the loss of a fetus after the 20th week. A stillbirth may be the result of one or more of many causes—placental abruption, prolapsed cord accident, severe Rh disease, severe fetal hypoxia, serious infection, diabetes, severe postmaturity syndrome due to placental dysfunction, congenital malformation due to either a genetic abnormality or as a result of a teratogen, and severe uteroplacental insufficiency (inadequate oxygen or nutrient supply to the fetus due to any cause). At times the cause is unknown.

If you have a history of stillbirth—it is best to see your doctor before pregnancy (if possible) or early in pregnancy to find out if there are any problems or identifiable causes for the stillbirth(s) that can be alleviated, treated or managed throughout pregnancy. The incidence of stillbirth has been significantly reduced in recent years because of early and excellent prenatal and perinatal care. Many of the problems listed above can be successfully managed today—as discussed further throughout the book.

The Bottom Line

Great strides have been made in the identification, management and treatment of maternal diseases and conditions, as well as Rh and ABO blood incompatibility, post-date pregnancy, multiple births, uterine malformation, placental problems and incompetent cervix. Also, more is now known and more can be done about the problems of prematurity, miscarriage (in certain situations) and stillbirth. The point is—being at risk for a problem pregnancy today means something very different than it meant years ago. Modern technology and greater knowledge have led to much better outcomes for both mother and baby—and there is even more hope for the future.

THREE

RISKS AFTER AGE 35:
A SPECIAL CONSIDERATION

The number of women over 35 having children has increased tremendously over the past 15 years. The percentage of those between 35 and 39 has risen by almost 50%.

Whatever the reason, there is a trend developing—more women are getting pregnant after age 30 and 35, many for the first time. Career goals, later marriages, financial considerations and the widespread use of more effective birth control methods have all played a role. Additionally, single women, now older but wanting to have families, are deciding to do so more often than ever before.

As maternal age has increased, serious questions have been raised about the safety and well-being of both mother and baby. Unfortunately, many of these concerns have been blown up out of proportion—resulting in the spreading of misinformation on a large scale and causing unnecessary alarm for women over 30 or 35. That is not to say the publicity about maternal age is all bad. It has made some people more aware of potential problems or at least encouraged them to seek more information. The problem is, much of what you might have heard has been overdone and exaggerated.

There *are* some special considerations of which women and their partners should be aware if the woman is over 30. With advanced maternal age comes a greater potential for certain serious birth defects. Some researchers also feel that women who put off pregnancy tend to be type A personalities (driving, success oriented, determined, hard working), and type A personality women seem to be prone to diseases such as hypertension (high blood pressure). Further increases in risk come from diseases that are more prevalent with advanced age—diabetes, vascular and kidney disease, hypertension and others.

Also, some older women have an increased intake of alcohol, smoke, are overweight or underweight, and exercise less frequently than younger women. But these are all generalizations. Many women who wait until later in life to have children are extremely physically fit, have no hereditary or underlying disease, do not smoke, drink moderately (or not at all) and are in the best of health. Certainly the majority of the over-30 female population falls somewhere in the middle in terms of general health, fitness and habits.

If you're considering pregnancy and are in your thirties (especially over 35), it's very important that you see a doctor for an overall evaluation before getting pregnant. This evaluation will help to determine if you have an underlying disease or problem that could worsen with childbearing or cause an increased risk for either you or your unborn child.

You should also take steps to change all correctable health habits and problems before pregnancy. Stop smoking if you smoke. If you are overweight or underweight, try to reach your optimal weight before becoming pregnant. Begin an appropriate exercise program to promote cardiovascular fitness if you are not already on one, but see your doctor before starting such a plan. Follow a well-balanced nutritional plan. Don't drink alcohol or use unnecessary drugs while you are pregnant or trying to get pregnant. Remember, if you happen to get pregnant and don't know it, smoking, drinking and poor nutrition can affect your unborn baby's health. It is during this initial stage—precisely when you are least likely to be aware of the pregnancy—that the fetus is most vulnerable.

Because risks may be increased for both the unborn child and the pregnant woman after she has reached her mid-thirties, there are some things you and your husband or mate will want to know before you decide to have a baby, or if you have found yourselves in this situation unexpectedly.

The concerns generally associated with an increase in maternal age are twofold: (1) the "environmental" effects due to the mother's physical aging and (2) the effect of aging (chromosomal problems) on the female germ cell (egg).

If you are over 35, in good health and have no serious chronic problems, the risk for you (discounting chromosomal risks) will not be appreciably increased over that for a younger woman. The point is—if you have stayed physically fit, are quite healthy and without any of these often age-related problems—then you would more than likely be able to physically handle the pregnancy well. (Therefore, your risk for problems—other than an increased risk for chromosomal abnormalities—would not be much greater than someone younger.)

Women after age 35 have an increased risk of developing toxemia of pregnancy (hypertension—high blood pressure—as a result of pregnancy). They usually do not have the stamina they did when younger and tend to have more age-related diseases, such as diabetes, heart and vascular problems, liver problems, kidney disorders, hypertension and others. It is also more difficult for the woman over 35 to get back into shape after pregnancy—unless she has maintained physical fitness throughout her life and becomes physically active as soon after pregnancy as possible. However, you should realize that as our bodies age there is less adaptibility to physical change. Pregnancy brings about physical change which some older mothers adapt to well, while others have more problems—particularly in getting back into shape once the baby is born.

Simply stated, advanced maternal age often means less flexibility of the body and more health-related problems. Many such problems can stress the woman's health during pregnancy and also affect the health and safety of the unborn baby. And multiple risk factors pose added risks for both the woman and her fetus. Part of the answer is to get into shape before pregnancy occurs. Once in good shape with all medical problems under control then go about getting pregnant.

When *trying to get pregnant*, follow your doctor's instructions for diet and exercise, and for the control of any chronic medical problems. Do not smoke. Do not take any medications (prescribed or over-the-counter) not approved by your physician who *knows* you are trying to get pregnant. Do not drink alcoholic beverages unless infrequently and in very small amounts. Try to avoid x rays unless absolutely necessary and make sure you tell the doctor you are trying to get pregnant (which means you already might be and don't know it). Try to stay away from industrial hazards and other chemicals which may cause fetal malformations. (For more information on all of the above recommendations, see Chapter 5.)

If you are *already pregnant* and over 30 or 35, make sure you follow a recommended nutritional plan, continue to keep tight controls on any chronic or potential medical problem, and follow your doctor's recommendations for prenatal visits. In this way, any chronic problem or other medical problem which may suddenly occur, can be identified and managed as early in pregnancy as possible. This gives you and your doctor a jump on the problem and a better chance to keep it under control. No matter where you are in your pregnancy if you haven't stopped smoking—do so. And be careful about alcohol consumption, medications and drugs.

Regardless of age, however, women with chronic disease can have successful, healthy pregnancies. Chances of success are greatly improved for the woman who is treated and carefully monitored throughout pregnancy—from the very earliest time pregnancy is suspected—by a qualified physician who is aware of her risks and attentive to potential problems.

The second concern with advanced maternal age is the effect of aging on the female germ cell—the ovum (egg). A female is born with all the ova, or eggs, she will ever produce. There are some 400,000 ova distributed in each of the two ovaries. Once a girl reaches puberty she usually releases one ovum per month, alternating from one ovary to the other. After the egg is released into the Fallopian tube, it is either fertilized by a male germ cell (sperm) or dies in 48 hours or so and then is eliminated from the body. A woman releases only about 400 of the eggs during her life—between puberty and menopause.

All the while, the other ova wait in the ovaries, aging through the years. As time passes there seems to be a greater potential for chromosomal damage, a greater possibility that an "accident of nature" will occur. An extra chromosome may come from the egg, or there may be incomplete chromosomal material because of faulty cell division or breakage. Unfortunately, such chromosomal accidents can have grave consequences for the baby. It is this risk of advanced maternal age that concerns most people.

Remember, the 23 pairs of chromosomes are the major "building blocks" of life and are composed of thousands of genes, which determine our basic makeup. The 23 pairs from the mother's ovum must meet with the 23 pairs from the father's sperm. The matching of chromosomes and the ordering of their genes dictate the physical and mental growth and development of the fetus. If chromosomal material is missing or displaced, or there is too much chromosomal material, entire body systems are seriously affected.

Thus far, a relationship between paternal (the father's) age and chromosomal abnormalities has not been clearly established. There is some speculation that paternal age may have an effect on sperm production and health, but this is only in the investigative stages.

Unlike the ova, which are all present in the ovaries at birth, sperm are produced continually throughout the male's life. That does not, however, eliminate the possibility of "chromosomal damage" in the spermatozoa. It simply excludes the problem of aging in the existing sperm, since new ones are continually produced.

The chromosomes in the sperm can break or rearrange their genetic material (translocate), and there can be too much or too little chromosomal material present. These problems can exist before sperm production or can happen during cell division as accidents of nature. As with the female germ cell, chromosomal problems in the sperm may be due to weakness in the chromosome itself, faulty cell division or damage due to something still unknown.

Again, this problem needs to be put into perspective. Of the more than 3 million infants born each year in the United States, the majority are healthy. Around 75,000 of these newborns will have significant birth defects. Many infants with birth defects will have conditions resulting from other than genetic or chromosomal causes, such as various problems the mother experienced during pregnancy; the use of alcohol, cigarettes and drugs; exposure to a large amount of radiation or certain chemicals; and some external environmental factors and their interactions with genes. (See Chapter 5 for more information on these possible causes.) The majority, however, have no identifiable cause.

To date, most babies with birth defects and genetic disorders are born to women under 35, because more women under 35 are having babies. However, the risk of having a child with a chromosomal disorder increases with maternal age, especially after age 35. When you compare the percentages, you find that the risk of a chromosomal abnormality increases from 2.5 per 1,000 births for women age 30 to 4.5 per 1,000 for women 35 to 13.7 per 1,000 for women 40.

Most chromosomal abnormalities are lethal for the fetus—they are incompatible with life and result in spontaneous abortion early in pregnancy. A small percentage of fetuses survive until birth with very serious defects, but many of these babies die in infancy. Of those who do not die, nearly all have severe deformities and do not develop normally.

Of greatest concern to women 35 years of age and older is Down's syndrome, seen in increased incidence with advanced maternal age. A chromosomal abnormality in which there is an extra chromosome (as discussed in Chapter 5), it jumps from one birth in every 885 for mothers 30 years old—to one birth in every 365 to one birth in every 12 for mothers 49 years old.

Couples facing the issue of pregnancy after age 35 may be at risk for hereditary or genetic disease other than Down's syndrome—

especially if such diseases are known in either partner's family. (Existence of hereditary or genetic disease in either partner's family indicates a risk for women and their partners under 35 as well.) For these couples genetic counseling aimed at identifying various risks for potential problems would be a very good idea. Ideally, genetic counseling should be done *before* pregnancy, but it can also be done during pregnancy. Most metropolitan areas have centers for genetic counseling, and if you are concerned, your physician can refer you and your mate. Counseling must include both partners in order to yield optimal results.

Today, various tests are available for prenatal diagnosis of chromosomal and other disorders, and many more will be developed in the future. Such procedures as amniocentesis (in which some of the amniotic fluid around the developing baby is removed for analysis); testing of the amniotic fluid or the mother's blood for abnormally high levels of a substance called alpha-fetoprotein; and fetoscopy (an investigational technique that allows the developing fetus to be directly viewed through a special instrument and even permits some of the baby's blood to be taken before birth) are all currently available. (Fetoscopy is still in its research stages, however, and is available at only a few major centers that perform clinical testing under very specific guidelines.) Section 2 details these and other tests and what they would tell you and your doctor.

The Bottom Line on Maternal Age

One thing is certain—every pregnancy has risks associated with it, whether the couple are older or not. While the majority of pregnancies are normal and produce healthy babies, any couple could find themselves facing the birth of a child with serious abnormalities, even though the risk is statistically low. Knowing how each partner feels and what options might be acceptable to each if they are faced with an abnormal test result will help the couple face these potential problems openly and realistically.

What's important to remember is that for the vast majority of couples facing pregnancy over the age of 35, the picture is anything but grim, in contrast to what many people would have you believe. You should be aware of certain increased risks yet not over-react to them. Most pregnancies in the over-35 group are not only without complications but generally very rewarding, and most will result in perfectly normal babies.

FOUR

TERATOGENS: DRUGS AND OTHER POSSIBLE CAUSES OF FETAL MALFORMATIONS

Let's set the stage.

Imagine. The uterus—warm, secure, protective. The baby—growing, cells multiplying, organs developing.

Imagine. A drink in the baby's forming hand, a cigarette hanging from its mouth, a pill floating in the warm liquid, ready to be swallowed. Exaggerated? Certainly. But in a very real way, these images tell the story.

A drug is any substance that affects the body or changes its chemistry. Alcohol, cigarettes, coffee, tea, cold medications, aspirin, laxatives and antacid tablets—all have properties that place them in the general category of drugs. Coffee, tea and cola contain caffeine, which speeds up the cardiovascular system. Tobacco products contain nicotine, which constricts or narrows the arteries and veins; when burned it produces carbon monoxide, which "steals" oxygen from the tissues and organs. Alcohol was one of the first painkillers identified, and it is still used liberally in medications today. For example, many over-the-counter cold and cough medications have alcohol in them. If taken in frequent or large doses, alcohol has the potential to damage cells and eventually destroy organs and tissues. We forget when we pop aspirin into our mouths that we are taking a "real" drug. With today's advertising our society has become drug-oriented—the "for-every-ill-there-is-a-pill" syndrome. We've become accustomed to taking medication without even thinking much about it. Advertising has drugged our sense of reason.

Drugs are only one example of a potential teratogen. (A teratogen is "anything which is capable of inducing malformation in the developing embryo," according to the *Faber Medical Dictionary*.) That would include any chemical, drug, physical agent, virus, bacteria,

54

environmental agent or "other" factor that alters the growth, form, development or function of the embryo or fetus. German measles, medications and drugs, alcohol, venereal disease, high doses of radiation, environmental agents and many other causes are included.

The science of teratology attempts to determine the causes of deviations, to identify the various mechanisms involved and their actions, and to deal with their manifestations. More is known today than ever before about teratogenic agents—but what we now know still represents the tiny tip of the iceberg. Much is still left to speculation and to further research.

Considering the statistics and the often life-long problems congenital defects can cause, you can see why so much emphasis is being placed on prevention—particularly of those that can be avoided—like many teratogens! The more you know, the better equipped you are to prevent some potential problems and take action against others. It would be fantastic if congenital defects due to teratogens could be wiped-out.

Exposure to teratogens during the fertilization and implantation period—that is, from the time of conception to around the second week of pregnancy, will more than likely destroy the developing organism. In this stage of gestation, cells are dividing and multiplying rapidly and are extremely vulnerable to any toxic influence.

During the embryonic period (the third week after conception to around 55 days), teratogenic agents can cause serious functional and developmental defects. This stage seems to be the most critical, because of the tremendous growth and organ formation that occur. This is also a stage when you may still be unaware of your pregnancy.

The fetal period (from around 56 days until delivery) is a time of continued rapid growth and development. Teratogens can still affect the developing baby, but since organ formation is completed, the risk is much less. It seems that the fewer the cells and the smaller the size—that is, the more primitive the embryo—the greater the teratogenic effect. The first trimester (three months) is a crucial period overall, and you should take every care to ensure the health and safety of the growing little being.

Alcohol

Fetal alcohol syndrome was identified in 1973. Prior to that no one said much about alcohol and pregnancy, because no one knew much about it. Birth defects possibly due to alcohol consumption were categorized under "source unknown."

Some research is worth noting. One study from the University of Goteborg in Sweden, published in 1979 showed that 33 percent of babies born to alcoholic mothers (who continued drinking during pregnancy) had fetal alcohol syndrome. Another 33 percent had some features associated with alcohol use during pregnancy. That means only 33 percent were normal.

Alcohol consumption and pregnancy is still one of those areas with a lot of questions and not many answers. Few studies have been done on the mild to moderate drinker and the effects of alcohol consumption on her newborn. Because of this, no one can tell you exactly how much drinking is too much, and how often is too often to prevent adversely affecting your unborn child. That means *you* must really make the decision yourself—for both of you.

The best recommendation is to avoid drinking during pregnancy altogether. If you must, though, a very rare drink might be prudent—but no alcohol would be better.

Some experts believe that something about the constitution of certain women—something in their genetic or metabolic makeup—makes them more susceptible to this problem. That could mean a few drinks for one woman might do nothing, while a few for another might be disastrous. Other experts contend that alcohol use must be chronic and in large quantities to be damaging. The truth is—nobody really knows.

There are many manifestations of fetal alcohol syndrome, and children with this problem share many specific characteristics. In fact, they look almost like brothers and sisters. Most have small birth weight and length, and 98 percent have facial abnormalities, such as small eyes, flat nose and unusual folds around the eyes. Skeletal defects include limitation of motion of the elbows, knees and hips and dislocation of the hips. Research shows that 50 percent of these babies have heart defects, and 30 percent have abnormal external genitals. Many have abnormal creases in their palms.

Postnatal (after birth) mental and physical growth and development is commonly retarded, and it is not unusual for the maturation of motor coordination to be delayed or for coordination to be impaired. "Failure to thrive" is also not unusual in these babies, and they are known to be hyperactive and irritable. These children seem to have difficulty adapting to life outside the uterus and so tend to have various problems in the perinatal period.

Some neurological and fine motor damage can last for weeks,

months, years or permanently. Also, infant mortality (death) rates increase in babies of mothers who are alcoholic or use alcohol in excessive amounts.

Fetal alcohol syndrome can be deceiving, because it doesn't appear to be an all-or-nothing phenomenon. Some children manifest one or two minor problems, while others have all the problems associated with it. That makes it doubly difficult to identify subtle cases. Where only growth impairment or mental retardation is identified, it is often suspected that maternal alcohol consumption may have been a factor.

We should point out that the use of alcohol as a treatment measure to control premature labor, when utilized late in pregnancy, for limited times and for very good medical reasons, is absolutely acceptable. The potential benefits of alcohol (given intravenously) in this situation far outweigh the risks. The risk of one exposure to alcohol is less than the risk of premature delivery and all its potential ramifications, as we discussed in detail in Chapter 2. (Alcohol and other drugs used to stop premature labor are discussed in Chapter 15.)

Again, the best advice is to avoid the use of alcohol if you're trying to get pregnant or are pregnant. You may not realize conception has occurred until several weeks into your pregnancy, and those first few weeks and months are vitally important and sensitive times for your baby's development.

Smoking

In 1957 connections between smoking and problems with pregnancy were first reported. Volumes of research have spanned the last few decades. Some questions have been answered, while others are left to speculation and to more research.

We know that smoking during pregnancy is associated with lower birth weight—"small for dates" babies. As birth weight decreases, it seems, the potential for problems usually increases. Smoking, in general, retards fetal growth. There also seems to be an increase in perinatal (around the time of birth) death—that is, stillbirth or death within the first month of life.

Mothers who smoke have a higher incidence of premature birth, and smokers tend to have more complications of pregnancy and labor.

Some reports have indicated persistent growth lags in the children of smoking mothers and lower reading achievement scores (learning ability) when compared to the children of nonsmokers. Although there has been criticism of some studies, statistics have shown that the overall outcome for infants of smoking mothers is not as favorable as that for infants of nonsmoking mothers.

Because of these factors women who smoke are considered in the "high-risk" group for potential problems. Obviously, if you're already at risk for premature delivery, you may be adding a great deal more risk to the situation if you smoke.

There is more. After birth the child may experience pulmonary and cardiovascular problems. Children of smoking parents are much more likely to develop respiratory problems such as bronchitis and pneumonia during the first year of life than the children of non-smokers—probably the result of so-called passive smoking.

When you add smoking to pregnancy—high-risk or not—you can be sure the toxic effects pass to the baby. As is true with alcohol, the placental barrier does not stop cigarette toxins from reaching the fetus. It appears that the more the mother smokes—more cigarettes or stronger ones—the greater the risk for problems. There is some concern about an expectant mother constantly inhaling cigarette smoke in smoke-filled rooms, as well. Either way, no one really knows how many cigarettes are too many, and how often is too often.

Although there is some question about the role a woman's physical makeup plays in this problem—that is, whether some women are more susceptible to having problems if they smoke than others—there is no way as yet to identify precisely which women would be at greater risk if they smoke.

Considering the associated fetal problems, it is best not to smoke during pregnancy—particularly if you are already at risk for other problems.

Drugs: Prescribed Drugs, Over-the-Counter Medications and Street Drugs

The bottom line—don't use any drugs without first asking your doctor, and then use them only when absolutely necessary. Sound harsh? Drugs should be taken carefully, only when necessary and as prescribed or recommended by a physician who knows you're pregnant. The reason is simple—any drug you take has a potential risk. No drug is absolutely safe. (Throughout the book "drug" and "medication" are terms used synonymously—chemicals meant to alter body function. When we mean illegal drugs we will use that term.)

With pregnancy there is an added risk of adversely affecting your unborn child—because he or she also receives some of the drug you have taken. There are some drugs known to be hazardous during pregnancy, some we're not sure about and others still being investigated.

To list all the drugs that cross the placental barrier would take page after page. It is accepted that almost all drugs (in some form or amount) cross from the mother to the fetus. That *does not* mean all drugs will cause serious harm to the baby. Some will. Some will not. There is still not nearly enough information for us to be sure about all (or even most) drugs. Therefore, cautious skepticism is a good approach.

In adults the renal and hepatic (kidney and liver) systems are fully mature and have enormous excretion and detoxification capabilities—they cleanse the body's blood and fluids of toxins, reducing adverse effects. Because the growing fetus is only in its developmental stages, the placenta takes over part of this detoxification function. With some drugs, the detoxification system protecting the fetus may work well, while with others it may be less efficient in removing toxins. Therefore, a drug might have a low risk factor for a mother but pose a potentially serious threat to the unborn child. The drug then becomes toxic or poisonous (teratogenic) to the fetus, who because of his or her immaturity, is unable to effectively deal with it.

Also, certain body organs and enzyme systems develop in the fetus at very key times in gestation. During these times developing organs are at special risk for damage from teratogenic agents, such as drugs. A drug taken early in pregnancy (the first 12 weeks are very special) may cause more serious or deadly effects for the unborn baby than if it were taken in the last months.

Prescribed Drugs

It's important for you to understand that, in certain situations, the use of a drug has a much greater benefit than its potential risk. When information about various drugs and pregnancy became available to the public, many women refused to take any medication, even if their doctors felt them necessary. Certainly their fears were understandable and appreciated, but in many cases the fears were unreasonable and misinformed.

For example, using certain antibiotics when an infection is present has potentially greater benefit to both mother and baby than the risk involved, provided the antibiotic is chosen wisely. Because serious infections can have adverse effects on the fetus, it is better to take the potential risk of using a medication than to leave the infection untreated. There are other equally important situations in which your doctor would prescribe drugs for you, and in which the benefits would outweigh the risks by a wide margin. If these arise, discuss the benefits and risks with your doctor in detail.

As you probably know, not all prescribed drugs are as safe as they were once thought to be. Hopefully, regulations and sound scientific principles will prevent future disasters of the type seen in the past when so-called safe drugs caused unexpected problems.

Every drug—whether it be morphine or aspirin—has potential associated risks, and some drugs carry greater risks than others. Also, what might be a risk for you may not be for someone else, which makes it difficult to generalize about risk factors.

The best way to judge the use of any drug is to determine its risk-benefit ratio. By weighing the potential benefits against the potential risks, as well as the necessity of using the medication, a conscientious decision can be made. (This applies to all of us all the time, not just during high-risk pregnancies.)

As an overview, the following drugs should *not* be used during any pregnancy: tetracycline, an antibiotic that causes abnormalities in the fetus's developing teeth and bones; aminopterin-methotrexate, used in cancer therapy; oral hypoglycemics, which change the level of sugar in the blood and are sometimes used to treat mild cases of diabetes; iodides, which cause newborn goiter (some over-the-counter cold medicines contain iodides, so read the labels carefully, or ask your doctor about which cold or cough medication is recommended, if any); and coumadin, an anticoagulant, or "blood thinner," which crosses the placental barrier (however, it may be useful and indicated in some situations with due consideration for the risk-benefit ratio). There may be some other drugs in which the risks outweigh the benefits during certain stages of pregnancy. Your doctor would be the best judge and would be up-to-date on continuing research in this area.

Over-the-Counter Drugs

When serious problems occur, they may not be the result of using prescribed drugs. A potential villain is the casual use of over-the-counter drugs, self-prescribed and self-administered, during pregnancy. One survey showed that a startling 80 percent of drugs used during pregnancy were self-prescribed. Another study found that 65 percent of pregnant women took drugs not prescribed by their physicians.

There are several potential problems associated with these drugs. First, some of these preparations contain combinations of several drugs, many of which have not been studied well in pregnancy. While *specific* hazards may not be known, the drugs may not have been proved safe during pregnancy either. Additionally, many of the ingredient drugs in the over-the-counter medications are not shown to be effective for the conditions for which they might be used. Why expose an unborn baby to a chemical unnecessarily, even if no definite hazard has been identified? With some preparations the culprit can be identified—for example the iodide in a cold medication or the aspirin in some pain-relievers. Often the problem involves the use of large quantities of medications for long time periods without the knowledge of the physician.

Again, we often forget what is really a drug. Vitamins are drugs and are potentially dangerous if taken beyond their recommended doses. Some items in health foods stores are drugs and should be approved by a physician before use in pregnancy. Cold and cough medications, aspirin, non-aspirin analgesics, laxatives, antihistamines, bronchodilators, hormones and alcohol are all drugs. The list goes on and on.

Remember, what may be safe for almost anyone else may not be safe for you, based on your genetic and metabolic nuances. What might seem harmless at any other time may suddenly be harmful during your pregnancy or at least during certain parts of it. And if you are already high-risk, it is best not to stack one problem on top of another when it can be avoided.

The best rule in every case is to *ask your doctor*. He or she knows you, your medical history, your risk factors and family history. Your doctor is following your pregnancy and so can best judge the necessity of using a certain drug and the risk-benefit ratio. If you have a question about any over-the-counter drug, call your doctor first and find out if the drug is safe before using it.

And if you are not using an effective birth control method or are trying to get pregnant, it is best not to use any kind of medication without first conferring with your physician. Because of organ development in the first few weeks of pregnancy, the fetus could be at risk while you may not even know you are pregnant. This may be the time to put up with some of the more minor or annoying discomforts rather than "fix" them with over-the-counter medicines.

Be sure to read all labels and use only the medications approved by your physician and only when absolutely indicated. It is a good idea to ask your doctor at your first visit what he or she recommends avoiding altogether, and what can be used for problems like headaches and colds when absolutely necessary.

Street Drugs

PCP, heroin, marijuana and other street drugs are difficult to study, because they are illegal. Since controlled studies are impossible, the effects of these drugs on the fetus are less well-known and are more guesswork than actual fact. Odds are that many of these drugs have potentially serious effects on the developing baby.

We know heroin causes growth retardation in babies and has a toxic effect on the fetus, who becomes addicted to it while in the uterus. After birth the infant may go through withdrawal, in which the baby becomes extremely jittery and upset, vomits, has diarrhea and may have convulsions over several hours to days. This withdrawal is a dangerous process that sometimes results in death if it is not recognized or controlled.

Although the specific effects of marijuana are not known and no direct evidence exists that its use will cause problems for the fetus, no one can say its use is harmless either. There have been concerns about the effects of marijuana use on sperm production, as well as the possibility of chromosome breakage in marijuana users, which could lead to problems at the time of conception. Although there have been sporadic reports of birth defects in children of marijuana users, the association of the drug with a specific kind of malformation has not been consistent. During pregnancy, there would be a risk of chronic hypoxia (lack of oxygen) to the fetus if marijuana was smoked frequently, because of the inhalation of carbon monoxide and other toxic products of burning.

PCP (phencyclidine or "angel dust") is one of the most commonly used street drugs. Its use during pregnancy has led to symptoms of drug withdrawal (vomiting, jitteriness, increased muscle tone and diarrhea) in two infants, as reported in 1981 (Strauss et al). PCP was found in the urine of both of these infants after birth.

It is vital that the doctor who is supervising a high-risk pregnancy know exactly what is happening in the pregnancy, including all drug use—both legal and illegal—by the mother. It is also essential that the doctor know about drug use by *either* partner before conception. Doctors do not usually report people for drug use. Since concern is for the health and well-being of the woman and the unborn child, truth and candor are vital in this situation. Also, some problems might be circumvented and others anticipated if a physician knows which drugs have been used and when.

Anticonvulsant Medications: A Special Problem

Certain medications used to control epilepsy can cause malformations in some infants if taken during pregnancy. Although all effects of the drugs are not seen in all exposed infants, upon careful examination of these infants, some subtle effects of the drugs are noted.

Fetal hydantoin syndrome is seen in infants exposed to phenytoin (Dilantin® and some other antiepileptic drugs) during gestation. With this exposure such effects as prenatal growth retardation, mental retardation and certain craniofacial (head and face) abnormalities can occur. Abnormal development of the fingers and toes (and their nails) is also possible.

Some children affected show only minor physical effects, but 5 to 11 percent of exposed children may be mentally retarded. There remains some question if all the abnormalities seen in children of women on phenytoin are due to the drug or if there is also some contribution from the epilepsy itself.

Another anticonvulsant, trimethadione, also produces problems of prenatal growth retardation and mental retardation as well as certain craniofacial deformities (these are different from those found in fetal hydantoin syndrome). Infants with fetal trimethadione syndrome are at increased risk for heart defects.

One of the drugs most commonly used for seizures, phenobarbital, has not been clearly associated with congenital deformities, but infants of mothers who were treated with high doses of this drug may show signs of medication withdrawal in the first days or weeks of life.

Because of the significant adverse effects that can be caused in the fetus, epileptic women should consult their neurologist before becoming pregnant to see if their drug regimen could either be changed or eliminated prior to conception. If that isn't possible, it's very important to consult an obstetrician, perinatologist or geneticist in order to understand the specific risks that may be present with the particular regimen of drugs being used.

If You're Taking the Pill

If you are taking birth control pills and miss a period or two, there are two possibilities: (1) amenorrhea—temporary cessation of periods or (2) conception. For those who have conceived while on the pill, there is a *very slight* risk of VACTERL syndrome, a complex of congenital deformities (vertebral, anal, cardiac, tracheo–esophageal, *r*enal and *l*imb defects) in the fetus. In this situation, discuss with your doctor the possible implications for your baby.

If you're thinking of getting pregnant, know you're already in a high-risk category and have been taking the pill, we recommend using another form of birth control for two or three months after stopping the pill as a safety precaution.

When you first stop taking the pill, two things might happen: You'll ovulate (and therefore be fertile) more or less "on schedule" in the next cycle, as expected; or you'll have a delay in ovulation for weeks to months—and you won't know when you are fertile. Since each woman is different, it's impossible to predict which way you'll react. If delayed ovulation occurs, it will be a little more difficult for you to know whether or not you may be pregnant.

A good guide to taking the pill is: If you miss a period, you may be pregnant, so immediately stop taking the pill and see your doctor—particularly if you know you might have missed one or more pills.

X ray During Pregnancy

The effects of radiation on the developing baby are still being studied, but patterns are beginning to emerge. The use of diagnostic X ray is relatively young (less than 100 years), and experience with high-dosage radiation to pregnant women and their fetuses is (fortunately) limited. Concern about background radiation and its long-term effects is quite new, and data are controversial.

That radiation can be harmful to the developing fetus is well-known. Radiation damages cells—can even kill them—and is especially harmful to cells that are dividing rapidly. Fetal tissues may be as much as 25 times more sensitive to radiation than adult tissues. The unborn baby is also more prone to direct cellular damage—resulting in serious deformity or death—early in gestation than later in pregnancy. It is probably most vulnerable in the first critical 10 to 12 weeks of gestation.

For purposes of comparison, it's important to discuss radiation dosage. The *rad* is a unit of radiation dosage most frequently used in comparison studies, although other terms may be employed. Diagnostic X rays—for example, routine chest X rays—usually result in mush less than one or two rads of exposure. Other common X ray tests, like intravenous pyelograms (IVPs), gall bladder series, and gastrointestinal studies, usually result in less than two to three rads of exposure to the fetus. High-dosage radiation—like therapeutic radiation used in cancer treatment or that received in Japan during World War II—is quite different, and may result in exposures in the thousands of rads. Failure to distinguish between low-dosage and high-dosage radiation leads people to serious overreaction to the use of X ray in pregnancy.

High-dosage radiation—conservatively defined as an exposure of over 25 rads to the developing fetus—has been associated with microcephaly (small head and brain) and mental retardation in infants. This effect is most pronounced if exposure is early in gestation, when the nervous system is developing most rapidly.

The incidence of spontaneous changes—mutations—in children of adults exposed to relatively high doses of radiation, while a theoretical risk, does not seem unusually high. Limited studies of the children of radiologists, for example, show no increased incidence of congenital defects. Further studies of workers in nuclear facilities will be valuable.

The amount of radiation a mother receives to her ovaries *before* conception and its effects is another area of concern. Here, cumulative dosage (that which builds up over the years) is probably important. Many studies have been done, and a few suggest an association between ovarian radiation and chromosomal defects. However, a great deal more research is needed in this area. One study cites an association between increased radiation to the ovaries and increased incidence of spontaneous abortion. Obviously, not all the data are in yet, but the current practice of shielding the lower abdomen in women (and the genitals in men) during X ray tests whenever possible is certainly warranted.

Research indicates there is an increased risk of childhood cancer in children of women who received diagnostic X rays during pregnancy, and many researchers believe the risk rises directly with increasing exposure. That is, the more films taken, the higher the risk. There is also a time association—early in gestation the risk for the fetus is greater than later. In large studies the risk of cancer developing in exposed children is 1.47 times greater than if there was no exposure.

Another perspective is worth mentioning. We know that the X ray dosage we receive is cumulative—it builds up over a lifetime. Starting before birth is getting a head start on accumulating radiation.

The best recommendation is to have a healthy respect for the known and unknown effects of X rays coupled with the knowledge that, for some women, diagnostic X rays are essential, even during early pregnancy:

1. Avoid "routine" X rays—for example, routine dental X rays, pre-employment X rays and those for chronic problems—during pregnancy. (You might also wish to avoid these during the latter half of your menstrual cycle if you're not using contraception or are trying to get pregnant, since you won't yet know you have conceived.)

2. Always question the need for X rays if you are or might be pregnant. Try to work with the doctor to decide if the relative risk, although small, is outweighed by the benefit. Ask if there are other ways to find out the same information.

3. Whether pregnant or not, ask for a lead shielding apron for your lower abdomen if X rays are to be taken and do not involve the lower abdomen. This helps you avoid buildup of X ray exposure to your ovaries.

Hyperthermia

Although the evidence is not conclusive, there is a suggestion that hyperthermia (increased body temperature) is teratogenic to the human fetus. This is an important consideration with the increased popularity of hot tubs and saunas.

In a small study (23 cases), six children had abnormalities seemingly associated with heat exposure—exposure to temperatures greater than 38.9 C (102 F). Abnormalities included growth deficiency; nervous system defects including small head, mental deficiency, small eyes and floppiness; and various developmental abnormalities of the face and head, including abnormal growth of the face, harelip and cleft palate, and ear abnormalities.

While further study is warranted, avoiding excessive heat exposure—especially in saunas and hot tubs and especially in the first trimester (three months) of pregnancy—would be prudent. (Exposure later in pregnancy would not be wise either, because of increased stress on you and the fetus caused by changing demands for blood supply.)

Environmental and Occupational Hazards

There is currently much concern (and rightfully so) about exposure to noxious chemicals in the environment. The possible teratogenic effects of such materials as carbon monoxide and other components of smog and insecticides such as DDT and malathion are currently unknown, and both short-term and long-term studies need to be completed.

While definite information is not available, caution is probably warranted. When at all possible, reduce or eliminate your exposure to these materials. If you've already had a known exposure or cannot avoid being exposed, discuss the possible implications for you and your baby with your doctor.

Polychlorinated biphenyls (PCBs) are a group of industrial compounds that has received much attention over the last few years. The compounds themselves have many uses, especially in the electrical industry, where workers—including women of child-bearing age—are subjected to occupational exposure. Besides occupational exposure, there is as much concern about contamination of water and soil—and therefore food—by PCBs in industrial wastes.

Some of the first data about the teratogenic effects of PCBs came from Japan, where an accidental contamination of grain oil occurred. Infants of poisoned mothers had low birth weights and increased skin pigmentation. Many of them showed slight but definite persistent neurological damage.

A serious contamination of water supply by PCBs occurred in Michigan in 1978. This spill, while of concern because of potential teratogenic effects, has raised other issues, especially regarding breast-feeding by exposed mothers. (PCBs are deposited and stored in adipose, or fat, tissue and are present and secreted in fairly high quantities in breast milk.) While recommendations are not firm, caution is in order.

It appears there is not a *serious* risk for teratogenicity from PCBs as long as a woman does not have occupational exposure to them. However, both pregnant and nursing mothers should probably reduce or eliminate dietary intake of fish from water known to be contaminated with PCBs and discuss other possible precautions with their doctor if they live in high-risk areas. Analysis of breast milk for excessive levels of PCBs is available in high-risk areas and might be advisable with known or highly suspected exposure.

Congenital Infections

Congenital infections—those acquired by the fetus from the mother, usually while it is still in the womb—have many characteristics in common in the newborn infant.

Infected babies are very often small and sick at birth. They have bleeding problems, jaundice, enlarged livers and spleens. Nervous system abnormalities, such as small or large heads and seizures, are common. There may also be abnormalities of the eyes, called "chorioretinitis," due to the infection.

Because these infections can mimic each other, babies who may have been infected are usually tested for all of these "types" of infections. Doctors refer to these teratogenic infections as "TORCHS" or "STORCH" infections—for toxoplasmosis, rubella, cytomegalovirus, herpes and syphilis. Herpes and syphilis will be discussed later because of their special characteristics as sexually transmitted diseases.

All these can be detected in infected infants by means of special tests. Unfortunately, treatment is now possible for only two of the infections (syphilis and toxoplasmosis). Drugs for herpes treatment are currently under investigation. But even with these treatable infections, the effects on the baby can be severe and permanent.

Most important, four out of five of these infections can potentially be avoided: rubella, toxoplasmosis, herpes and syphilis.

Rubella

Before rubella vaccine became available some 15 years ago, most people got this disease (often called "German measles" or "three-day measles") when they were children. For most of them it was a very mild disease. In fact, about half had no signs or symptoms, and the other half had only slight fever, aching, swollen glands and a mild rash, which lasted one to three days.

Rubella is also a mild disease for adults, including pregnant women—high-risk or not. In fact, until 30 or 40 years ago, no one ever dreamed such a common, mild "childhood disease" could be so devastating for a developing fetus.

A viral disease, rubella is transmitted to the fetus from the infected mother. No one knows exactly how or why this virus specifically affects the developing fetus, but it does. Once contracted, there is no treatment.

Statistics show that when susceptible women (those who have not had rubella infection before) are exposed to rubella during the first three months of pregnancy, up to 50 percent of their babies can be affected by congenital rubella. Defects such as congenital heart problems, deafness, cataracts and microcephaly (small head) and mental retardation are common with congenital rubella. If exposure comes after the first trimester, the risk of major problems diminishes markedly, but certain problems such as mild mental retardation may still occur.

The good news: If you've had rubella or been immunized against it, either in childhood or adulthood long before pregnancy, there is nothing to worry about.

A simple blood test (called a "rubella titer") is now routinely available to determine whether or not a person has had rubella—or is immune to it.

Recently, many states have enacted laws that require women to be tested to determine if they are immune to rubella before they are married (just as they require a syphilis test of both partners). A rubella titer is also routinely perfomred during the first few months of pregnancy by most doctors.

The association between rubella and congenital defects spurred the development of rubella vaccine, which has been available since the mid-1960s. This vaccine, made of modified live rubella virus, is routinely recommended for children after the age of 15 months and *certainly should be given just before puberty to girls who have not had it before*. It can and should be given to nonpregnant adult women who are not immune to rubella—with certain precautions (which will be discussed below).

What can you do about the problem of rubella and your pregnancy? First, be sure you know whether or not you're immune to this disease. Even if you think you've had the disease or were vaccinated against it, it's best to be absolutely sure. See your doctor long before pregnancy occurs and have your rubella titer checked instead of waiting until you're already pregnant.

If you have been exposed to rubella or think you may have been and might be pregnant—see your doctor immediately. He or she can determine whether or not you are at risk. Your doctor would want to talk to you and your partner about the risks and options if you have been exposed, are not immune and are pregnant.

Vaccination against rubella during a high-risk pregnancy (or any pregnancy) is generally not recommended. Remember, the vaccine contains a dose of the live rubella virus that has been changed to make it safer. The concern is that the vaccine itself could possibly cause congenital infection and malformations. That's why a woman is always asked if she might be pregnant before the vaccine is ever given.

It is highly recommended that *pregnancy be prevented* for several months after vaccination against rubella. (A precaution: Early pregnancy may not be recognized right away, so it's best to make sure you are immune *long* before trying to get pregnant.)

Because they do not yet know they are pregnant, some women are inadvertently vaccinated against rubella while in the first few months of pregnancy. There really hasn't been enough research and study thus far to determine whether or not vaccination in such cases causes serious problems.

In the early 1970's, the Center for Disease Control (in Atlanta) collected data on 317 women who had been inadvertently vaccinated against rubella either soon before or after conception. None of the infants (147) who were term showed any clinical signs of the rubella vaccine virus-related congenital malformation or infection. However, 43 percent of the women in this study (138) decided not to take the risk and had therapeutic abortions. In these women the vaccine was found to have reached the fetus in 5 percent to 10 percent of the cases. It would seem prudent, then, to avoid vaccination while you're pregnant or might be pregnant, as a safety precaution.

Therefore, if you're thinking of getting pregnant—find out if you're immune to rubella. Take every precaution not to be exposed to people with the disease if you are at risk. And if you've been exposed or might have been exposed to someone with the virus and are pregnant—contact your doctor immediately for consultation.

Cytomegalovirus Infection

Cytomegalovirus (CMV) infection during pregnancy is a possible cause of fetal infection and subsequent congenital abnormalities. Like rubella and toxoplasmosis, this infection has its most devastating results if the baby is infected during early pregnancy.

Caused by a virus, the infection resembles infectious mononucleosis in adults and children. However, the usual blood test for mononucleosis is negative, and the disease is most often not positively diagnosed. CMV infection can be passed by direct contact between people or may be acquired from blood transfusions. Many people—both adults and children—have had this disease without noticing it and have few if any permanent effects from it. Because it is often unrecognized, its exact incidence is not known.

A fetus infected with congenital cytomegalovirus, on the other hand, may be seriously ill at birth. The symptoms include anemia, bleeding problems, life-threatening swelling and liver damage. Brain abnormalities—such as microcephaly (small head and therefore small brain) or hydrocephalus (abnormally large amount of fluid in the head)—seizures, mental retardation and/or cerebral palsy may occur. There is no known cure or prevention for this devastating infection.

Cytomegalovirus probably accounts for severe disease in 1 out of 1,000 births, and the risk to the fetus is probably limited to fetuses of women who are having their first infection.

Women in the reproductive age group can be tested to see if they have had the infection in the past. If they have antibodies against the virus, indicating previous infection, they are probably at low or no risk for fetal abnormalities. However, if they have no antibodies and may become pregnant, they should not work in newborn nurseries, especially for high risk infants, where many babies may be shedding this virus.

Toxoplasmosis

Blood tests show that many adults have had an infection called "toxoplasmosis," but few ever knew about it. Caused by a parasite, the disease is acquired through contact with cat feces (or cat litter) and by eating raw meat. Although the infection may cause a flulike illness, the adult often experiences no symptoms and has no permanent effects from it.

On the other hand, toxoplasmosis in pregnancy can cause severe problems for the developing fetus. As with other teratogens, this transplacental infection (gotten from the mother via the placenta) has its most devastating consequences very early in pregnancy—during the time of fetal organ formation in the first trimester.

Infants infected with toxoplasmosis may manifest a variety of problems. Most are small for dates at the time of birth and are sick enough for some type of intrauterine infection to be suspected. Others, though, may have less obvious problems at birth, and the infection is not diagnosed until developmental problems become apparent in childhood.

The long-term effects of congenital toxoplasmosis are severe and permanent. There may be abnormal brain growth detected early in infancy—microcephaly and hydrocephalus. Mental retardation, seizures and cerebral palsy occur frequently, and blindness due to toxoplasmal infection of the eyes (chorioretinitis) is not unusual. Although treatable in both adults and infants, the disease goes untreated most of the time because it is not recognized.

You may reduce your risk of contracting toxoplasmosis in pregnancy by not eating raw meat and by not handling cat litter if you have a cat.

Sexually Transmitted (Venereal) Diseases

A venereal disease is simply an infection caused by a bacteria or virus and sexually transmitted from one person to another. But there is nothing else simple about it.

Traditionally when venereal disease (VD) was discussed, people were referring to syphilis and gonorrhea. These diseases have become so prevalent that they are epidemic. Another fact has rapidly emerged—there are other sexually transmitted diseases that are just as damaging to the health of adults and unborn children alike, and these "new" diseases are also tremendously common.

Syphilis and gonorrhea are serious health problems and are reportable diseases—meaning that a physician who treats a person who has either disease must give the patient's name to the local health department. The person with the disease will be contacted and asked to reveal his or her sexual contact(s), so those individual(s) can also be treated. Although this sounds cruel and humiliating, its purpose is really to protect unsuspecting people who might never know they have a sexually transmitted disease—until it's too late.

It's important to realize that some types of sexually transmitted disease are "silent threats"—they don't cause symptoms in some people who have them.

Anyone who knows or suspects that he or she has a sexually transmitted disease should be examined by a physician as soon as possible. This is especially important for pregnant women, since many of these diseases can infect and harm the unborn fetus.

Syphilis

Historically known as the "great imitator," syphilis can affect nearly every organ system in the body. Its signs and symptoms can be very subtle, especially after the first stage of the disease, and are often not recognized. Unfortunately, the disease also has devastating effects if it occurs in the developing fetus.

An affected infant may be ill at birth, with bleeding problems, liver problems, skin rashes and pneumonia, and be smaller than expected for the length of the pregnancy. He or she may develop a serious nasal problem (called "snuffles") and may have inflammation of the coverings of the bones, causing pain, as well as bone and cartilage deformities.

The spirochete often invades the brain, the nervous system and the eyes, resulting in permanent damage. Treatment of the disease is effective in preventing the spread of the germ but does not stop the disease from leaving scars and permanent damage.

Insidious is a good description for this infection in adults. Frequently asymptomatic (producing no signs of illness), it may go unrecognized until its later stages when serious damage has already been done. This could be as long as months and even years after the first stage of the infection.

Syphilis is transmitted sexually (except in newborn babies, who acquire it from their mothers). In the adult the first signs of the disease usually occur 10 to 90 days after exposure. A sore called a "chancre," most often located in the genital area, is usually the telltale sign. The sore is normally hard but not painful and disappears regardless of treatment. A chancre may not be noticed in a woman, because it can be on an unexposed genital area. However, the bacteria remain, and the disease continues in a latent or hidden form for months to years. Later, skin rashes, difficulties related to the nervous and cardiovascular systems, and joint problems develop.

We need to emphasize that this destructive disease can go entirely unrecognized and may be detected only after a sexual partner is diagnosed or upon routine screening/testing (such as is done at the time of marriage, employment at some jobs and sometimes during pregnancy).

Presently, syphilis responds well to penicillin, erythromycin and tetracycline in prescribed dosage routines, and these (except tetracyclines) have no known adverse effects on the fetus or small child. On the other hand, untreated syphilis can have very serious, permanent effects on exposed unborn/newborn infants. When you weigh the risk factors, the scales tip heavily toward treatment during pregnancy.

Death, blindness, retardation, disability—all can result from syphilis. But here's the vital thing to remember: Most problems can be prevented by *early* recognition and treatment of the disease. The embarrassment and unpleasantness some experience when seeing a doctor for possible sexually transmitted disease is real. But it's worth the temporary discomfort to prevent serious, permanent damage to the unborn baby and the often hideous long-term effects it can have on a woman if left untreated.

Candidly, if your husband or mate believes he has come into contact with someone with venereal disease, he should be checked immediately and you should be told promptly so you can see your doctor right away. Conversely, if you have been exposed, see your doctor as soon as possible and tell your partner—for his protection and safety. Although this is a very sensitive subject for most couples, it is also an area about which you must be frank and responsive, emphasizing first the health and safety of each other and that of your unborn children.

Gonorrhea

The gonococcus is a bacteria similar to several others that can cause diseases such as meningitis. This bacteria, though, is transmitted through sexual contact with someone infected with it.

In the male this infection produces disturbing symptoms. Men experience burning with urination, irritation and pain, and discharge from the penis. Because of these discomforts, men usually seek medical care immediately. The disease is then diagnosed and treated.

Unfortunately, the situation is different for women. Women can carry gonorrhea and not even know they have it. For them there may be no symptoms or signs of infection. They can, in effect, harbor the organism indefinitely, passing it on to others through sexual contact.

In some women, gonorrhea produces a serious infection called "pelvic inflammatory disease" (PID). The infected woman is seriously ill, with abdominal pain and perhaps joint swelling and a skin rash. This kind of infection can lead to tubal damage and ultimate sterility. (Some feel there is almost an epidemic of sterility as a result of the epidemic of gonorrhea in recent years.)

Gonorrhea can cause problems for the unborn child of a pregnant woman, as well. The bacteria are harbored in the area of the cervix and can infect the baby during vaginal delivery. There is also some evidence to suggest a baby can be infected when the woman's membranes (water) have been ruptured for a prolonged time before delivery.

The major effect on the newborn baby is a serious eye infection called "ophthalmia neonatorum," or neonatal conjunctivitis. This appears two to seven days after birth and can result in blindness if not treated. Other forms of gonococcal infection are possible but are less common than the eye disease: septicemia (generalized infection), arthritis and meningitis.

The eye infection of newborns can be very effectively prevented with silver nitrate or antibiotic eye drops applied to the baby's eyes within two hours of delivery. Other methods of prevention are possible but are used less often. Most states, recognizing gonorrhea as a common disease (not restricted to certain groups of people) and realizing its effects on newborns if untreated, require that some form of eye prophylaxis (preventive treatment) of newborn infants be carried out at birth.

Unfortunately, there is no foolproof way for a woman to know she has gonorrhea without a culture, and often little evidence is available to tell her doctor she has it either. Part of the detection is based on the reporting of contacts of men with the disease. However, subtle symptoms of unusual vaginal discharge or more generalized problems may tip off a very perceptive doctor or nurse.

In pregnancy gonorrhea may disseminate (spread) to the rest of the body and result in a skin rash, a swollen joint, fever and generalized illness. If not treated, this infection can progress rapidly and destroy joints in a matter of hours or days. Although this generalized spread of the gonococcus bacteria can occur at other times, it is more common during pregnancy.

The saving grace for people with gonorrhea is the mandatory reporting system for the disease. Although it may be embarrassing, it is better to know the disease might be present than to suffer the damaging consequences.

Herpes

Two types of herpes virus infections have thus far been identified— as you might expect, "type 1" and "type 2." Because there are two types, a great deal of confusion has resulted, along with some very reasonable concern and fear. The diseases are quite different, however, and have different manifestations and different long-term consequences. Type 1 herpes virus causes a minor ailment, which usually manifests itself as fever blisters. Herpes simplex, type 2, in contrast, is generally a very painful disease and is, in fact, the most common of the sexually transmitted diseases today.

Type 1 herpes virus causes blisters in the area of the mouth—

the typical "fever blister." This infection is contagious and is acquired through contact with the fluid from the blisters. Although
a person who has the virus does not always have a fever blister, the
virus still lives in the cells around the mouth. Stresses such as fever,
sun exposure, infection, tension and menstrual periods have been
associated with causing a new blister. Herpes type 1 can also occur
in other areas of the body, generally above the waist, with unusual
exposure.

Type 1 herpes virus infections have been reported in newborn
infants, but they are not usually as serious as type 2 infections.
However, caution should be exercised and direct contact with active
lesions should be avoided for the newborn. It is best to cover any
lesions and not allow nursing if lesions are present on the breast.
Handwashing should also be practiced before contact with the
baby.

Type 2 virus, often called "genital herpes," usually resides in the
tissues of the genital tract—the penis in males and the vagina or
vulva in females. It is transmitted from one person to another
through sexual contact—it is solely a venereal disease except in the
newborn. Although much less common than lesions on the genitals,
herpes blisters can occur on the skin below the waist and are almost
always caused by type 2 rather than type 1 herpes virus.

The primary infection in a woman usually causes painful vul-
vovaginitis—inflammation of the genital area with intensely painful
ulcers—which last for one to three weeks. There is no effective
treatment or cure now known for the disease, and the only thing
that can be done is to provide pain relief. The virus must run its
course, and when it has, the symptoms disappear.

But this is not the end of the problem. The virus lies dormant
in the tissues, only to become active at another time. It is very
contagious when the ulcers are present. When there are no ulcers
present, the probability of getting the disease from someone who
carries the virus is not great, but the use of a condom during
intercourse is highly recommended even at these times. Use of a
condom better protects both male and female from infection if the
partner may be carrying the virus in an unseen area.

Unfortunately, the newborn does not do well with generalized
herpes virus infection. That does not mean that all babies of women
with type 2 herpes infection die or have serious problems. It does
mean, however, that there is a risk of infecting the infant. If the
mother is experiencing a primary (first) infection while pregnant,
the risk to her baby is even greater.

It appears the newborn is at greatest risk of contracting the infection during vaginal delivery—when the mother has active disease (lesions in the vagina or on the genitals). If the newborn comes into contact with the virus during vaginal delivery, generalized infection may take place within the next few days.

But transmission to the baby during delivery isn't the only way he or she can be infected. There is some suggestion that babies can be infected inside the uterus after the membranes have been ruptured for over four hours and even a (rare) possibility that they can be infected when the membranes are intact.

On the positive side, when the disease is active, C-section (cesarean birth—through the abdomen) delivery appears to protect the newborn from infection if performed before the membranes are ruptured or within four hours of their rupture.

If the baby is infected, there are many possible results. Systemic disease in the newborn primarily damages the nervous system. Although the disease appears at or shortly after birth, and some babies develop blisters, only half of the cases will be recognized because of skin and other manifestations alone. As many as 88 percent of babies who are clinically ill will have serious central nervous system (brain) damage, and many of these will die.

Although no one really knows why, statistics show that active herpes simplex 2 infections may be more common in pregnant women than in nonpregnant women. About 1 in every 100 pregnant women will manifest the infection clinically. If the expectant mother gets this virus infection at or after 32 weeks of gestation, there is a significant risk of infection to the infant during the birth process.

The risk of spontaneous abortion is clearly increased in this situation, and there may be a risk of serious fetal deformities when the disease has its onset in the earliest stages of fetal development. The woman and her partner should have a frank discussion with her doctor about the risks and options in this situation.

There is no way to color these statistics. They are alarming. It is highly recommended to avoid sexual contact with someone with this infection during pregnancy. If you or your husband or mate at all suspect either of you may have herpes simplex 2, it's important that you communicate that possibility and each see a doctor immediately. Protection (like the use of a condom) is always recommended when having intercourse with a person who has this disease, whether it's active (lesions present) or not.

Streptococcal (Strep) Infections

The term "strep" is often used synonymously for all infections caused by a group of bacteria called streptococci. In fact, there are several groups of beta streptococci (referring to laboratory characteristics of the organisms), and two of them—group A and group B—cause serious problems in the newborn. (One of them—group B—can be a sexually transmitted disease.)

The most commonly known streptococcus bacteria is group A beta strep. This bacteria usually causes the infection known as strep throat, and it most often results in difficulties for older children and adults. In addition to throat infections, this germ is implicated in some skin infections in older children, scarlet fever, some cases of kidney disease, and—if not treated early enough—rheumatic fever. Group A strep can cause some problems of infection in the newborn infant and in the mother who has just delivered. However, group A strep is much less common and worrisome than infection caused by group B strep.

Group B beta strep infections (sexually transmitted) are probably the most common cause of fatality due to infection in the newborn infant today. This bacteria is harbored in the male and transmitted to the female, although its passage is not always just sexual. Pregnant women are usually spared infections of the upper genital tract that lead to sterility, but as many as 4 percent to 26 percent of pregnant women will be harboring this dangerous bacteria in their lower genital tracts. The problem is—this infection rarely has symptoms in the woman. Sometimes a problem with her newborn is the first indication of the presence of this infection.

Group B strep infections in the newborn can be very serious, resulting in a very high fatality rate due to pneumonia and meningitis. The infection has also been associated with premature delivery, stillbirth and spontaneous abortion. It seems to be more common in premature infants than in term babies, although it is still not known whether it might be implicated as a cause of premature birth, or if these babies are just more susceptible to the disease.

The most devastating manifestations of this infection occur within hours of birth—usually within the first two days of life. The newborn infant shows signs of sepsis (overwhelming generalized infection), respiratory distress (breathing difficulties) and shock. When these serious symptoms occur, the mortality rate is as high as 70 percent to 90 percent.

A second type of group B strep infection may not surface until ten or more days after birth. A newborn with this type of infection has a better chance of survival than the newborn with the "early" form of the disease, but 15 to 30 percent still die. This "late" strep infection usually results in meningitis, and leaves its victim with a very high likelihood of neurologic damage.

Although massive doses of penicillin can be used to destroy this bacteria in the ill newborn infant, there is no good way to anticipate that a baby might have a problem with a strep infection. Even if treatment is started immediately when the signs of the disease are recognized or suspected, the chances for the baby are not very good.

Identification of the group B strep germ is accomplished by means of a special culture to grow this bacteria in the laboratory and identify the type of strep germ present. Some institutions routinely culture pregnant women and newborns for this disease, although the impact of this action on the early recognition and eradication of the germ is still unknown.

Chlamydia

In recent years there has been some evidence suggesting that cases of "nonspecific urethritis" in men and "nonspecific vagnitis" in women might be caused by an infection with chlamydia organisms, which are very small, somewhere between bacteria and viruses in size. Such infections can be treated with an antibiotic, erythromycin, when recognized. Laboratory methods are now available to identify this organism but are very expensive.

These infections, like the others discussed in this section, are transmitted sexually. Their effects on the fetus and newborn are treatable and less serious than those of most of the sexually transmitted diseases.

A common result of chlamydia infection for the newborn is an eye infection that appears about 5 to 14 days after delivery. Another manifestation is a combination of pneumonia and an eye infection occurring within the first two months of life. These infections last a long time even when treated but, once recognized, can be controlled with appropriate antibiotic therapy.

The Bottom Line on Teratogens

As you can see there is a whole array of potential teratogens. It is important for you to be aware of these and do all possible to avoid them. It is often helpful to tell your husband or partner about these potential hazards to you and your unborn baby. This is particularly important when it comes to smoking, drinking and medications, where support and understanding are helpful. Often a man will quit smoking when his wife is pregnant or is trying to become pregnant, because she needs to quit. Your husband or mate can also remind you about not drinking or support you when friends insist you join them in a few drinks. When it comes to sexually transmitted diseases, honesty is vital, as is an understanding of what the disease can mean to your unborn child. It may be particularly important for you to ask your husband or mate to read this chapter and others—indeed the entire book—to learn more about high risk pregnancy in general and problems you can avoid in particular, for the safety and well-being of your child.

FIVE

WHAT EVERYONE SHOULD KNOW
ABOUT BIRTH DEFECTS

"Is my baby okay?" is usually the first thing a new mother and father ask at the birth of their child. That same question is still asked by almost all parents today. The difference? Years ago there was no way for doctors or expectant parents to know if the baby had a genetic or chromosomal abnormality or other birth defect— until the baby was born. Even if something was suspected—there was no way to verify or discount this suspicion. Today, genetic counseling and various diagnostic tests are available for parents whose babies may be at increased risk for certain abnormalities that can now be detected early in pregnancy.

A Perspective on Birth Defects

Of the more than 3 million babies born in the United States every year, some 200,000 or more will have some type of birth defect. About 20 percent of these infants will have a minor to major inherited problem, while the other 80 percent will have problems caused by a combination of factors. Some of these problems can be anticipated before conception, and some others can be detected early in pregnancy. However, the majority result from unexpected events or accidents that occur later in pregnancy or during labor and delivery.

Parents and potential parents should also be aware of abnormalities that result from a single accident of nature or some influence at certain stages of fetal development. These accidents of nature can affect genes or chromosomes on which they are located and problems can occur. Other accidents of fetal development that have little or nothing to do with the genes or chromosomes can cause minor to major fetal problems.

Genes and Chromosomes: The Blueprints of Life

The human cell itself is almost unbelievable—but the human gene (a unit of DNA) is virtually incomprehensible. Just imagine—no fewer than 50,000 genes (tiny blueprints of life) are found in each human cell. To appreciate the size of one gene, consider the fact that we cannot even see the human cell with the naked eye, and yet at least 50,000 genes are housed in each cell's center! To put this into perspective—picture the size of a pinhead. If we were to cover this surface with a single layer of cells, there would be (in total) more than 2 million genes on that pinhead. The DNA of the cell—with its thousands of genes grouped into 46 chromosomes—is probably the single most powerful material in the world, and yet so tiny!

It is difficult to imagine that anything so very tiny is actually responsible for dictating inheritance. These miniscule blueprints of life—called "genes"—determine characteristics as simple as eye and hair color and as vital as body structure and brain power. Indeed, these genes determine the size, purpose and function of every living cell!

To put the importance of genetics into perspective, each of us receives a unique makeup from our parents at the moment of conception—when the germ cells (ovum and sperm) join together. At conception the genetic material from the mother (contained in the ovum) and that from the father (carried in the sperm) combine to form a new, unique mixture of genetic material. From this moment on, that one-of-a-kind genetic material, made up of a special chemical called "DNA" (deoxyribonucleic acid), duplicates itself over and over and over again to make up the entire body. Each cell of the body formed after conception will have exactly the same genetic composition and blueprint as that first cell (except the new human being's germ cells—ovum and sperm—which will be discussed later).

All cellular activities are directed by the DNA, found in the center of the cell. It is in the DNA that all genetic information is stored. When cells of the body are not duplicating themselves, the DNA looks very similar to a tiny ladder twisted like a corkscrew. Scientists call this shape a "double helix." To reproduce, the DNA ladder basically "unzips"—leaving the same genetic information on each half; then, in a highly complex procedure, special enzymes attach to each half of the DNA and rebuild it to complete the new second half of each ladder. This splitting and rebuilding of DNA results in two identical sets of DNA having the very same genetic formation within the cell. The cell itself then splits into two cells— with each cell being genetically identical to the other.

Each time a cell divides, its duplicated DNA arranges itself into units called "chromosome"—tiny structures that contain specific segments of the DNA. Each cell of a normal person will have 46 chromosomes (in 23 pairs) except the reproductive (or germ) cells. The ovum and the sperm (the germ cells) have only 23 chromosomes each. If you think about it, this makes perfect sense: Once combined at conception, the 23 chromosomes from the mother and the 23 chromosomes from the father equal the 46 chromosomes needed to form the new cell. Thus the fertilized egg will contain the now unique blueprint of genetic material for the next new life.

Of the 23 pairs of chromosomes in the human cell, 22 are matching pairs and are called "autosomes." The 23rd pair of chromosomes, called "sex chromosomes," determines the sex of the new person. The normal female has two identical sex chromosomes, called "X" chromosomes (one from mom and one from dad). The male, on the other hand, has only one "X" chromosome (from mom) and a smaller "Y" chromsome, which is the male chromosome (from dad). Therefore, the ovum carries only "X" chromosomes, but the sperm can carry either an "X" or a "Y" sex chromosome. That means the father will determine the sex of the baby.

As noted, each of the germ cells—ovum and sperm—must contain only half of the usual 46 chromosomes, one from each of the 23 pairs. This happens through a special kind of cell division called "meiosis" or "reduction division." Each ovum then contains 23 chromosomes, including one "X" (female) chromosome. Each sperm also has 23 chromosomes, including either an "X" (female) or a "Y" (male).

After the joining of sperm and ovum, the newly fertilized cell divides rapidly, duplicating its genetic material and forming organs and tissues. As the embryo turns into a fetus, organs and tissues become more complex—but the genetic code remains the same, directing all function and general growth and development.

As we have previously discussed, each chromosome contains thousands of units called "genes," now known to be composed of segments of DNA. Genes, like the chromosomes on which they are located, are paired. Every gene pair is responsible for a single characteristic, function or metabolic process in the body. Each parent contributes one gene of every pair. The theory of how genes determine inheritance was developed based on the work of Gregor Mendel, a monk who studied plants extensively in the mid-1800s. Mendel observed that when he cross-pollinated the plants he was studying, he could predict with some certainty what characteristics the offspring plants would have. His work led to the concept of "gene dominance," which subsequently has been supported again and again by the work of later scientists.

"Mendelian inheritance" (obviously named after Mendel) is based on the principle that certain genes are dominant over others—they are, in essence, "stronger." The characteristic determined by the "dominant gene" would be expressed, or seen, in the offspring where only one gene of that type was present in the gene pair. A trait controlled by a "recessive gene," on the other hand, would not be expressed unless both genes of the pair were identical. An offspring who inherited one dominant gene and one recessive gene would show the dominant characteristic. The exact genes inherited—called the "genotype"—will determine the visible characteristic—called the "phenotype." To simplify this—essentially the *genotype* represents the "cause" and the *phenotype* represents the "effect." (These are terms you may hear from a geneticist or genetic counselor.)

These terms can be more easily understood if we look at a simplified example of dominance in humans. Suppose the letter *B* represents brown eye color and *b* represents blue eye color. If brown (*B*) is dominant, then only one *B* gene is needed for the child to have brown eyes. If blue (*b* is a recessive trait, a child would need to inherit a *b* gene from each parent in order to be blue-eyed. A child with *BB* or *Bb* genotype would have brown eyes (the phenotype), but only a child with the *bb* genotype would be blue-eyed. The recessive gene must therefore be present in a "double dose" in order to stand out or be apparent.

These same types of combinations (recessive and dominant) are possible for each of the other gene pairs. When you also consider that certain characteristics are determined by more than one gene pair acting together, even greater variation is possible. If you then add the effects of environment to the basic genetic potential, the possibilities become almost infinite. These interactions account for the uniqueness, the one-of-a-kind genetic makeup that is so typical of people—even those in the same family.

Often people are confused about the role of the genes and the role of the chromosomes—since both are the material of inheritance. People generally find it difficult to understand the difference between a genetic defect and a chromosomal abnormality—and therefore assume these terms are interchangeable. In actuality, the terms are distinctly different and represent totally different problems. To put this into perspective, it is important to remember that a gene pair (one gene from the mother and one gene from the father) will determine a specific trait, characteristic or problem. Because many genes make up a chromosome, when something goes wrong with the chromosome, the problems which result usually affect many body systems—not simply one trait, characteristic or problem.

The best analogy may be a building. The *chromosomes* would be represented by the major beams of steel which are responsible for holding up entire sections of the building. Supported by these major beams are hundreds of smaller pieces of steel, wood and glass—*the genes*—which determine the size, shape and function of certain areas of the building. If a ball were thrown through the window, the window would break but the building would not collapse. If a tree fell on the roof, part of the roof might be destroyed but the building would stand. Even if a more serious incident occurred, such as the floor caving in (a major catastrophe)—the building would still stand. But, if a major beam was somehow damaged, for example, broken in half—that entire section of the building—the walls, the windows and the floor—would all be damaged or destroyed as well. The problem could be quite extensive depending on which major beam was damaged—even to the point of the total collapse of the building.

Genetic Disorders

Certain human abnormalities are the result of inheriting a single defective gene or a faulty gene pair. Some genetic disorders are extremely rare, while others are common enough for you to have heard about them. Each year more genetic disorders are uncovered, and more of them are able to be diagnosed before birth as well as afterward.

Three types of genetic disorders are commonly seen:

1. *Autosomal dominant conditions,* in which a child manifests

an abnormal trait as a result of having inherited "a single defective dominant gene" located on an autosome

2. *Autosomal recessive disorders*, in which a child manifests an abnormal trait as a result of having inherited "a pair of defective recessive genes" located on an autosome

3. *Sex-linked recessive defects*, in which a child manifests an abnormal trait as a result of having inherited "a defective recessive gene located on a sex chromosome" (rather than on an autosome)

Each of these groups of genetic disorders, which will be discussed in the following subsections, has unique features that allow geneticists to make predictions about the way they are inherited, as well as about the mathematical likelihood of the defect's occurring in any particular pregnancy.

Autosomal Dominant Conditions

An autosomal dominant trait is passed on to a child directly from a parent with that trait. Only one gene of the gene pair (located on one of the 22 pairs of autosomes) needs to be defective in order for the child to show signs of the abnormality. This means, then, that if you were able to look at a large family, you should be able to trace the defect back through each generation: Each child with the disorder should have a parent with the problem.

Because each child with an autosomal dominant condition should have a parent with the same problem, you might assume that autosomal dominant defects would not be lethal—and much of the time you would be correct. A person with a very serious autosomal dominant abnormality would probably not be able to have children, so the genetic disorder would go no further in the family. However, the situation is not quite that simple.

In some families two parents with totally normal genes will have a child who has a condition usually known to be inherited as an autosomal dominant trait. Even with careful searching, however, no sign of the abnormal condition can be found in either parent's family. A "gene mutation"—a spontaneous change in the child's DNA—can account for this phenomenon.

In other families the situation may appear on the surface to be similar. Two seemingly normal parents have a child with an autosomal dominant disorder. However, upon careful examination of one of the parents, one or more subtle signs of the genetic disorder are found, and often a search through that parent's family will uncover even more individuals with incomplete forms of the problem. The condition is autosomal dominant, but the way the condition expresses itself can vary. This phenomenon is called "incomplete penetrance." This family condition may only be detected if a child is born with the "complete" problem and may otherwise go undetected.

It is extremely important to know if a usually dominant trait was due to a mutation or, in fact, was passed to a child from a parent who may not have known about his or her abnormal gene. In this way, the genetic probabilities about future children can most accurately be determined. The point is, the parents with truly normal genes will have no more than a chance risk (like all other couples) of having another child with the defect, because the defect resulted from a chance mutation. The parent who actually has an abnormal gene will continue to pass the defective gene on to subsequent children 50 percent of the time (that is, there is a 50 percent possibility of each child's not having the defect and a 50 percent risk of each child's having the defect). Furthermore, in the case of the mutation, the affected *child* will then be able to transmit the faulty gene to his or her *own* children 50 percent of the time but will in all likelihood be the only affected family member in his or her own generation. Because the brothers and sisters of the affected child do not carry the abnormal gene, *their* children will not be at risk for the defect (any more than any other person).

The following are among the more common *autosomal dominant conditions:*

- Achondroplasia (a form of dwarfism)
- Familial polydactyly (a condition in which the child has extra fingers and/or toes)
- Hereditary spherocytosis (an abnormality of the red blood cells that makes them fragile)
- Neurofibromatosis (a disease in which there are varying numbers of nervous system and skin tumors)
- Tuberous sclerosis (another nervous system disease involving multiple tumors)
- Adult-type polycystic kidney disease (a condition in which multiple cysts are found in the kidney, often leading to kidney failure later in adult life)
- Familial polyposis and Gardner's syndrome (two similar disorders in which multiple tumors are found in the intestines, with a tendency for these polyps to become cancerous)
- Huntington's chorea (a degenerative brain disease)

A look at some of these conditions in more detail will not only explain what they are but will also illustrate some of the general characteristics of autosomal dominant traits.

Achondroplasia is one form of dwarfism in which the arms and legs are very short in proportion to the head and trunk of the body. The cartilage at the growing ends of the bones does not function normally. While this type of dwarfism is usually inherited as an autosomal dominant trait, there is also a high rate of spontaneous mutation. Therefore, two parents can have a child with this form of dwarfism without either of them having any features of dwarfism. Achondroplastic dwarfs, on the other hand, can pass on the gene for dwarfism to their children, even if their own problem resulted from a gene mutation (because the mutant gene has permanently become a part of their own genetic makeup).

Both *neurofibromatosis* and *tuberous sclerosis* are diseases inherited as autosomal dominant traits. They are both diseases that primarily affect the brain or nervous system because of the growth of tumors in the brain and involve unusual skin lesions and tumors elsewhere, as well. The severity of both can vary widely. The skin manifestations of the diseases may be very obvious and disfiguring or so subtle that no one is aware of their presence. While mutation is possible with these diseases, it is usually possible to identify subtle indications of the disease in one parent and in other family members.

Familial polyposis is a problem in which a person develops multiple tumors (polyps) of the intestines, usually not recognized until adolescence or adulthood. *Gardner's syndrome* is a similar problem involving multiple intestinal tumors but is also associated with tumors of the bone, as well. Patients with either of these autosomal dominant diseases are at risk for developing cancer in the intestines. *Adult-type polycystic kidney disease* is a problem in which multiple cysts of the kidney ultimately lead to poor kidney function and even kidney failure. *Huntington's chorea* is a devastating disease of the nervous system that does not manifest itself until its victim is in his or her twenties or thirties. The person's motor and intellectual functions deteriorate over a period of 10 to 30 years.

These four diseases (familial polyposis, Gardner's syndrome, adult-type polycystic kidney disease and Huntington's chorea) share certain characteristics that do not apply to some of the other dominant diseases. First, the genetic nature of the disease may not be apparent from its earliest signs in a person, and its presence in previous generations of the family may not be known. In addition, the person with the disease may have already had children before his or her own disease was diagnosed. This often leads to intense guilt and worry on the part of these parents, whose own children may develop the diseases at a much later stage in life.

With some autosomal dominant diseases, as with other genetic diseases, knowing that they may occur can allow early diagnosis and treatment. For example, an infant at risk for *hereditary sphero-cytosis*, a disease in which red blood cells are very fragile, may need blood transfusions and treatment for jaundice as a newborn. Later, removal of the spleen may result in relieving him or her of nearly all the symptoms of the disease (but he or she can still transmit the gene to his or her children). This type of intervention allows for the control of some other dominant conditions, as well.

Autosomal Recessive Disorders

Most of the common, serious genetic diseases are recessive traits. That means in order for a person to inherit the problem, he or she must receive a defective gene for the trait or problem from *each* parent. The person who has only one abnormal gene (recessive) and also has a normal gene (dominant) in the pair that is stronger than the abnormal gene does not have the trait or problem but "carries" it and can pass it on to the next generation *if* his or her mate carries the same abnormal gene. Two parents who each carry an abnormal gene could have several children who would not inherit the trait or problem. In fact, most people do not even know they are carrying an abnormal gene unless they have an abnormal child or there are others in their family who have affected children.

Statistically, when both parents carry the same abnormal reces-sive gene, there is a 25 percent risk in each pregnancy that the fetus will inherit both of the abnormal genes and have the recessive disease or disorder. Another 25 percent of the time the fetus will inherit a pair of normal genes—it will not have the recessive disease and will not carry the recessive gene, either. There is a 50 percent risk that the fetus will inherit one normal and one abnormal gene—the child will be normal but will be a "carrier" of the abnormal recessive gene.

With each person having 50,000 or so genes, all of us more than likely carry one or more abnormal recessive genes. What determines whether a child has an autosomal recessive disease is (1) whether *both* parents carry the recessive gene, and (2) whether an ovum containing the abnormal gene is fertilized by a sperm that also carries the same abnormal gene.

The risk of inheriting an autosomal recessive trait is increased when parents are closely related. When there is blood relationship—called "consanguinity"—there is an increased probability that the couple will share some of the *same* recessive genes. The closer the relationship, the greater the risk, and the more likely that the union will bring out the undesirable recessive traits in a family's genetic makeup.

There are hundreds of diseases caused by *autosomal recessive genes*. Some of these are quite well known—because they are relatively common. Others are much rarer—and their specific biochemical causes have just recently been discovered.

Some of the more common autosomal recessive diseases are:

- Cystic fibrosis (a disease in which there are usually problems with digestion and with chronic, progressive lung disease)
- Phenylketonuria or PKU (a defect in the way the body uses protein, in which buildup of abnormal products leads to mental retardation)
- Galactosemia (a defect that prevents a child from properly metabolizing milk sugar and results in liver disease, cataracts and ultimately mental retardation)
- Tay-Sachs disease (a serious nervous system disease in which a child seems normal at birth but then deteriorates over the next few years and dies, usually before the age of 5)
- Sickle cell anemia (a type of anemia that is caused by a defect in the red blood cells and leads to their early destruction)
- Beta-thalassemia (a type of anemia caused by an abnormal kind of hemoglobin)

In addition to these more common single-gene disorders (that is, involving a single gene pair), many more rare metabolic diseases are recessively inherited. Many of them, like PKU and galactosemia, are associated with mental retardation, as well as with a variety of other symptoms and signs. In fact, in a study of mental handicaps in England in the 1960s, significant mental retardation was found in 3.1 persons out of every 1,000. In 14 percent of these, the cause was a single-gene defect.

Over the past 15 to 20 years, biochemical tests to detect as many as 75 to 80 of these recessive inborn errors of metabolism have been developed and can be performed in large medical centers or special laboratories across the country. Since all but a few of the recessive metabolic diseases are rare, mass screening of all babies (in the newborn stage or in early infancy) for all of these diseases is not practical. However, if a problem is suspected in a baby, the testing—which is done on samples of blood, urine or occasionally other body tissues can be performed. Theoretically, most of these same genetic disorders could potentially be diagnosed prenatally, as well, through amniocentesis (as will be discussed in Chapter 11). Prenatal diagnosis would be wise if a couple had had a previous child with one of the recessive inborn errors of metabolism. Sometimes prenatal diagnosis might be warranted if one of these diseases had been found in other relatives of either parent, as well, particularly in nieces or nephews.

Phenylketonuria (PKU) is a metabolic disease in which protein breakdown is defective. Abnormal chemicals build up in the body and can also be found in the urine. This disease, which can now be treated with a special diet with encouraging results, leads to severe mental retardation if not treated very early in infancy. Extensive research findings accumulated in the 1960s led to a simple test in which urine could be analyzed to detect this abnormality. Several years later an even more accurate test, which could be performed on a drop of dried blood, was developed. By law this blood test is now performed on all newborns in all states in the United States in order to detect this recessive disease, which occurs in approximately one out of every 1,600 births. Identification of newborns with PKU allows them to be treated with the special diet beginning as soon after diagnosis as possible. Treatment within days to weeks after birth is most successful in completely preventing or reducing the degree of mental retardation from the disease.

Standard newborn screening now includes not only PKU (a metabolic disease) but also galactosemia (another autosomal recessive metabolic disease) and hypothyroidism (a sometimes genetic endocrine disease), both of which can be treated successfully, with reduction or prevention of the mental retardation that is inevitable if no treatment occurs. As other screening tests are developed that are simple, reliable and cost-effective, they may become routinely used. Screening tests are most valuable and desirable for diseases that can be successfully treated early in infancy—as is the case with PKU, galactosemia and hypothyroidism.

With certain recessive traits the carrier of the trait, who has one dominant normal gene and one recessive abnormal gene, can be detected by special laboratory testing. Sickle cell disease, beta-thalassemia and Tay-Sachs disease are three diseases for which carriers can be detected through special blood tests. Genes for these three diseases each occur in particularly high frequency among a certain group of people

Sickle cell disease is a condition in which the hemoglobin is abnormal. It is most commonly found among the black population. *Beta-thalassemia* is another disease involving an abnormal hemoglobin and is most common among certain groups of Mediterranean origin. These blood diseases can be partially treated or controlled, but cannot be completely cured. *Tay-Sachs disease* is a degenerative condition that occurs among Jewish families, primarily those of Eastern European ancestry. There is no known treatment for this disease, which ultimately results in death, usually before a child reaches the age of 5.

These two factors—easy detection of the carrier state and a relatively limited population in which the defective genes commonly occur—make screening reasonable for those who may carry the specific gene. Work on techniques to detect the carriers of other genetic diseases is continuing. For example, techniques to detect the carrier state for *cystic fibrosis*, one of the most common genetic diseases, are being studied. It would be a major breakthrough to be able to detect carriers of this gene, which is found in about 1 in 20 people. Cystic fibrosis occurs in one out of every 1,500 to 1,600 births. Each year the ability to control some aspects of this disease improves, but it still causes serious disability and death for nearly all of its victims.

Sex-Linked Recessive Defects

With sex-linked recessive defects the abnormal gene is located on a sex chromosome rather than on an autosome. For some reason these genes are located only on the "X" chromosome. The "Y" chromosome seems to contain only genes that determine or relate to maleness.

Two of the best known sex-linked recessive diseases are *hemophilia*, a disorder in which there is little or no factor VIII, a blood component required for clotting, and *Duchenne-type muscular dystrophy*, a progressive muscle disorder. These and other sex-linked disorders are carried by the mother but affect male offspring who inherit the recessive gene nearly 100 percent of the time.

As with other recessive genes, the defective genes located on the "X" chromosome can be masked by a normal dominant gene or another "X" chromosome. Because a female has two "X" chromosomes (one from each parent), she will usually be normal. A male, on the other hand, has only one "X" chromosome (from the mother). If it contains an abnormal recessive gene, the male will be abnormal—because there is no normal gene on a corresponding sex chromosome to balance the abnormal one.

Therefore, sex-linked recessive genes are usually passed from a carrier mother to her children. If a carrier mother and a normal father were to conceive, the risks of the child having a recessive disease depends on the child's sex. If the child were female, she would have a 50 percent chance of inheriting the abnormal gene (that is, of becoming a carrier like her mother) but would not have the disease itself, because she received a normal "X" chromosome from her father. If the child were male, he would have a 50 percent chance of being normal (if he inherited the normal "X" from his mother) and a 50 percent chance of having the recessive disease (if he inherited the abnormal "X").

Other features of sex-linked recessive inheritance deserve comment. A father with a sex-linked recessive disease—for example, hemophilia—does not pass on his *disease* to his children. The abnormal gene would not be passed on to any son, because the father contributes only a "Y" chromosome, not an "X." All of his daughters, on the other hand, would receive his abnormal gene on the "X" chromosome, and so would be carriers of the abnormal gene.

Hemophilia and other sex-linked recessive disorders are rare in females but can occur if a carrier mother and an affected father were to conceive. With this combination all daughters would have at least one recessive gene. The risk for having an affected daughter—one who received an abnormal gene from each parent—would be 50 percent. With this kind of union, 50 percent of the sons would have the disease and 50 percent would be normal.

While exact prenatal diagnosis of an affected child is still not possible for the sex-linked recessive traits, it is becoming increasingly possible to detect the carrier state in some of these disorders. This is helpful in counseling, because occasionally these diseases occur as a result of mutation. Prenatal diagnosis of the sex-linked diseases is limited only to the determination of the fetus's sex. Knowledge of the fetal sex allows a decision to be made if it is male—based on the 50 percent risk of a male child's having the disease. While termination of a pregnancy may not be a viable option for many families, especially when the fetus has only a 50 percent risk of being affected, this is currently the only possible way to reduce the incidence of most sex-linked diseases. However, work is presently being done in recombinant DNA to find answers to some of these problems, and the future looks hopeful. Work on trying to identify these sex-linked disorders during early pregnancy also continues.

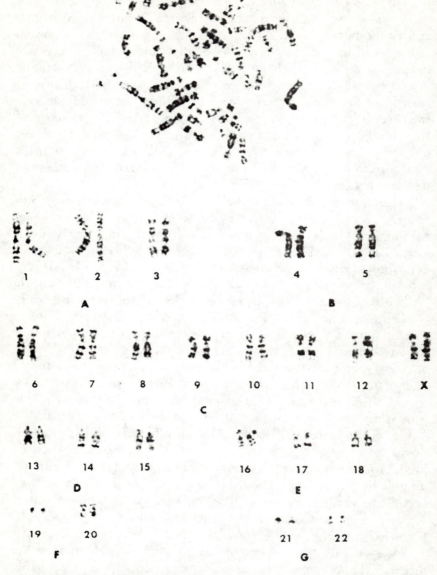

KARYOTYPE OF FETUS WITH NO CHROMOSOMAL ABNORMALI-TIES: The chromosomes (at top) are from the nucleus of a single cell and are shown arranged (below) according to their shape and size. Arranged (categorized and numbered) this way, the chromosomes can be carefully analyzed and compared to known "normals." Geneticists can then determine whether or not a chromosomal abnormality is present. The female fetus (note the two "X" sex chromosomes) has no chromosomal abnormalities. Amniocentesis and advances in genetics have made this type of analysis possible.

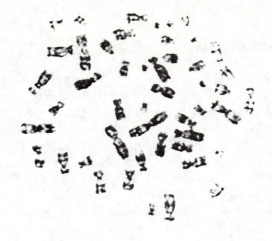

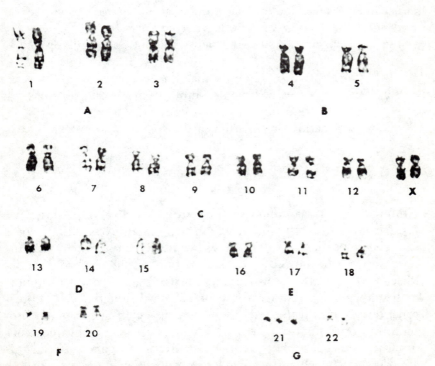

KARYOTYPE OF FETUS WITH DOWN'S SYNDROME: In this karyotype we can see an imbalance in chromosomal material called "Trisomy 21" (Down's syndrome). Note the three chromosomes at the 21st chromosome instead of the normal pair. The fetus is a female identifiable by the pair of "X" sex chromosomes.

Chromosomal Abnormalities

Chromosomal abnormalities can be of many types and can lead to serious, often life-threatening defects in affected fetuses. Because chromosomal defects most often involve many genes—rather lengthy segments of DNA—the fetus usually has abnormalities in more than one body system. Certain physical traits tend to occur in patterns, presumably because of the close association of their various genes on the chromosome. These combinations of defects—of either malformations or malfunctions—are called "syndromes."

When a chromosomal problem is suspected, a chromosome analysis, called a "karyotype," can be useful. A karyotype is a photograph of the chromosomes from a cell in which they have been arranged in a specific way according to size and shape. With a special technique called "banding," individual genes on chromosomes in the karyotype can be outlined, allowing even more precise study of these carriers of genetic information.

Types of chromosomal abnormalities include those involving:

1. Duplication of an autosomal chromosome
2. Breakage, reattachments, duplications or deletions of portions of autosomal chromosomes
3. Duplication or omission of the sex chromosomes

Duplication of Chromosomes (the Trisomies)

Among the most common of the chromosomal abnormalities are the trisomies—conditions in which there is an extra chromosome in each cell of the body. Trisomies can involve either the autosomal chromosomes (discussed in this sub-section) or the sex chromosomes (discussed in a later sub-section). Most often this kind of abnormality results from an error called "non-disjunction." Non-disjunction occurs during reduction division when one pair of chromosomes does not split, leaving a pair of the same chromosomes in either the egg or the sperm. If fertilization occurs between this abnormal germ cell and a normal one, the embryo will get all three chromosomes of a matching set (called a "trisomy") rather than two. This extra genetic material results in specific abnormalities, depending on which chromosome is involved.

By far the most common trisomy is *Trisomy 21*—triple representation of the 21st chromosome—most commonly called "Down's syndrome." This trisomy most often results when the 21st chromosome in the egg remains doubled during reduction division because of an error in distribution of genetic material. While this accident can occur in any pregnancy, the risk becomes progressively greater with advancing maternal age (see Chapter 3 for more details).

In general, babies born with Down's syndrome survive. However, 13 percent to 18 percent experience severe mental retardation and death. Those that survive will suffer both mental and physical effects. In fact, the characteristics of Down's syndrome are so distinctive that it is easy to identify these children from among a large group of children. Physically, they tend to have shorter hands and fingers than normal; the bridge of the nose is flatter, as is the contour of the face, particularly in profile; the corners of the eyes slant upward, and the lower eyelid is fuller; the tongue usually protrudes a little, and the ears are smaller; the children tend to be shorter, overweight in later years and have a degree of impairment in their coordination. Around 40 percent will have or develop a heart defect in the first few months or years of life.

Mentally, those with Down's syndrome will range from having very serious mental deficiency to having an IQ of perhaps 60 or so as adults. Essentially, the extra 21st chromosome changes the development and potential of the brain. It is impossible to say which child will achieve greater mental development and which will experience severe mental retardation.

However, experts who have worked with these children on into adulthood say that most children and adults with Down's syndrome are happy, charming and teachable to a certain degree. They do have limits to their ability but should be given every opportunity to reach their mental, physical and psychological potential. Although these children tend not to walk until around the age of 2 to 5 years because of muscle laxity, most can be taught to feed and dress themselves. Many parents care for a child with Down's syndrome at home, while others place him or her in a home for special care or an institution. This is a decision for the family involved and should be based on their needs and those of the child.

Down's syndrome, like other chromosomal abnormalities, can be identified early in pregnancy through amniocentesis (discussed in Chapter 11). Finding that a fetus has Trisomy 21 leads to a serious dilemma for many couples. Since Down's syndrome is not curable and its effects are well known, some couples choose to discontinue the pregnancy by abortion, while other couples choose to continue the pregnancy. This, too, is very much an individual choice and must be made based on the couple's religious beliefs and personal feelings. The point is, abortion is not an answer for some people. This does not mean that prenatal testing for Down's syndrome and other chromosomal abnormalities is useless. Prenatal verification of Down's syndrome often allows a couple to prepare for the needs of the baby and adjust to the situation.

Usually the most important aspect of prenatal diagnosis, however, is to reassure a couple that the fetus does not have Down's syndrome or some other chromosomal abnormality. Remember, the vast majority (greater than 99 percent) of fetuses do not have a chromosomal abnormality. Therefore, prenatal diagnosis is very often just the thing that is needed to relieve the parents' built-up anxiety or fear that something may be wrong with the baby. This is particularly important for women over 35, who have a higher incidence of Down's syndrome babies. It is quite a relief for them to know the fetus does not have a chromosomal abnormality, and they can continue the pregnancy without worrying about it.

For those interested in a very fine book on Down's syndrome, there is one available by the late David W. Smith, MD, and Ann Asper Wilson, titled *The Child with Down's Syndrome (Mongolism)*. This is an excellent resource that clearly explains Down's syndrome, its causes, characteristics and the experiences of couples who have a child with Down's syndrome. It is highly recomended for those interested in knowing more about others' expereinces and is especially helpful to couples who may be facing the birth of a baby with the problem or even to those whose child has Down's syndrome. Another recommendation for those of you who may be facing the birth of a child with Down's syndrome is for you to visit some of the special centers where children with Down's are taught or ask your doctor if there is a couple with a baby or child with the problem whom you could talk to and see. It is also useful to talk to your minister or rabbi or anyone else whom you trust and whose counseling may be of some help.

Two other trisomies—Trisomy 13 and Trisomy 18—tend to have more serious consequences for the fetus than Trisomy 21. These two abnormalities usually result in death at an early age. Trisomies of other autosomal chromosomes invariably result in fetal death. Trisomies of the sex chromosomes ("XXX" or "XXY") result in viable fetuses, as will be discussed later in this chapter.

(Another problem of the chromosomes occurs when a full chromosome is missing. When this happens with autosomes, it is called "monosomy," and the fetus does not survive. Spontaneously abortion generally results early in pregnancy—usually during the first trimester. However, babies can survive with monosomy of the "X" chromosome—a condition that will be discussed later in this chapter.)

Chromosome Breakage

Breakage of chromosomes during division and subsequent rearrangement of chromosomes has been known to be possible for many years. It has only been since the most recent techniques of chromosome study were developed that the extent to which such breakage occurs has been appreciated. Chromosome breakage in a normal individual is probably common but does not lead to serious consequences as long as the normal amount of genetic material is present. However, breakage can have profound or more subtle effects on the normal person's offspring, depending on what happened to the broken chromosome.

Translocation—attachment of all or nearly all of a broken chromosome to another chromosome—is a common result of chromosome breakage. When this happens, it is possible for the sperm or ovum to receive a "double dose" of all or most of this chromosome—one normal chromosome plus a translocated one. When fertilization occurs, the result is a translocation trisomy, in which the fetus has only 46 chromosomes, but one actually contains the genetic code for two chromosomes. (If on the other hand, the fetus had received only the translocation chromosome, he or she would not be abnormal, because the translocation is "balanced" and there would not be an excess of genetic material.) Nonetheless, he or she would be at increased risk of having children with translocation syndromes, because the abnormal chromosome would be passed on, along with a normal chromosome from the mate's germ cell.

Approximately 4 percent of Down's syndrome infants have translocation trisomy, and of these about one-third have one parent who is a balanced translocation carrier. Most translocation Down's syndrome infants are born to young parents. In Trisomy 13, as many as 20 percent of the affected infants have a translocation trisomy.

Small pieces of a chromosome may break off and be lost, leaving one arm of a chromosome shorter than normal. Such an omission (called a "deletion"), where passed on during cell division, results in less than the usual amount of genetic material. Likewise, breakage, then reattachment of an extra small piece of one chromosome to another, results in a slight excess of genetic material called a "duplication." With increasingly sophisticated methods of chro-

mosomal analysis and banding, more and more deletion and duplication syndromes are being identified each year. These disorders
may be suspected when an infant or child has unusual physical
features or abnormalities. The types of defects the child has will
depend upon which chromosome is abnormal. It has been noted
that deletions or duplications can be found in some children with
certain types of tumors. In particular, such genetic associations
with malignant diseases should be suspected if the family shows
repeated occurrence of the same tumor.

Several types of rearrangements of chromosomes after breakage
are possible and, again, would be suspected in unusual-looking
children or those with abnormal development. Breakages may be
"mended" by the formation of "ring chromosomes," in which broken ends of the DNA-containing structures are joined in a circle.
In other accidents the sequence of genes in a chromosome may be
reversed during a break and reattached.

One principle application to the breakage of chromosomes is
important to keep in mind: The greater the imbalance in the amount
of genetic material—too little or too much—the more serious the
defect is likely to be. This is especially true in terms of neurological
development. On the other hand, a person with balanced genetic
material (even if it is arranged in an unusual way)—for example,
a balanced translocation carrier—is often normal in both appearance and intellectual function.

Sex Chromosomes

The possibilities for *structural accidents*—duplication or loss—of the
sex chromosomes are varied and often confusing. Understanding
some basic background information about normal sexual differentiation and development should make this area more understandable.

As mentioned previously, the genetic makeup of an individual—
including genetic sex—is determined at the moment of conception.
However, that genetic sex may have a variety of effects on the
fetus's actual body characteristics and organ development. In its
earliest stages the human embryo has the capacity to develop features that look either male or female, regardless of its genetic sex.
The embryological origins of male and female sex organs are the
same. What, then, makes a person look "male" or "female"? Several
factors can interact—namely, the genetic sex (that is, the "X" and
"Y" chromosomes) and other influences (such as hormone exposure).

Research strongly suggests that the embryo will undergo development and differentiation to look "feminine" unless influenced otherwise. The presence of a "Y" chromosome in the genetic makeup stimulates the developing embryo to differentiate into what looks "male"—what could have been the labia change into the scrotum; the would-be clitoris enlarges to become a penis, and changes occur so that the urethra (the opening from the bladder) is located in it; what would have been the uterus and vagina fail to develop further and almost disappear; and the gonads—testicles—move from inside the abdomen (where the ovaries usually stay) to the outside, into the scrotum. Without the "Y" chromosome—whose only function seems to be to control and determine maleness—the embryo would look female. In order for normal sexual differentiation and development to occur, the female, then, must have two "X" chromosomes (the "XX" genotype), and the male must have one "X" and one "Y" (the "XY" genotype).

As is the case with autosomes, sex chromosomes can undergo *errors in reduction division* resulting in abnormalities. Monosomy (omission) of one "X" chromosome (abbreviated "XO") results in a well-known condition called "Turner's syndrome." Girls with this syndrome are short, have poor development during adolescence and are sterile. They may share some typical characteristics that make unrelated girls look much like sisters. Monosomy for the "Y" chromosome is lethal—these fetuses spontaneously abort early in gestation.

Errors in reduction division can also lead to a fertilized ovum containing an extra sex chromosome. There are several possible results, each involving babies with characteristic features: "XXX," "XYY" or "XXY." The *"XXX" girl* most often looks normal but may have delayed emotional and physical development. The *"XYY" male* (sometimes referred to as a "super male") may be completely normal, but some controversial studies suggest that this extra "Y" chromosome is associated with excessive aggression and criminal behavior. The *"XXY" male* has a group of features referred to as "Klinefelter's syndrome." These males are very tall, tend to be somewhat mentally retarded, and have small testicles that produce very little male hormone and few if any sperm.

Another group of accidents involving the sex chromosomes may lead to "confusion" in sexual development—the child may even show features of both male and female development. Often these types of syndromes result from "sex chromosome mosaicism"—the presence of two separate kinds of cells.

Some of the sex chromosome disorders are quite common, while others are very rare. About 1 in 600 males will have an extra chromosome—either "XXY" or "XYY"—while Turner's syndrome ("XO") occurs in about 1 in 2,000 girls. These kinds of defects of sex chromosomes are almost always random "accidents of nature" and are not transmitted to children of the affected person, because most individuals with sex chromosome disorders are unable to have children.

Chromosomes are not the only factors that influence the embryo's differentiation into a "male" or "female." Hormone influences—especially during the embryological stage of development—can also cause "confusion" in sexual development. If a genetic female embryo is exposed to an excessive amount of malelike hormone—because of either an abnormality of the adrenal gland or administration of hormone to the mother—the fetus may become "masculinized." Her genitals might look male or might be ambiguous (that is, they might have features that are both male and female). Similar types of problems can occur in genetic males whose bodies might not respond correctly to the masculine hormones that are present: A genetic male may look completely feminine from the outside. These disorders of sexual maturation are relatively rare and are sometimes called "intersex" syndromes.

Congenital Defects Due to a Combination of Factors

Certain common fetal malformations definitely occur more commonly in some families than in others, but they are not inherited in a pattern like a single-gene disorder, nor do they involve an identifiable chromosomal abnormality. These types of congenital malformations (defects present at birth) probably result from a combination of hereditary and environmental factors—so-called *multifactorial or polygenic inheritance*.

There are many disorders that fit into a pattern of multifactorial inheritance:

- Congenital hip dislocation and dyplasia (a spectrum of conditions in which the hip and its socket do not develop properly)
- Cleft lip (harelip) with or without cleft palate
- Clubfoot deformities
- Neural tube defects (spina bifida, anencephaly and encephalocele)

- Pyloric stenosis (overdevelopment of the muscle at the outlet of the stomach, causing vomiting in young infants)
- Some heart malformations
- Some childhood cancers

It has been observed that if a couple have a child with one of these malformations, they are at increased risk for having another child with the same disorder. The risk of the couple's having another defective child after the first one is about 3 percent to 5 percent. If they have a second affected child, the risk is even greater for future children, rising to 10 percent.

The exact way heredity interacts with the environment is not known. No specific chromosomal or biochemical abnormalities have been detected in such cases, and likewise the nature of the environmental impact is not constant. It might involve the intrauterine environment, drugs, radiation—or none of these. Perhaps in the future the relationships will be more clear. Neural tube defects and childhood cancers can be used to illustrate the interactions between genetics and the environment in producing defects.

While many congenital defects are inherited and are present from the time of conception, others develop during gestation. Some of these are amenable to some form of intervention, while others are not, depending on the nature of the accident or influence when it occurred. Problems such as congenital hip dislocation and dysplasia, and clubfoot deformities, which result from crowding, as well as defects due to teratogens or blood vessel accidents, seem to develop in response to the intrauterine environment.

Neural Tube Defects

One of the most well-studied groups of multifactorial disorders is the neural tube defects—congenital malformations in which the development of the nervous system is faulty. Very early in the embryonic development—in the 4th week after conception—the embryo's nervous system (which starts as a flat, platelike structure) folds over to form a neural tube. The failure of this tube to close results in a neural tube defect.

There are three basic kinds of neural tube defects. The most severe, *anencephaly*, is the complete or partial absence of the skull along with a primitive, underdeveloped brain. As many as 50 percent of anencephalic fetuses are spontaneously aborted, and others are stillborn. Those who are born alive usually die within a few hours of birth. In another type of defect, *encephalocele*, the brain and its coverings protrude out through the skull, usually at the back of the head. Some infants with this defect survive beyond the newborn period, but they are almost always severely retarded and neurologically handicapped.

Spina bifida is the most common of the neural tube defects seen in surviving infants. In this defect, the spinal cord along with nerves and their coverings protrude from the lower back, because the bones of the vertebral column failed to close around the cord. The spinal cord and membranes are "open" 90 percent of the time, and 10 percent of the time the defect is covered by a full layer of skin.

Spina bifida most often leads to serious neurological disabilities, including paralysis and lack of sensation of the legs and lower body, lack of bowel and bladder control, frequent urinary infections and deformities of the legs. Frequently *hydrocephalus* ("water on the brain") develops as a complication of spina bifida and is often associated with a major mental disability.

No one knows what causes neural tube defects or exactly how common they are. In the United States there are about 1 to 2 cases per 1,000 newborns—3,000 to 6,000 births each year. While there is some genetic component to the inheritance of these defects (if a couple have a child with a problem, there is a 3 percent to 5 percent risk of their having another child with the problem), certain environmental factor(s) (which remain unknown) are thought to be partially responsible.

Neural tube defects can be detected during early pregnancy. They are associated with abnormally high fetal levels of a substance called "alpha-fetoprotein," which can be measured in the amniotic fluid and maternal blood. Presently, studies are being done to determine the usefulness of measuring the alpha-fetoprotein in the mother's blood to detect an abnormality. Ultrasound is also being used to identify any visible defects. (For more information about detection of a neural tube defect in a fetus, see Chapter 11.)

Genetics, Environment and Childhood Cancer

Recent observations and studies have lent increasing support to older ideas that certain childhood cancers occur more often in some families than in others. In a Tokyo study in the 1960s, for example, congenital malformations were found in 41 percent of childhood cancer patients but in only 13 percent of the control group. Results of other studies have confirmed the association of some congenital defects with childhood cancers. While all of the risk factors are not known, there are associations between some chromosome disorders (for example, Down's syndrome), susceptibility to radiation, many drugs and a whole host of other factors yet undiscovered. Further research and observation will clarify exactly which of the many possible factors has a major impact on cancer, and when and how that impact is expressed.

Uterine Constraint

Over the past few years there has been increasing interest in the study of the effects of crowding inside the uterus—external pressure or constraint—on the developing fetus. It has become more and more clear, based on studies by the late David W. Smith, MD, and his students and colleagues, that intrauterine crowding can have both temporary effects and profound, long-term effects on the fetus.

The most common type of crowding in the uterus happens even with normal babies, who often become crowded after the 35th week of gestation. Before that, the amniotic fluid forms a cushion around the baby, but as the pregnancy advances, the baby grows much faster than the uterus. At this time the baby tends to find a position that gives the most room—most often the cephalic or "head down" position, which allows the baby's legs the greatest freedom.

As fetal growth continues, pressures on the fetus, whose bony structure is somewhat soft and pliable, tend to "mold" the baby's body. The result is often bowed legs, turned-in legs and feet, arms and legs that cannot be straightened and a long, almost pointed head—the look that is commonly thought of as "a normal term baby." And normal it is.

When these pressures of crowding happen only in the last few weeks of pregnancy, the effects on the baby are usually temporary. When the constraint is removed, the deformed area returns to the normal, non-constrained shape. Therefore, most babies' heads become round and "normal looking" within a week or so of delivery, and legs and feet become less curved over a few months. Pressures that were present for longer periods of time leave longer-lasting problems—but most will become normal in several months to years.

When pressures occur earlier in fetal development, the results may be more long lasting or severe. For example, congenital hip dislocation or dysplasia—abnormal development of the hip socket leading to actual dislocation of the joint in some cases—is often seen in breech babies. About 50 percent of children with congenital hip dysplasia were in the breech position, where unusual pressures on the hips prevent normal hip socket formation. Similar factors might be associated with so-called clubfoot and other deformities of bones and joints.

Deformations—either temporary or more permanent—can be associated with one or more of the following:

- First pregnancy (the uterus is not as "stretchable" as with later pregnancies)
- Small size of the mother
- Very small pelvis
- Malformation of the uterus (for example, bicornuate—two-horned—uterus and others)
- Uterine fibroids (which take up space in the uterine cavity and make its shape irregular)
- Multiple fetuses (crowding as well as unusual pressures of the fetuses on each other are possible, especially as the pregnancy advances)
- Oligohydramnios (too little amniotic fluid, for whatever reason)
- Unusual fetal position (breech, face and others)
- Engagement of the fetal head in the pelvis too early in gestation

With some of the defects that seem to be at least partially caused by constraint, there is some tendency for the mother to have another child with the same type of deformity. Congenital hip dysplasia and some mild to moderate deformities of the feet and legs are sometimes seen over and over again in families. However, most of the deformities due to constraint do not happen again in subsequent pregnancies unless the same causative factor is present. Factors such as the shape of the mother's pelvis or a uterine malformation that cannot be repaired might cause the same type of pressures to be exerted on a fetus in any pregnancy.

While many of the deformations caused by constraint inside the uterus—that is, caused by a totally normal fetus's being "crowded" or in an unusual position—will need special treatment, the results of treatment are often excellent. In fact, just delivering the baby—because the pressures on the fetus's body have been removed—is often all that is needed to allow the baby's shape to return to normal.

In other situations where the baby's defect may be more complex, results may not be as good. This is especially true if the baby has an underlying malformation that leads to further deformation inside the uterus.

This sort of combination of factors might be seen, for example, with a fetus whose kidneys do not form at all—so-called renal agenesis. With no kidneys, no fetal urine can be made, and the amount of amniotic fluid around the baby is therefore low, because fetal urine makes up part of the amniotic fluid. This oligohydramnios limits the growth space for the fetus—produces constraint— and is associated with poor fetal lung development. Consequently, the fetus will not only have no kidneys but will also have lungs that will be unable to support life outside the womb. He or she will have unusual external body features from the pressures of crowding during fetal development, as well. The underlying malformation (the lack of kidneys) along with its serious consequence (the lack of lung development) prevent the baby from surviving outside the uterus. Thus, a serious fetal *mal*formation can lead to an equally serious *de*formation.

Blood Vessel Accidents and Related Problems

Interruption of the fetal blood supply—whether as a single, devastating accident or as a chronic problem—can have major effects on a fetus. Both the severity and the timing of the lack of blood flow—and therefore the lack of oxygen and tissue nutrients—influence what the final result for the fetus will be.

The most common types of interruption of blood supply to the developing fetus happen in late gestation as a result of uteroplacental insufficiency—the failure of the placenta to meet the oxygen and nutritional needs of the fetus. The common effects in late pregnancy are intrauterine growth retardation if the interruption is ongoing and fetal distress (see Chapter 12). Long-term damage to the brain and other organs can result if the lack of oxygen is severe and if intervention is not successful.

Actual vascular malformation or interruptions of blood supply in the fetus itself may also cause congenital malformations. Newly developing fetal blood vessels may be damaged in a variety of ways, leading to temporary or permanent loss of blood supply to an area of the body. Such factors as a blockage of a blood vessel by outside pressure or a clot inside an artery may lead to permanent damage.

Disruption of blood vessels may be seen in twins and in other multiple pregnancies. Twins who share the same placenta may have abnormal communications between their blood vessels, and unequal blood flow might result. One twin then gets more blood than the other during the pregnancy—and the fetuses develop differently. The twin who gets more blood—and therefore increased nutrients and oxygen—will be larger than the other, often by a great margin. Sometimes the reduction in blood supply to the second twin is so severe that it cannot survive. At other times, the discrepancy is not so severe, but one twin will have problems at birth because of too much blood (called "polycythemia"), while the other will be anemic.

Sometimes vascular interruptions are related to accidents, such as very early rupture of the fetal membranes (the amnion), with later scarring by tissues called "amniotic bands." If these fibrous scarlike bands are stretched across a part of the fetus's body or encircle a leg, for example, a deformity will result. The part whose blood supply has been cut off by the band will not develop normally. Often these amniotic bands are clearly visible at the time of birth and need to be surgically corrected. Clubfoot deformity is sometimes thought to result from this type of diminished blood supply along with long-lasting pressure on the developing foot in some cases.

Birth Accidents

Complications in late pregnancy and birth accidents (unexpected complications around the time of delivery), account for a large number of permanent defects in children. Most often, these kinds of accidents result in damage to the nervous system, either temporary or permanent, and may be related to difficulties in the delivery of the baby, as well as to other factors.

Asphyxia of the baby—the combination of lack of oxygen and buildup of carbon dioxide—can result from any number of problems in late pregnancy and around the time of delivery. Once delivered, the baby may need assistance to support his or her breathing and heartbeat. The effects of hypoxia (lack of oxygen) can be temporary or may be more permanent and associated with mild to severe brain damage, seizures (convulsions), cerebral palsy and developmental problems. (Fetal distress and hypoxia are discussed in detail in Chapters 12 and 13.)

Damage to specific nerves may happen with difficult deliveries and, again, may be temporary or permanent. *Brachial palsy*—paralysis of an arm or hand due to pressure on or stretching of the nerves that supply the arm—may happen with the delivery of a large baby, or if an extreme amount of pulling is required during the delivery. This kind of paralysis may affect the whole arm or just the wrist and hand and may be complete or partial.

Likewise, pressure on the facial nerve, which is located close to the skin just in front of the ear, may lead to *facial palsy*, a weakness or paralysis of the muscles of one side of the face. Facial palsy may happen without a known cause or may result from a difficult forceps delivery. When it is associated with forceps use, it is most often temporary and disappears within several weeks to months. (Some other cases of brachial and facial palsy are known to result from pressure or damage to these nerves and their blood supply before birth, during fetal development.)

Genetic Counseling: Is It for Us?

As previously noted, one of the greatest fears of any woman or couple concerning a pregnancy is whether there will be something wrong with the baby. While this is a worry for almost all women and their partners, it is of particular concern for women who are contemplating pregnancy at an older age (or find themselves over 35 and pregnant), those who have had an abnormal child previously and those with known hereditary disease in the family. For these people, genetic counseling may be very valuable.

Genetic counseling is a complex process involving the careful gathering of information, followed in some cases by prenatal testing, and then the determination of the risks for the couple. It can be time-consuming and stressful for a couple.

There are many situations in which genetic counseling is very useful:

- When there is known hereditary disease in the family of either parent
- When one or both partners have had a child with a birth defect
- When either parent has had a child with a chromosome problem
- When pregnancy occurs or is planned, and the mother is older (over 35 years of age)

The genetic counseling process involves several steps and requires the participation of *both* partners. The first step involves a long interview of both partners by either a geneticist (a physician with special training in hereditary diseases) or a genetics associate who is specially trained in the counseling procedure. The interviewer will ask for very detailed information about any problems that have occurred in either partner's family. Bring as much information as possible with you to this interview—names, relationships and *any* known medical information—about relatives for as many generations as possible. Ask older members of the family for this kind of information, and be sure to include as many distant relatives as you can.

The geneticist will want to learn as much as possible about known or suspected problems in your family. He or she will want to review

Pedigree

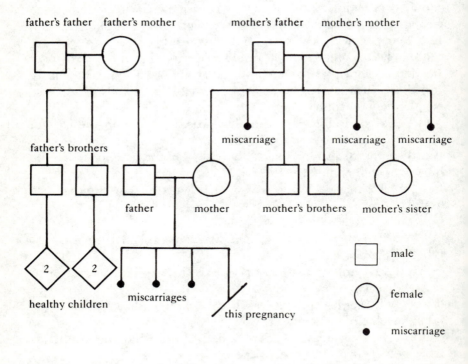

PEDIGREE: After diagramming this pedigree (family tree) the geneticist would analyze the information further to see if there is any possible hereditary basis for the miscarriages experienced on the mother's side of the family. In addition to analyzing a potential genetic link, the geneticist might also recommend that the mother be examined carefully to see if there is any structural or other physiological reason for the miscarriages, if she had not already had this kind of examination.

any medical records available on any family members with birth defects or who are suspected of having any hereditary disease. If you have a child with a birth defect, that child may be examined, and various diagnostic tests may be recommended.

Based on the information you have given, the geneticist will prepare a *pedigree*—a family tree that shows all the members of the family, with the problems and their relationships. The pedigree can then be used to help the geneticist see any patterns of heredity in the family and use what is known about genetics to get a preliminary idea of your potential problems.

Depending on the reason you are having the genetic counseling, certain tests on you and your partner and perhaps on others in your family might be suggested. For example, if you have a child with a chromosome defect, a blood test on you and your partner might be useful to see if one of you is carrying a translocation chromosome. Or if there is a history of sickle cell disease or Tay-Sachs disease or some other autosomal recessive disease in the family but not in your own children, a blood test might determine whether one or both partners are carriers. (If you have a child with one of these problems, this would not be necessary since you already know that the child got one recessive gene from each parent.)

If you are already pregnant, testing of the fetus might be useful. The geneticist may suggest and arrange an amniocentesis (see Chapter 11) for chromosome analysis or other metabolic studies. If you have had a child with a neural tube defect, a blood test for alphafetoprotein might be done as a screening test (also discussed in Chapter 11). Ultrasound may also be recommended to determine both fetal age and to detect any possible visible defects (see Chapter 10). Fetoscopy may be needed to try to look at the fetus or to obtain blood or tissue samples for further diagnostic tests. See chapter 20.

After all this information has been collected, you and your partner will have another meeting with the genetics counselor to review the data. The geneticist will explain the pattern of problems in your family and discuss any potential risks for you and your future children in great detail. He or she will answer any questions you have about the information that has been collected.

One of the most important facets of the genetic counseling process is making sure you understand your risks (if any) and, if there are risks, your options. If you are already pregnant and are carrying a fetus who has a diagnosed abnormality or potential abnormality, you will need to know as much about the defect itself as possible— how serious it is or could be, what can be done about it, and what you and your child could expect for the future. You will also want to know about your options to either continue the pregnancy or terminate it, so you and your mate can make the best decision for you and your family, based on solid, accurate knowledge as well as on your own ethical and religious beliefs.

If you are not yet pregnant, your counseling session would be different. It would focus on your risks if you were to become pregnant, as well as on what diagnostic tests, if any, would be recommended in any subsequent pregnancy. You would also receive information about your options—birth control, if needed or desired, as well as alternatives if you were to conceive a child with a problem.

The purpose of the counseling is to share as much information as can be known with you and your partner—about both your family's risks for inherited disease or congenital problems and your possible choices if such problems occur. It is vital that you get any and all questions answered—even if they are embarrassing, frightening or seem "stupid." When issues as important as the health and well-being of your future children and your family are at stake, no question is unimportant or trivial.

If you think you need genetic counseling or want more information about it, ask your doctor about where you can get information and whether you would or might benefit. Genetic counseling centers are available in all major cities and are usually found in major medical centers and perinatal centers. You can get information about your nearest genetic counseling center by contacting your local/regional office of the National Foundation–March of Dimes or writing the March of Dimes Birth Defects Foundation, Box 2000, White Plains, NY 10602. You may also obtain information from the National Genetics Foundation, Inc., 9 West 57th Street, New York, NY 10019.

The Bottom Line on Birth Defects

All parents are concerned about the possibility that their children may be born with a serious, lifelong problem. When considering the number of absolutely healthy babies born each year in contrast to those with insignificant to major abnormalities—you can see that the majority of the time, the odds are in your favor for having a healthy child. However, for those whose children (for whatever reason) are at increased risk for a genetic defect, chromosomal abnormality, congenital defect or birth accident—one or more forms of surveillance or detection may be recommended (i.e. genetic counseling, amniocentesis, ultrasound, etc.)

In this way, potential problems can be identified before pregnancy, others detected early in pregnancy and still others identified as the pregnancy progresses. At times this allows for intervention where possible—and where not possible—allows parents to prepare for the child's needs.

SIX

PROBLEMS ANY WOMAN MAY EXPERIENCE DURING PREGNANCY

Potential problems mentioned in this chapter are risks for all pregnant women but are especially applicable to women already identified as high-risk. Every couple should know about these. In high-risk pregnancies it's even more important that these be taken into consideration, because it's sometimes easy to over-react when a benign symptom appears. Knowledge of major, minor and inconvenient problems gives everyone a better idea of when to be concerned, when to call the doctor, or when it's merely a normal part of pregnancy and nothing more.

Aches and Pains

Many types of aches and pains trouble women during pregnancy. Back pain is particularly agonizing for some. It is often related to the changes in posture necessary to keep your balance as the fetus grows inside the uterus and extends out in front of you. (Carrying even a ten-pound sack of flour out in front of you for a short time will illustrate this graphically!) It may also be related to stretching of the ligaments of the back and pelvis.

Pain due to this relaxation of the pelvic ring (the bones and soft tissues) may also be experienced as lower abdominal discomfort. This relaxation of tissues is nature's way of anticipating delivery and is thought to be a result of the secretion of a special hormone. Stretching of the supporting muscles and ligaments of the uterus is an additional culprit. Your doctor may call this type of discomfort "round ligament pain."

Increase in Body Fluid

Some of the other perplexing discomforts (aches and pains) of pregnancy are related to an increase in body fluid. Some swelling, especially late in pregnancy, is expected, because the size of the uterus prevents the blood from draining from the tissues as efficiently as before pregnancy. On the other hand, serious swelling is *not* normal and may signal a problem, especially during the last three months. Report this to your doctor.

Puffiness of the hands and feet causing tight shoes and rings is bothersome. Sometimes swelling of the hands and fingers becomes great enough to produce numbness and tingling. This phenomenon is called "carpal tunnel syndrome" and results when swelling puts pressure on the median nerve, which runs through the underside of the wrist to the hand. Swelling is thought to be the cause of various aches and pains in other parts of the body, as well. If it becomes a great problem for you, talk to your doctor for advice.

Leg Cramps

Leg cramps are very common during pregnancy, and often calcium supplementation, whether through diet or through calcium tablets, may be helpful. Never add calcium to your diet or take tablets without your doctor recommending it, though. When cramps occur (most often at night), they can be relieved by stretching the cramping muscle. Usually this can be accomplished by extending your leg or foot and then pushing your foot against resistance.

Stretch Marks

Stretch marks can't be prevented—unfortunately. No cream, ointment, or exercise can stop these small tears in the skin from developing or make them disappear. Women get varying numbers of stretch marks—some get only a few and others end up with many—usually related to the amount of extra weight or growth. Stretch marks are most common on the abdomen, breasts and buttocks and are more prevalent and troublesome for fair-skinned women (especially redheads) than for those with darker complexions.

Although the presence of stretch marks is upsetting, especially for those who like bikinis, the marks won't always look as bad as you think they do at first. With time—usually 6 to 12 months after the stretching of the skin has stopped—the marks fade and become more like the color of the surrounding skin.

Loss of Firmness or Tone

The loss of firmness or tone of the abdominal muscles after pregnancy is worrisome for most women. Because of the growth of the uterus during pregnancy, the abdominal muscles will not be as tight as you might like after delivery. The so-called pot belly that results can usually be conquered through routine exercises to effectively increase the muscle tone again. Exercise should begin as soon after delivery as possible (your doctor is the best judge of the timing), since the longer you wait before reconditioning gets started, the more likely it is that the muscles will stay lax—that the pot belly won't disappear and the abdomen will sag.

Breast Enlargement and Tenderness

Breast enlargement and tenderness is a normal part of pregnancy and takes place in preparation for milk production. Although it can be very disturbing if you bump into something, there is really nothing you can do to prevent the everyday, normal discomfort and tenderness. Wearing a support bra will usually help during pregnancy and while nursing.

If you intend to nurse your baby (and this is very beneficial, even if done for only a few weeks or months), you may want to begin nipple toughening and stimulation in the latter half of pregnancy. Roll the nipples gently between your thumb and first finger several times a day. Exposing the bare nipples to sunlight for no more than 10 to 15 minutes a day helps to toughen them. Avoiding excessive washing with soap and water, which removes some of the natural skin oils, and using a bland ointment on the nipples are often recommended, as well.

Many women worry about the *shape and firmness of their breasts* after pregnancy and nursing. For some, the loss of that which is considered attractive in this society—firm, round breasts—of being less attractive to husband or mate can be very distressing.

For others, the change is hardly noticeable. How important and how disenchanting this is depends on the individual woman. Discussing this fear openly is often helpful.

Flushing and Other Effects of Hormones

Sudden flushing and feelings of warmth are the source of many complaints during pregnancy. These sensations are normal and probably result from the effects of estrogen, as do other common annoyances, such as small spiderlike red marks under the skin (called "spider angiomas") and red, warm palms (called "palmar erythema").

Many pregnant women develop an increase in skin pigment over the face—forehead, cheeks or the entire face—during pregnancy. This is called the "mask of pregnancy" and is thought to be related to hormonal changes. Unfortunately, in some women this increased pigmentation may not fade completely after pregnancy is over. In this case cosmetic coverage can be used.

Shortness of Breath

If you think about it, you can probably understand why it is common for women who are pregnant to have episodes in which they feel short of breath and are aware of a rapid heartbeat. There is increased demand upon your body during exercise (walking, going up stairs, housework, etc.) because of the additional weight and the increased blood supply to the fetus. This occasional shortness of breath is normal. If, however, the shortness of breath is severe and continual, call your doctor immediately.

Increase in Saliva and Hair Loss

Two complaints not easy to explain are an increase in the amount of saliva and hair loss during pregnancy. The increase in saliva, often associated with a metallic taste in the mouth, is called "ptyalism." This may cause nausea but should not cause worry.

Loss of hair, although obviously frightening to some, is usually subtle and noticeable only to you. Don't worry if this happens—the hair will usually grow back after delivery.

Dental Problems

Many women have problems with decay or deterioration of the teeth during pregnancy. This may be related to the fetus's bone growth and development, which places increased demands on the mother's calcium supply. See your dentist before pregnancy, if possible, and regularly during and afterwards. Omit X rays whenever possible, and be sure to tell your dentist you're pregnant. Do all you can to keep your teeth in the best possible shape to avoid often costly and uncomfortable corrective work later.

Change in Vision

Another side effect a woman may experience during gestation is a change in vision. This may result from a general increase in the amount of liquid in her body and is usually normal. Because of this frequent difficulty, the nine months of pregnancy are not a good time to have your glasses checked or changed.

If the problem is very bothersome, be sure to tell your doctor, especially if it is during the last three months of pregnancy, when visual problems might also signal toxemia. Women with diabetes, hypertension and some endocrine problems should consult the doctor if they experience visual changes. While most of the time these will be nothing to worry about, your doctor may wish to examine you to be sure.

Heartburn

Many women experience heartburn throughout pregnancy, and it often gets worse as the pregnancy advances. In fact, for some it might be the first hint of pregnancy, overshadowing the other telltale signs.

As the uterus gets larger during pregnancy, it pushes up on the stomach and causes its contents and its acid to regurgitate into the esophagus. When the acid touches these sensitive tissues, it causes a burning sensation. This can be relieved by antacids, but these should be used only with your doctor's approval. Heartburn can also be helped by eating small, frequent meals rather than large ones and by not lying down immediately after eating.

For women with heart disease, heartburn can cause a great deal of anxiety, because it can be confused with chest pain starting in the heart. They should not hesitate to call the doctor to make sure it actually is heartburn and to discuss steps to help relieve the discomfort.

Gas and Constipation

Gas and constipation are frequent complaints of pregnant women. Eating foods high in fiber with plenty of bulk and increasing fluid intake will usually help. Do not use laxatives unless you discuss this with your physician and he or she agrees.

Stuffy Nose

A stuffy nose is a nuisance to many pregnant women. Although its exact cause is not known, it seems to result from increased circulation to the membranes of the nose. But it's nothing to worry about. Although this problem is irritating and bothersome, try *not* to take any medication to reduce the swelling, and never take drugs—including those you can buy without a prescription—without checking with your doctor.

Tiredness

Tiredness is a very common affliction of the pregnant woman, and interestingly, for many it seems to be more acute during the first trimester (three months) than later in pregnancy. Some women report a loss of energy and a desire to sleep a lot. A change in hormones may play a role in these feelings of fatigue.

Planning to rest every day could be of benefit, although this does not work for all women. Some women identified as high-risk are advised to rest more often than others or to stay off their feet. If you are asked to do this, it is for your benefit and that of your unborn child.

Faintness and Light-headedness

Some women feel faint (off and on) during their pregnancies, and others actually faint or lose consciousness temporarily. Light-headed feelings and faintness may result from poor diet, low blood sugar or anemia. In some cases, especially late in pregnancy, these feelings may occur when a woman is lying on her back. This is caused by the pressure of the uterus on the large blood vessels that return blood to the heart and brain.

In all cases, when you feel dizzy or faint, immediately lie down *on your side*, and keep your head at the same level as or lower than the level of your heart. If you have not eaten recently, get something to eat or drink, as well.

Notify your doctor *immediately* if you ever lose consciousness. It's wise to mention episodes of light-headedness or faintness during routine prenatal checks, or sooner if these are frequent, since your doctor will want to make sure there is no potentially serious underlying reason for these episodes.

Vaginal Discharge

A possible minor problem for some women is an increase in vaginal discharge. Vaginal discharge can be anything from a nuisance to ruptured membranes. Usually, slight changes in vaginal secretions are due to increased mucus production and engorgement in the pelvic area. If however, there is itching, burning or a particular bad odor, an infection is probably the culprit.

Infections are rarely a serious problem but can be terribly uncomfortable if left untreated. For the sake of comfort and safety, it's best to have your physician check to see if an infection is present. This is especially important if you might have been exposed to a sexually transmitted disease (venereal disease), or if your partner has any genital sores or discharge from his penis. .

Worth mentioning here is the difference between mucus discharge and ruptured membranes, better known as "your water breaking." First of all, ruptured membranes do not occur during the first trimester (three months) of pregnancy. When the membranes rupture (break), there is usually a "gush" of water from the vagina. For some women this event can be confusing, however, since the so-called gush is more like a trickle.

Unfortunately, many women are reluctant to call the doctor, because they're not sure whether their membranes have ruptured or not. If you're not sure, don't hesitate to call. It's better to be certain than to worry unnecessarily about whether the baby is on the way or a problem exists. It should be mentioned that prolonged membrane rupture can lead to an increased risk of infection for both mother and baby.

Morning Sickness

The trials of morning sickness are very well known and have been regarded as the first sign of pregnancy. Certainly, morning sickness (that whole array of unpleasant symptoms) to most women is a telltale, overt sign that pregnancy may have occurred. This is confirmed when coupled with a missed menstrual cycle or two.

In some cases the "off and on" sensation of having a touch of the flu, not feeling well or bouts of dizziness arrive even before the first period is missed.

No one denies the fact: Morning sickness isn't pleasant and can be downright miserable. It can place additional stress on a woman identified as high-risk, because she is often fearful something is wrong. Although the condition got its name because so many women experience problems in the morning (probably due to lack of food for so many hours), it can occur at any time of the day.

The best part of morning sickness is that it's usually self-limited. The vomiting and bouts of nausea are most often restricted to the first three months of pregnancy, when a woman's body is adjusting to the pregnancy and its hormonal changes. Since the symptoms of morning sickness rarely continue past the third month, it's important to see your doctor if the problem persists. This is especially true if you are high-risk otherwise, since an additional problem like severe morning sickness may require treatment for your safety and that of your growing fetus.

Much of the time the symptoms of morning sickness are exaggerated by a lack of sufficient food intake or are the result of a lengthy period of time between meals. Drinking small volumes of liquids frequently and eating a few crackers now and then helps, but this should be approved by your physician. Some high-risk women (particularly those with diabetes or hypertension) need to maintain special diets.

We would like to emphasize one point. There is no basis for the argument that claims morning sickness is an overt sign a woman does not want a pregnancy. Myths develop in medicine, as in any other area. *This* is a myth and is simply not true. In most cases women feel very badly about getting sick or complaining about it.

Most physicians are very understanding and aware of how uncomfortable morning sickness can be. Don't feel badly about discussing your problem with a doctor and asking for advice. Hopefully, your family and friends will also be sympathetic, understanding and supportive about this gnawing problem of pregnancy if it occurs.

There is, however, a serious side to the problem of morning sickness. Some women are so miserable that steps must be taken to alleviate their severe symptoms. When the vomiting and nausea become so excessive that they threaten the mother's nutrition or fluid and salt balance, the use of medication may be considered. A doctor might be even more concerned if the mother is already at risk for other problems and want to alleviate the threat morning sickness could cause to her health and that of her baby. (In *extremely rare cases* even hospitalization and intravenous, or IV, feeding might be necessary.)

As discussed earlier, since all drugs reach the fetus in some form and amount, it is wise to avoid taking any drug during pregnancy unless the potential benefit outweighs the possible risk. When a pregnancy is already high-risk, all care should be taken not to add any other potential problems. But when morning sickness is severe, the relative risk of using a widely tested, prescribed medication to control vomiting may be warranted, as compared to the dangers of continued vomiting.

Benedectin®, a drug prescribed to control severe nausea and vomiting, is often used early in pregnancy. First marketed in 1956, the drug was reformulated in 1976 to eliminate one ingredient said not to add to its effectiveness. According to the *FDA Drug Bulletin* (March 1981), Benedectin® is prescribed for an estimated 10 percent to 25 percent of pregnant women in the United States, usually in the first trimester of pregnancy.

Because of Benedectin®'s widespread use in pregnancy and public concern over a lawsuit that raised the question of the drug's association with birth defects, the FDA's Fertility and Maternal Health Advisory Committee evaluated unpublished and published epidemiologic studies to determine the drug's safety. Their investigation found that information now available showed no increased risk of birth defects with Benedectin® use. It did, however, cite two studies that left "residual uncertainty" and suggested that surveys of Benedectin®'s use be continued.

The studies reviewed by this committee were exhaustive. In fact, this drug has been studied better than any other anti-nausea drug used in pregnancy and appears to be relatively safe for both mother and fetus. Its use, however, is recommended only when the nausea and vomiting have not responded to conservative treatment measures (such as eating and drinking small amounts frequently, as recommended by your doctor), and when symptoms become a *serious threat* to the mother's well-being and that of the fetus.

Anemia

Anemia is a condition in which a person's blood has fewer than the usual number of red blood cells. It can occur during pregnancy and is most often caused by the increased iron demands of the fetus and the necessity for the mother to expand her blood volume. Your doctor will often recommend or prescribe tablets containing iron to prevent or treat this problem, but do not exceed the dosage he indicates.

Other causes of anemia are possible, and your doctor will want to identify these. Routine, periodic blood tests during pregnancy help to detect this problem.

The Bottom Line on Some Problems in Pregnancy

It is very important for those identified or potentially high risk to know what problems any pregnant woman may possibly experience. Many of the problems discussed in this chapter are minor to moderate irritations, inconveniences and other temporary discomforts. Others are more serious, need evaluation and sometimes management or intervention. It is always best to know about these problems all women face when pregnant. It gives you a means by which you can often identify potentially serious developments early while still recognizing minor discomforts that are not a cause for worry.

However, if ever in doubt about a symptom or if ever really uncomfortable, do not hesitate to call your doctor and ask if this is something worth seeing him or her about. Sometimes a simple phone call or a visit to the doctor (where indicated) can relieve a great deal of unnecessary anxiety and worry.

SEVEN

SEX, EXERCISE AND DIET DURING PREGNANCY

Often women feel they can do little to help make a pregnancy safer. This is far from the truth. As we discussed in Chapter 4 (Teratogens), women can and should do all possible to avoid certain drugs, chemicals and other agents that could possibly cause fetal malformation. You also have control over other aspects of everyday life—diet, exercise and sex—often taken for granted. These are important areas of consideration which sometimes require special attention during pregnancy. There are also areas where myth, assumption and misunderstandings flourish. Often women casually assume that their activities must be totally restricted because of pregnancy. On the other hand, others assume that they need not restrict anything.

It's important for us to take a close look at the importance of a sound nutritional plan, in what situation sex is not advisable and what role exercise should or should not play in your pregnancy. These are areas over which you have control and where your efforts can make a difference.

Sex during Pregnancy

The question of whether or not it is safe to have sexual intercourse during pregnancy has been of concern to couples over the years. Many old wives' tales have been spun, and legend has it in some parts of the world that sex during pregnancy is evil. Some people say that sex during pregnancy is dirty or harmful or that the pregnant woman, if she's "normal" and will be a "good" mother, isn't interested in it and doesn't enjoy it. Others will insist that men don't find pregnant women appealing and sexy, or that having sex will always harm the baby.

All of these statements are false—because they are generalizations. For the most part, having sexual intercourse during pregnancy is a very personal decision. Each person's feelings may be different, and the couple involved must make the decision themselves—if there is no medical reason not to have intercourse.

Indeed, many men confess that they find their wives even more appealing and sensual when pregnant. Some women will tell you their sex drive increases when pregnant, while others say it diminishes.

In any case there are two important aspects that need to be considered when it comes to sexual intercourse during pregnancy: (1) the safety of the mother and the unborn baby and (2) the feelings and comfort of the couple.

Scientifically speaking, there is no solid evidence available that shows that sexual intercourse during pregnancy causes problems. On the other hand, there have been some real concerns raised— although these possible risks are still theoretical, and much more study needs to be completed before a definitive answer can be given.

There is some evidence suggesting that certain bacteria can be transmitted through intercourse, causing serious uterine infections potentially harmful to the mother and unborn baby. Also, the mechanical aspect of intercourse may activate a substance called "prostaglandin," which stimulates uterine activity or contractions. Seminal fluid also contains prostaglandin, and this may theoretically stimulate uterine activity. Orgasm itself has been shown to cause prolonged and sustained uterine contractions.

Does this mean the fetus could spontaneously abort, or that premature labor could be started? One study published in the *New England Journal of Medicine* (November 29, 1979) suggested that sexual intercourse one or more times a week during the last month of pregnancy was associated with a higher frequency of uterine infections and infant deaths than when women abstained from intercourse during the last month. The important words here are "suggested" and "associated with." Further, these data were collected between 1959 and 1966, when less was known about the treatment of uterine infections as well as about premature labor.

No one has an absolute answer. Most experts agree, however, that women at high risk for premature labor, those with a poor pregnancy history, women with other high-risk factors, and those shown through pelvic examination to have premature "ripening" of the cervix (meaning it is dilating early) should abstain from sexual intercourse and orgasm (that is, from any type of sexual stimulation) after the 20th week of pregnancy.

If on the other hand, there is no reason to expect a high risk for premature labor, and there are no other risk factors for you, there is presently no known reason for abstinence throughout pregnancy. If this is your first pregnancy, there is no easy way (because of the lack of a pregnancy history) to gauge your risk—the risk for premature labor in a first pregnancy is unknown.

To set the record straight, first talk with your doctor about sex during *your* pregnancy. He or she knows you, your medical history, your present physical condition and any potential risks you may have. Doctors, in general, will respect and appreciate frank questions regarding sexual activity. Part of quality patient care involves answering difficult questions and relieving anxiety brought on by lack of information or misinformation.

If your doctor feels there is no contraindication for sexual intercourse, orgasm or sexual arousal, the decision lies with you and your partner. The personal feelings of both the man and the woman involved are most important in this situation. If having intercourse is mutually satisfying, a couple should not be uncomfortable because of what's been said by friends or relatives. Communication is the key. If as the pregnancy progresses, sex becomes more physically difficult, either partner should feel free to express this. Problems usually arise when communications stop, when people listen to others who mean well but don't know the personal feelings and preferences of the couple or when either partner fears that any type of sexual activity will hurt the baby or the expectant mother.

Prevent or alleviate these problems by talking with your doctor when you find out you're pregnant. Ask if you have any risk for premature labor or other potential problems that could be worsened by sexual activity, intercourse or orgasm. And if your partner is not with you during the visit, be sure to tell him what the doctor said. He, too, needs to clearly understand the facts as they pertain to *you* and *him* and *this* pregnancy. As you progress through the pregnancy, reaffirm your doctor's original recommendations by asking if sexual orgasm and intercourse are still safe.

Your doctor may recommend abstinence from intercourse, sexual excitement or orgasm during the last month of pregnancy—even if you have no known risk factors. It's always best to ask questions and get answers rather than to be fearful and anxious.

Meanwhile, research will continue, and more will eventually be known about those at high risk for premature labor and the relationship, if any, to sexual intercourse, sexual excitation and orgasm.

Nutrition and Diet

If you talked to an architect, he or she would tell you that the foundation of any building is probably the most important structural factor in its design and construction. The support must be laid solidly in place, brick by brick, to achieve the highest degree of stability. And so it is with our bodies. Cells, particularly in those first nine months of life within the womb, are multiplying, building cell upon cell like little bricks, one on top of the other and side by side. This building of cells, organs and systems is the foundation for constructing the human edifice.

You can see why there is such concern about nutrition during pregnancy. The old truism "you are what you eat" is applicable to the fetus, too—as an individual. But the unborn child has no control over what he or she will "eat." Only the expectant mother can control the diet of the growing and developing little being. Because of this, it is important for you to know exactly what you should and shouldn't eat.

Unfortunately, the subject of diet in pregnancy has produced numerous evangelical advocates for one nutritional "miracle plan" after another. In general, these advocates are relying on testimonials for a plan's effectiveness rather than on sound medical fact. That's why you find hundreds of diets claimed to be the "best" for the pregnant woman.

You will also find that different doctors will prefer variations on certain nutritional plans during pregnancy. In most cases, however, the plan a qualified physician gives you to follow will be based on what science does and does not know, and not on a new fad that promises to "deliver the healthiest baby you've ever seen."

We honestly don't have all the answers about diet and the nine months of pregnancy. While medical science now knows a great deal, many questions are still unanswered.

In reality, the nutritional plan necessary to promote health and safety during pregnancy is very easy to follow. It doesn't rely on any particular listing of specific foods to be consumed each day of the week or during certain stages of pregnancy. It *does* rely on simple, basic nutritional principles.

THE FOUR BASIC FOOD GROUPS

DAIRY PRODUCTS
(for example)

Whole milk
Lowfat milk
Skim milk
Evaporated milk
Buttermilk

Cheddar cheese
American cheese
String cheese
Jack cheese
Other cheeses

Cottage cheese
Yogurt

Ice Cream

Other milk products

MEATS AND OTHER PROTEINS
(for example)

Beef
Pork
Veal
Fish
Lamb
Poultry
Liver

Eggs
Nuts
Peanut butter

FRUITS AND VEGETABLES
(for example)

Dark Green Vegetables:

Spinach
Broccoli
Brussel sprouts

Fruits:

Oranges
Lemons
Apples

Prunes
Grapes
Dates
Raisins
Papayas

GRAINS AND CEREALS
(for example)

Whole or enriched:

Wheat breads
Rye breads
Sourdough

Asparagus
Cabbage
Dark leafy lettuces
Peas
Green beans

Yellow Vegetables:

Carrots
Squash
Potatoes
Bean sprouts
Corn and hominy
Pumpkins
Mushrooms

Peaches
Pears
Plums
Grapefruit
Apricots
Figs
Bananas

Citrus fruit juice and other
    fresh juices (no artificial
    sugars added)

Mangos
Tangerines
Strawberries
Other berries
Cucumbers
Tomatoes

Other breads
Cereals (hot or cold)

As well as:

Wheat germ
Rice
Tortillas
Crackers
Pastas (including noodles, macaroni,
    spaghetti, etc.)

Proper diet during pregnancy means following a consistent, well-balanced nutritional plan. Daily specific servings from the four basic food groups (shown above) *represent a "balance" of proteins, carbohydrates and fats, as well as essential vitamins and minerals.* Because certain chronic diseases and some problems during pregnancy require or are often better controlled or managed by a specific special diet—and since all women are different—nutritional plans are tailor-made to meet each woman's individual needs. Therefore, the number and size of servings from each food group and those foods your doctor may emphasize more than others will very much depend on your own nutritional needs and any necessary dietary restrictions you may have during pregnancy. *Make sure you ask your doctor questions if you do not understand the specifics of the dietary plan he or she recommends for you.*

The plain fact is, it always makes sense to eat a well-balanced diet—especially while pregnant, for your sake and that of your unborn baby. Such a diet contributes to your health and well-being. A balanced nutritional plan involves the following:

1. Using the four basic food groups as a general guide and eating recommended portions every day (see Table 00).
2. Eating enough calories to gain between 20 and 25 pounds during the nine months of pregnancy.
3. Having enough iron in your diet to maintain your own good health and that of your unborn baby. (Many doctors recommend and prescribe iron supplements or vitamins including iron, to ensure that there is enough iron available for extra blood production during pregnancy.)

But it *does not* mean going on a reducing diet while you're pregnant. Carbohydrate restriction in particular can be dangerous to your unborn baby.

Presently, there is no evidence that prenatal vitamins are essential or helpful. We do know that when a woman is taking prescribed vitamin supplements, her unborn baby does not have any vitamin deficiencies. We also know that if certain vitamins and minerals are not in an expectant mother's diet, certain maternal deficiencies do occur.

If taken as prescribed, vitamins are not harmful to the mother or fetus. Excesses may be harmful, however. Do not take vitamins or supplements not prescribed by your doctor, and don't take more than the amount prescribed or recommended.

Megavitamins are vitamins packaged or taken in large doses—and they are drugs. Do not take megavitamins or begin any special vitamin program without the approval of your doctor. The old saying, "if some is good, more is even better," doesn't apply here. This is also true of iron tablets or supplements—take them only as directed.

A note of caution. If you have small children already, be especially careful to keep all vitamins, supplements and iron pills—as well as other medications—out of their reach. Many accidental poisonings occur each year because young children take pills. And iron pills can kill! Remember, small children are curious, and may think pills are candy. Do all you can to assure their safety.

You have probably also heard a great deal about the importance of extra protein in the diet during pregnancy. Another fallacy.

Studies show that pregnant women only need to consume a normal daily requirement of protein. However, high protein consumption (70 grams to 100 grams per day) probably will not harm you if you prefer more protein in your diet. You need not be as concerned about the intake of protein as you should be about the intake of carbohydrates.

Some women remember the days when a restrictive diet was recommended during pregnancy—meaning carbohydrate restriction. This was popular because of the belief that toxemia could be prevented or controlled by restricting sugar and starch intake. (Toxemia during pregnancy manifests itself as hypertension—high blood pressure—which can cause problems if not controlled.)

Recent studies, however, show that carbohydrate restriction does not prevent toxemia. New studies further show that restriction of carbohydrates may result in a greater incidence of lower intelligence levels and physical underdevelopment of babies. In fact, women who gain less than ten pounds during pregnancy have a serious risk for stillbirth, premature birth or having a baby who is undergrown and not fully developed.

While you should remember not to restrict your carbohydrate intake during pregnancy, do not go to the other extreme, either. Your emphasis should be on meeting the *minimum daily requirement* necessary for optimal health and safety for you and your unborn baby.

One point worth mentioning: Many women experience constipation during pregnancy, especially toward its end. It usually helps to add more fiber to your diet, in the form of leafy vegetables or bran, plus fruit. Adding more liquids helps too. *Do not use laxatives—* unless you have talked with your doctor, and he or she recommends their use. Laxatives are medicines, even though you can buy them in any drugstore or supermarket. Like all medications, their use during pregnancy should be greatly limited or avoided, except when recommended by a doctor who knows you are pregnant.

What about too much weight gain during pregnancy? In most cases, a weight gain of over 25 pounds means adipose tissue (fat) is being added to your body. Being overweight is unhealthy, even during pregnancy, so your doctor will want to weigh you at every visit throughout pregnancy to make sure you are gaining the right amount—not too little and not too much.

If you're gaining too much weight, it may be that you are eating more than your necessary daily requirements of carbohydrates (starches and sugars), protein and fats. In other words, the servings are too big. You and your doctor will be the best judge, and you will be able to find a workable solution together.

Women interested in losing weight should always do so *before* pregnancy occurs. This allows for better cardiovascular fitness and general good health. If you become pregnant and have not gotten around to starting that diet—don't start one while pregnant. And don't go on a restrictive diet while you are trying to get pregnant, because you may conceive and not even suspect it. Dieting during this time could put the developing fetus at risk, because the first trimester is a very important period of cell and organ development.

In any case, be sure to talk with your doctor if you have questions concerning diet before and during pregnancy. If you have a chronic disease or problem (for example, diabetes) that requires a special dietary regimen, it is especially vital to discuss the best nutritional plan for you *before* conception occurs (if possible) and throughout the course of the nine months.

Exercise and Pregnancy

If you've ever started an exercise program, you know how sore you can get and how long it takes to condition your body to the new stresses placed upon it. With pregnancy there are enough changes taking place inside your body that it would be unsafe to suddenly add strenuous exercise to which you are not accustomed.

The point is, the type and amount of exercise recommended depends on each individual woman and what she is used to routinely performing, as well as her stage (fourth, sixth, eighth month) of pregnancy. In any case, your physician will be the one best informed as to your present and continued physical condition. You should talk with him or her about the kind of exercise you have been doing routinely, and what amount and type of exercise would be recommended during the various stages of your pregnancy.

Certain risk factors require modification of activity during pregnancy. If you have a placental problem or a chronic condition such as hypertension, diabetes, heart disease or certain others, you will no doubt be advised to refrain from any activities and remain more or less sedentary during pregnancy. In these situations, short leisurely walks are often recommended. (In some situations bedrest is necessary and the doctor will recommend *no* physical activity.)

Most doctors agree that even those women with no added risk factors during pregnancy should refrain from all *strenuous* exercise, including running, and should substitute less active routines. There is a very good reason for this. Vigorous exercise shunts blood away from the uterus to the muscles used in the exercise. This is normal, but it creates a potential problem during pregnancy. This shunting of blood could compromise the fetus, because the mother's blood provides the fetus with oxygen and nutrients necessary for well-being and growth. Additionally, strenuous exercise may put undue stress upon the mother's already stressed cardiovascular system.

Again, some moderate or mild exercise is good unless there are specific contraindications. Golf, swimming, moderately active tennis and walking are reasonable during the first part of pregnancy for women who are used to being active. During the second half of pregnancy, if all is well, walking is a healthy way to maintain cardiovascular fitness while still staying within the guidelines for your health and that of your unborn baby.

Your doctor should be your source of information about what is best for you. Make sure you are honest about what you are used to doing and how you are feeling as the pregnancy progresses. If you have a chronic condition, be especially sure to check with your doctor about *all types* of exercise, and what amount of exertion you can tolerate without causing or aggravating potential problems. (Remember, exercise in this case refers to all forms of exertion—including housework and other "usual" activities.) It is essential that you be careful not to overextend yourself if you are at risk for problems that could be aggravated by excessive exertion.

The Bottom Line on Sex, Exercise and Diet During Pregnancy

Finally, we want to emphasize the fact that during pregnancy many of the everyday activities that we simply take for granted (diet, exercise and sex), may need to be modified in order to optimize your pregnancy outcome. The exact modification will be dependent on your particular circumstances and needs and those of the fetus. Your doctor will be your best resource and able to adjust your recommended activities and nutritional needs based on the time in your pregnancy and your physical well-being.

EIGHT

COMPETENT OBSTETRICAL CARE: PROMOTING MATERNAL AND FETAL HEALTH

Competent obstetrical care is important to all pregnancies but particularly vital for those pregnancies already identified or potentially high risk. We know that minor to major problems can occur at some point during any pregnancy which will suddenly put the pregnancy in the high risk category. We also know that 60 percent of high risk problems can be identified very early in pregnancy with appropriate and routine evaluations. The other 40 percent will be identified at some point later in pregnancy or during labor and delivery.

With early detection when a problem occurs, careful management and necessary intervention, many complications can now be readily controlled. Excellent obstetrical care is particularly vital for women with a chronic disease or condition, those 35 years of age or older— and in fact, for anyone identified as at increased risk for potential problems. Consistent, regular and (where indicated) specialized obstetrical care does play a significant role in promoting a safer, healthier pregnancy, with optimal results. What this does is give you and your doctor a jump on a problem before it worsens or allows for special evaluations to be ordered if a problem is suspected.

Pre-pregnancy Visit

Although done less often than is desirable, a "pre-pregnancy evaluation" by your doctor is highly recommended if you know you would be or suspect you might be at increased risk for problems during pregnancy, labor or delivery. In fact, a pre-pregnancy visit is always a good idea, whether you are potentially high-risk or not.

This visit allows for the identification of any existing problems concerning your health and well-being. It should include a comprehensive physical assessment—a complete medical history, a detailed examination and some laboratory studies. Your gynecological status history and past pregnancy history, a gynecological examination and a Pap smear are important aspects of this pre-pregnancy visit. Of particular importance would be any physical problems or underlying disease that should be brought under tight control before pregnancy occurs and/or managed and treated during pregnancy. You may also want to ask your doctor if he or she recommends genetic counseling based on both partners' family histories.

This pre-pregnancy evaluation also gives you an opportunity to discuss any concerns and questions you or your partner might have about pregnancy, your well-being and that of a future child. The doctor will be able to recommend any vitamin supplements considered necessary, as well as a sound nutritional plan and safe exercise program, and reinforce the things you should avoid while trying to get pregnant.

One significant issue to discuss is how to "date" your pregnancy if it occurs. Dating a pregnancy—estimating when you will deliver—is particularly important if you may be high risk. Many tests and treatments that might be deemed necessary later in the pregnancy are based on the gestational age (number of weeks since conception) of the fetus. These various procedures (discussed in Section 2) are less useful or even potentially useless if dating is not accurate.

It is fairly easy for your doctor to date a pregnancy if you keep careful records of your menstrual cycles while trying to get pregnant. Your doctor will want to know the exact date your last menstrual period started, if it was lighter or heavier than usual (which may indicate for some women that pregnancy has already occurred), and how long your menstrual cycle usually is (24, 28, 30, 32, 35, etc., days between periods).

Pregnancy dating is based on calculations made from the time of the start of the *last normal* menstrual period. The length of the pregnancy can be estimated based on the knowledge that ovulation—and hence fertility—occurs about 14 days *before* the start of a menstrual period. If your normal cycle is 28 days, then you would probably ovulate around 14 days after your last period began. If your normal cycle is 50 days, on the other hand, you would then be most likely to ovulate about 36 days after your last period began.

The ovum is probably only susceptible to fertilization during a few hours of any given cycle, but sperm capable of fertilization may remain in the genital tract for several days.

All it takes to accurately date your pregnancy when it occurs is to carefully mark a calendar. Note the day your menstrual period starts, and the day it ends, as well as any other information—it was lighter, heavier, shorter, longer than usual. Do this for several cycles (several months), so the average length of your cycle can be determined (28, 32, 35, etc., days between periods). This information should be carefully noted if you're trying to get pregnant or are not taking any precautions to prevent pregnancy. In this way, you'll be able to answer all your doctor's questions and enable him or her to more accurately date your pregnancy. This information is very important as the pregnancy progresses.

You should also ask your doctor during this visit at what point he or she wants to see you if you think pregnancy has occurred. It is advantageous for anyone who has missed a period to see her doctor within four weeks of the missed period. With high-risk problems, the doctor will decide when it would be most beneficial to you to determine if you are pregnant, based on your own unique needs.

There are a few other noteworthy considerations regarding the pre-pregnancy visit. If you have been using oral contraceptives (the "pill"), it's always best to wait two or three cycles after you've stopped the pill before trying to conceive. If you have been using an IUD (intrauterine device), have it removed two or three cycles before trying to become pregnant. In these situations, use a diaphragm, contraceptive foam or cream, or a condom (as directed) during the two- or three-month wait.

Also check to be sure you are protected against rubella (German measles)—either because you have had the disease or because you have been immunized against it. A blood test called a "rubella titer" will give you the most definite answer about your rubella status. If you are susceptible to this infection and need to be immunized, be sure to avoid getting pregnant for at least four months after you have had the immunization.

Make sure you ask questions and express any concerns you may have at this pre-pregnancy visit. You can optimize your chances of a healthier pregnancy and reduce any avoidable risks by being as informed as possible. If you have a chronic disease, make sure you request special instructions (if any) to keep it under control while trying to get pregnant and when you think you might be pregnant.

What If You Miss a Period?

Remember that missing a period does not always mean you are pregnant. It should, however, be the first thing that comes to mind if you ordinarily have very regular menstrual cycles—especially if you have not been using contraception. (As you know, pregnancy occasionally occurs even with conscientious use of a contraceptive method.)

For many women, the earliest sign of pregnancy can be exaggerated premenstrual problems: fatigue, irritability, urinary frequency, nausea, breast tenderness and enlargement, fluid retention, possible lack of appetite, uncomfortable abdominal cramping or a funny metallic taste in the mouth.

Pregnancy testing is not accurate until two weeks after the missed period. Home pregnancy tests, while probably accurate, rely on the unknown skill and ability of the technician—in this case, you. Whether you use a home pregnancy test is up to you, but when you go to your doctor to be examined, he or she may want to verify the test result anyway.

If you have missed a period, then waited two weeks, and have some of the symptoms mentioned above, you should make an appointment to see your doctor. In some cases, especially when a disease such as severe diabetes, heart disease, hypertension, etc., is involved, the doctor may wish to evaluate you at specific intervals while you are trying to get pregnant.

First Prenatal Visit

When you go to the doctor's office, you may be asked to complete an extensive questionnaire, even before seeing the doctor. This is a screening process that provides information important to your physician—particularly in identifying your risk for certain problems based on your medical history and maternal history.

You will also have several laboratory tests during this visit, either before or after seeing the doctor. You will be asked to give a urine specimen called a "clean catch," meaning an uncontaminated specimen. Be sure to follow the instructions carefully and, if you don't understand, ask questions—before you give the specimen. (Otherwise, you will probably need to give another specimen, and that costs additional money.) Your urine will be analyzed for pus cells, protein, blood and sugar (called "routine urinalysis"), and a culture (for infection) may be done.

Your doctor will also want you to have several blood tests (for which only a single blood sample needs to be drawn, however): a complete blood count, blood typing and testing for your Rh group, antibody screening and a test for syphilis. If you have not previously been checked for rubella immunity, this test would also be done.

You may be given a pregnancy test either before or after you see the doctor. Some physicians want to talk with the patient about symptoms beforehand, while others prefer to know the results of the pregnancy test before seeing her. If the physician can diagnose the pregnancy with the physical examination alone, a pregnancy test will not be necessary.

There are several different kinds of pregnancy tests, but all require special examination of either blood or urine. One takes only a few minutes for results to be available. Another test takes two hours and is more accurate. A third takes an entire day for results but is the most accurate of the three types. There are different reasons for using each of these tests. For your information, some things can interfere with the accuracy of pregnancy tests: aspirin, other salicylates (aspirin related compounds), protein in the urine and various barbiturates. Repeating the test or changing to a different type of test may be necessary if the results are questionable.

If it has been eight weeks or more from your last period, your doctor can pretty much determine if you are pregnant through physical and pelvic examination alone. However, he or she may want to perform a pregnancy test to verify the findings. He or she will also want to "date" your pregnancy, so be sure you have all the information necessary to do this—the date of your last normal period and the usual number of days between your periods.

The doctor will also ask you about your medical history and your daily habits. He or she will want to know if you are taking any medications, what your eating habits are, if you smoke and how much, and if you drink alcohol and how much and how often. He or she will want to know the details of any other pregnancies you might have had.

Your doctor will also want to know about certain diseases or problems you or your partner's relatives may have had or have. During this first visit, it may be wise to have your husband or mate with you, since a complete family history involves both sides of the family. This information gives the doctor some idea if there would be an increased risk of potential problems for your baby.

At this time the physician may prescribe vitamin supplements for you and discuss nutrition and other aspects of prenatal care. Some doctors even like to explain the various choices you might have for delivery or recommend prenatal classes for you and your husband or mate.

This is a good time for you to ask about the cost of care. Most physicians are not reluctant to discuss charges, and most have a payment schedule that is to be met before delivery. If you have questions about costs, don't hesitate to ask. Also, new insurance laws may allow most of the costs to be paid by your insurance company, depending upon the type of coverage you have.

What Happens after the First Visit?

Generally speaking, your doctor will want to see you every four weeks up to the 24th week of pregnancy (about the sixth month) if your pregnancy is progressing well. You may need to be seen more often if there are concerns about your pregnancy, if careful management is necessary, or if you are at risk for a problem early in pregnancy.

Routinely, prenatal checkups involve an evaluation of your blood pressure; a review of any symptoms, problems or questions you might have; a check of your weight gain; and a urinalysis to measure sugar and protein. The doctor may listen to the baby's heart sounds with a special device called a "Doppler" at around 9 or 10 weeks and with a standard stethoscope or the Doppler beginning at around 18 to 20 weeks. Uterine size will be checked and can be determined in several ways. Some physicians simply use a tape measure, while others prefer to use a special calibration device. (This is merely a matter of the physician's personal preference.) The uterus is measured to detect abnormal growth or extra fluid and even to determine the possibility of twins.

Hemoglobin (or a similar measure for anemia) is usually rechecked around 28 to 30 weeks into the pregnancy for all expectant mothers. If you are Rh negative, your doctor will want to follow your progress especially closely to check for possible antibody formation. This means additional blood testing around the 20th, 28th and 34th weeks.

Around the seventh month and thereafter (28th to 36th weeks), your doctor will schedule you for more frequent checks. He or she will usually want to evaluate your progress at least every two weeks and often every week during the last month or until you deliver.

The doctor may perform a vaginal examination at certain intervals during your pregnancy. This examination tells him or her about the condition of the cervix—which is important to delivery. He or she will make note of any unusual thinning, flattening, softening or dilatation of the cervix. (These events normally begin in the last month or so before delivery.)

What About Fetal Movement?

Usually around 18 weeks of gestation, you will begin to feel movement from the fetus. Sometimes this movement seems like thumping or even gurgling in the intestines. As time passes, the movement becomes much more distinct. The fetus has sleeping time as well as awake time, when he or she is most active. Actually, the unborn baby will move several times even within a period of half an hour. Most fetal activity is felt late in the evening, often when you're trying to sleep!

Most women get used to the feeling of fetal movement and even forget it's taking place. It should be noted, however, that a marked decrease in fetal activity that lasts for more than several hours might mean something is wrong. Call your doctor if this happens.

Individual Variations and Schedules

There is no right and wrong way when it comes to visits to your doctor, as long as you follow your doctor's orders. You may be seen only every four or five weeks if all is well. If you have a chronic disease or problem, or need more frequent evaluations because a problem has surfaced, your physician may wish to see you more often than every four weeks, even during early pregnancy. Some women who need to be monitored closely see their physician weekly, even in early pregnancy, and daily for special tests in the last stages of pregnancy.

Some doctors do things at different times than others. Some may feel, for example, that it's important to perform a vaginal examination at every visit to check the cervix, while others may feel this is necessary only at certain intervals. Don't be concerned if your doctor's schedule of visits or routine is different from the one described here or is different from that of a friend or relative.

Be sure to ask questions if you don't understand the recommended routine, tests or their results or the recommended procedures. As a patient—it is your right to know.

NINE

PSYCHOLOGICAL EFFECTS OF A HIGH RISK PREGNANCY

Any discussion of high risk pregnancy would be incomplete unless it included not only the medical facts as they are known today, but also the possible psychological effects on mother and/or father, as well as other family members. In general, all expectant mothers tend to share common needs, concerns and fears. Expectant fathers, too, have needs and share concerns and fears about the pregnancy.

Some women and men experience little anxiety or stress while awaiting the arrival of a new family member—other than the usual off-and-on apprehension that comes with almost all pregnancies. Couples worry about whether all will go well, but often they say little about this thought. Others feel real pain, stress, fear and frustration. Most people do not realize that whether they are experiencing the more commonly shared concerns and needs or the more painful fears or problems—they are not unique. In other words—many other people have and do experience varying degrees of concern, stress and anxiety—and certainly everyone has needs. Sometimes discussing mild to major fears and needs—better equips parents to deal effectively with them. This is particularly true in many high risk pregnancies where stress can be greater if not put into perspective.

Fears and Concerns Common to High Risk Pregnancy

With all pregnancies (as we discussed) everyone has some concerns and fears. Essentially—being identified as high risk for a problem pregnancy—may "intensify" feelings and apprehensions. It may also lead to many misconceptions about the pregnancy and at times overreaction.

Rather than review all we have already talked about in this chapter, we will focus on the key issues of concern to those experiencing a high risk pregnancy.

Why Me?

Asking "Why Me?" is a perfectly normal thing when faced with potential problems during pregnancy. Women with chronic conditions such as diabetes, hypertension, heart disease and other problems who really want children cannot help but be frustrated and wonder why they "got stuck" with a chronic health problem which may jeopardize their well-being or that of their potential children. Others, too, with an increased risk of having children with certain chromosomal problems or inherited conditions—also ask "why me?" Unfortunately, there are no acceptable answers to this question.

It is often better to seek solutions—rather than to continually torture yourself by wondering why. As we have discussed throughout this book, so very much more can be done today than ever before to turn the odds in favor of a successful pregnancy for those at risk for problems. Early detection of problems, careful medical management and treatment (where necessary), have resulted in excellent outcomes for the majority of high risk pregnancies.

Even for those with an increased risk for chromosomal problems or the possibility of passing on some other inherited problem—genetic counseling and amniocentesis can at least give these couples more information about the risks or lack of risks for their offspring. Certainly there is no catch-all answer—but at least more can be done and more questions answered.

In this way, you can ask "what can I do to make pregnancy safer for me and my potential children," which is a more active and positive attitude than not getting past "why me?," which is passive, not constructive and can only make you feel helpless and worse. Pursuing an active role in the decision-making—assessing the risks (if considering pregnancy) or determining what you can do to lessen the risks and help manage the potential problems (if already pregnant)—is vital to both your physical and psychological well-being.

It is important too for your husband or partner to get actively involved in the decision-making and understand the risks and what special role he can play in helping you lessen and manage potential problems. Whether a chronic medical condition—or a potential genetic problem from the father's or mother's side of the family or from both sides—both partners need to realize that no one is "at fault." Feelings of fault or blame have no place in any of this. The best thing any couple can do is to move beyond the questions of "why" or "blame," (which can do no good and only cause more hurt and pain), to an active role in making decisions best for them.

Understanding the Reason(s) for the High Risk Status

As we have previously discussed, misconceptions and misunderstandings can lead to undue and unreasonable stress, worry and anxiety during high risk pregnancy. It is therefore very important that both you and your husband or partner *really* understand why the pregnancy may be considered high risk (if you become pregnant) or is considered high risk (if you are already pregnant). It is also vital that both of you understand what modern medicine has to offer to make the pregnancy safer for you and your unborn child. Although not all anxiety can be totally alleviated—knowing both the risks and what can be done to protect mother and unborn baby—can greatly lessen the stress. Not knowing the *real* situation simply intensifies fears that often have no basis.

You may have heard some people say that it is actually best not to know the risks or the procedures, etc., when it comes to health or medical needs. This philosophy has proven to be false time and time again. Not knowing what is going on can most often be an agonizing experience and only opens doors to exaggerating things way out of proportion. People tend to do well when they *know the facts*, what can and cannot be done, and what certain risks mean and do not mean to them. We find that most women and their husbands or partners are relieved to know exactly what is going on at all times. When couples know the risks and what can be done— they handle the situation quite well. Therefore, close communications between you and your partner and between the two of you and your doctor are vital. Misconceptions can be stopped short— before they cause undue stress. It is important that everyone have as clear a picture as possible of the situation—how the pregnancy is progressing, how mother and unborn baby are doing and what management and treatment may take place in the future, if any is necessary.

Therefore, it is important that you and your partner learn all you can about potential risks before pregnancy and during pregnancy, as well as what role modern perinatal medicine plays in assisting you in protecting both yourself and unborn/newborn baby.

Fear of Having an Abnormal Child

All expectant parents (or those considering having a child) are concerned about whether the child will be normal—or will have a minor to serious abnormality. Most parents admit they worried about this possibility (although statistically remote) during the pregnancy, but said little or nothing about this fear. It is therefore natural for this fear to be intensified during high risk pregnancy. Although there is no way to totally reassure parents that all will be well, we can say that the vast majority of high risk pregnancies are safe and successful today. This does not mean that things do not go wrong, but that (in general) the odds are in favor of mother and child.

The best thing expectant parents can do is to find out all they can about the potential for the baby having some kind of abnormality. Again, genetic counseling would be recommended before or soon after pregnancy occurred (and possibly amniocentesis) for those who have reason to believe that their children would be at increased risk for a chromosomal genetic disorder or if they already have had an abnormal child. Although genetic counseling cannot give absolutes in every case—but the statistical probability that a problem, condition or disorder will be inherited—this information is very important and helpful. Also, amniocentesis cannot tell doctors if the baby is perfectly normal—but it can tell them if certain detectable problems exist. Ultrasound can also be used to verify structural abnormality or to reassure parents that all seems to be well. There is no way, however, to reassure parents that the baby does not have brain damage or certain other problems.

We should mention that genetic counseling itself may be stressful for some couples. Sometimes the couple has difficulty understanding: the concepts involved in genetics; what the statistical probabilities for certain characteristics or problems in their offspring actually mean to them; and simply *what* is being said to them. This can cause more confusion and misunderstanding which can result in greater anxiety—the opposite of the desired effect of genetic counseling. If amniocentesis is recommended to identify chromosomal abnormalities and certain genetic and metabolic disorders or to reassure parents that their fears have no basis—this can also be somewhat stressful for expectant parents. It is the waiting period that tends to be the real cause of stress. Amniocentesis cannot be performed until the 15th to 17th week of pregnancy and parents must then wait another 20 to 30 days for results. This waiting period—a time of not knowing—can produce anxiety and stress.

Once the results are available the couple can relax if no detectable problems are identified (which is the case in the greatest number of couples). If an abnormality is identified, on the other hand, the couple experiences another emotional crisis. Shock, anguish, horror, guilt and denial are common initial responses. Depending on the seriousness of the abnormality, the couple may need to make some very difficult decisions. If a very serious problem is identified before birth, the couple may choose to terminate the pregnancy, or prepare for the medical and other needs of the baby, or decide whether they can care for the baby at home or find a suitable facility to take care of the baby. These are all very difficult decisions and must be made on an individual basis.

If you are faced with difficult and painful decisions, you and your partner may find it helpful and supportive to talk with your minister, rabbi, priest or other religious leader. A frank discussion with your doctor about the possible extent of the abnormality, what it may mean to your and the baby's quality of life may also be helpful. Talking to other parents who have had a child with the same problem can also give you another perspective to consider. It is best to find out as much as possible from a variety of sources before making a decision. Once you have all the information you need then you can better decide what is best for all family members.

If you are suddenly faced with a serious, unexpected abnormality when the baby is born—the same recommendations hold true. First you should find out all you can about the extent of the baby's problem, what it means to your baby and the child's future, and what the medical and daily needs and demands of the child will be. With this information you can better decide whether you can meet the baby's needs at home or if the baby will have more demands than you can handle.

It is highly recommended that you and your partner talk to the social worker at the hospital where the baby was born. These professionals can be very supportive in helping parents work through their grief, shock and feelings of blame or denial. Sometimes when parents are really hurting—they find it difficult to talk to each other about their feelings and their pain. Often an objective but sensitive professional can be very helpful in opening the lines of communications between couples and in supporting both parents as they work through their feelings together. Hospital social workers also have information about community and parent support groups which may be invaluable resources for you and your partner. Most of these groups consist of parents with children with the same or similar problems and provide emotional support as well as an open forum for expressing feelings, fears and the everyday problems experienced by parents who care for children with either chronic or serious abnormalities.

No matter how serious the problem, it is important that neither parent blame the other or oneself for the problem. No one is to blame in these situations (at least most of the time) and no one should try to carry that guilt. It is also vital that you and your partner talk openly about how you are feeling so that tensions and stress do not build up needlessly. Talking things out is certainly not a "cure-all" but it can make a major difference in how each partner relates to the other and helps each of you to be as supportive as possible.

Fear of Losing the Baby

Everyone has off-an-on fears that something will go wrong during the pregnancy or soon after delivery, and the baby will die. During high risk pregnancy this fear may be a little more intensified—depending on the reason for the high risk status. Again, it is helpful to remember that the vast majority of babies—high risk or not—do quite well and are healthy. Others who do need special management and treatment also do well, in general, today. Although we wish we could say that all problems can be cured or managed and no unborn or newborn babies die—that would not be honest. But we can say that fetal and newborn death is becoming more and more rare each year—as advances are made in technology and more is known about how to identify, manage and treat serious problems in both the fetal and neonatal stages.

However, for those who do lose a baby—these statistics provide little comfort or solace. The death of a baby is terribly painful and difficult for parents and other family members. Everyone feels helpless when this happens and there is no easy way to make parents feel better. Everyone needs to go through a grieving process and to work through the grief and pain. Sharing your feelings of loss and sorrow with your husband or partner is very helpful for both partners. Besides your doctor, the social worker at the hospital may also be an invaluable source of support to help you better deal with the grief and loss you are experiencing. Groups of people who have also lost children can be found in major cities and some smaller cities as well. These groups are supportive because they consist of people who have experienced a similar loss and know what you are going through.

One important point—one or both parents (at times) may feel responsible or somehow to blame if their baby dies. These feelings of guilt are in no way beneficial to parents and usually have no basis in fact. Often a serious abnormality, serious respiratory complications due to prematurity or another serious problem are to blame and the baby simply cannot survive. With some genetic defects, half of the defective gene pair comes from *each* family, not just one. It is important to remember that no one is to blame and everything that could have been done was done. Medical science simply does not have all the answers and even heroic attempts to save a baby are at times not successful. The real positive point in all of this is that the tragic loss of a child is becoming more rare today and because of advances made in the last ten years in particular—the vast majority of babies are born healthy—and others with minor to major problems now live quality lives because of intervention not possible until a few years ago. Although knowing this does not help parents at the time, most couples who have lost a baby go on to have healthy babies in the future.

The best thing to remember is that there is every reason for optimism when it comes to high risk pregnancy today. Discussing the possibility of losing a child is never easy—but not discussing it would be dishonest. No one likes to think about this slim possibility, but everyone *does* think about it. It is vital that expectant parents not blow this out of proportion and worry unnecessarily about it. Although unexpected and sudden events can occur throughout pregnancy and during the neonatal period, in general, your doctor will have a good idea about how the baby is doing before birth if careful management, testing and monitoring of the baby's condition are being performed for those at risk for potential problem (discussed in more detail in Section 2). After the baby's birth, too, doctors will be giving you status reports on the baby's condition—particularly if he or she needs intensive care in a special nursery.

You can be assured that parents are no longer kept in the dark about how the baby is doing or if there are real reasons for concern before or after birth. Therefore, if you are unduly stressed worrying about this—talk to your doctor openly about your fears. He or she cannot make any guarantees about the baby's total well-being, but can tell you if there is any reason for you to be alarmed or prepared for certain possibilities.

For those who have already lost a baby or experienced a spontaneous abortion (miscarriage), the fear of losing a future baby may be greater. Again, the best thing anyone can do is learn about the risks, continue to have open discussions with your doctor and be optimistic unless the doctor feels there is concrete evidence for *real* concern or tells you little can be done about a known serious problem.

Women Over 35

Often a woman over 35 years of age is having her first—and possibly only child. In this situation, stress can result if the mother and/or her partner become overly concerned about advanced age and pregnancy. Because of the increased risk for chromosomal abnormalities, amniocentesis is often recommended. This too can produce a dilemma for some couples, if a serious problem is identified. Do they feel terminating a pregnancy is the best answer for them or not? Could the woman conceive again safely or not? What can expectant parents do to better safeguard the mother and unborn baby, and to obtain maximum results?

As we discussed in Chapter 3, a healthy woman over 35 who is in good physical shape really has no greater risks for problems (other than chromosomal abnormalities) than the woman considered low risk. Genetic counseling and amniocentesis—may be recommended for women over 35 years of age—but other than those, the most important aspects of care are to follow your doctor's instructions throughout pregnancy and not become overly concerned about the baby unless the doctor feels there is real reason for concern. In other words—adding unnecessary stress and anxiety is not healthy or helpful. If you or your partner become overly stressed worrying about the baby—talk to your doctor to see if there is any indication of a serious problem. Again, the doctor cannot make any guarantees, but may be able to alleviate some unreasonable fears and lessen others.

Financial Considerations of High Risk Pregnancy

Although people do not like to talk about finances—when it comes to high risk pregnancy—medical bills can be very costly. Some insurance policies may cover the majority of costs for close management, necessary diagnostic testing and special treatment or intervention. Other insurance policies are not as financially helpful. Finances can be the basis for stress and this potential problem needs to be looked at reasonably.

Too often expectant parents say little about the financial burdens some high risk pregnancies may place on them. They think this sounds petty or heartless. It is not. If your insurance coverage is not that helpful or you have no insurance—you should seek alternatives *before* a serious financial problem occurs. Many hospitals and doctors are willing to work out a reasonable payment schedule. Also, the social worker at the hospital where you will deliver may be able to direct you to governmental or private programs which may be of some service to you.

The important thing is to be honest with yourself about where you stand financially, what you can reasonably do and when you need help. The cost for quality care is not inexpensive and many doctors are quite aware of this potential problem. Do not allow yourself to go under financially before seeking assistance or working out a payment schedule.

This also applies if the baby is in need of special (intensive) care for a prolonged period of time. Check with your insurance company to see what would be covered. If it appears that you may experience a financial drain, seek possible solutions immediately—before the expenses get out of hand. Again, the hospital social worker may be able to refer you to possible community resources that may help offset costs. If not, make arrangements with your doctor and the hospital so that you are not unreasonably stressed because of financial pressures.

Although financial considerations do not sound like realistic sources of stress—they really can be a significant issue that causes problems in the relationships of new parents. If this stress continues to intensify and is left unattended—it can cause real problems—particulary if there are other little family members to consider and the impact of a financial drain can harm them as well. It is therefore important to work out some solutions before a situation gets out of hand.

Having Other Children—The Risks and Rewards

If a couple has had a child with a genetic disorder or other problem, has experienced a miscarriage, lost a child for another reason or the mother experienced serious problems during pregnancy—they usually want to know if they dare try to have another child or other children. This decision-making process may be very stressful to parents.

It is impossible to make a generalized statement about this since every situation is different. The best thing for parents to do is have a frank discussion with their doctor. The doctor may recommend genetic counseling, special diagnostic tests to determine any underlying problem(s) in the woman or consultation by other specialists to evaluate what happened before and what the risks are for the same or similar problem(s) occurring again. Gathering all the possible information and working closely with experts in maternal-fetal medicine (where indicated) will give parents the tools to make this important decision.

The vast majority of couples are usually told that the odds are good that they can have a safe pregnancy and a healthy baby. Others decide to try again knowing the mother and unborn baby will need to be closely monitored, managed and possibly treated throughout pregnancy. And, some couples decide that adopting a child is a safer and more acceptable alternative for them.

The Bottomline on Stress, Anxiety and Concerns

Whether it be the commonly experienced off-and-on concerns or anxiety or the more fearful stresses of some situations, knowing the facts, keeping the lines of communications open, being honest about your feelings, fears and needs is the best medicine. Your doctor can be an invaluable resource in helping lessen or totally alleviate undue concern. Most problems occur when a couple does not know what is happening and fear what could happen. Other couples do not fully realize what can be done to intervene if problems occur—because they fail to ask questions or do not receive adequate answers to their questions. If your doctor recommends that you and your partner talk to the hospital social worker—this may be very useful in helping you with your fears and stresses. Make sure you ask questions and ask for help if you feel you may need it. It is also vital to remember that with proper medical management and intervention, the majority of high-risk pregnancies have very successful outcomes.

The Working Mother

Women who have been working must make decisions about their new role. Sometimes the answers are clearcut but other times the situation is much more complex and causes concern and confusion. Should you go back to work after the baby is born? If so, when? Should it be fulltime or parttime? Who will care for the baby (and your other children if you have other children)?

Some women have *no choice but to return to work* because of financial needs. Particularly in today's economy many women must help in the support of the family—at least on a parttime basis. Single mothers most often carry the burden of supporting the new baby and themselves and must return to work. In these situations, the greatest difficulty is finding a dependable babysitter or reputable child care center that can meet your needs and whose fees you can afford. At times, though, this is not the greatest problem. This need to return to work may be stressful to both partners or the single mother—particularly if the mother wanted (or her partner wanted her) to stay home for a longer period of time or to make motherhood a fulltime profession. This situation may put a strain on the couple's relationship or pressure on the single mother.

Other women, however, *wish to return to work* after a certain period of time and can make arrangements for the baby's care with a relative or friend or can afford a child care center. Some women feel they are (and they may actually be) better mothers because they work. Many mothers feel frustrated and bored if at home all day long and require another interest as well as the opportunity to excel in their field of expertise. Children generally do well if they sense that their parents (*both* mother and father) are happy at what they are doing and spend "quality" and "reasonable amounts" of time with them.

The decision to work or not to work must be made on a very individualized basis, which makes it impossible to make generalizations. Some women do quite well as fulltime or parttime working mothers while others are unhappy about the situation. For those who must work because of financial considerations but are upset that they cannot spend more time at home—it is helpful to remember that in most situations the quality of time spent with a child often outweighs the amount of time (as long as the amount of time is reasonable and all the child's needs are being met). Again, all women, their needs and wants and those of their family are different. What is good for one mother and one family is not for another and vice versa, so there is no way to say what is "best" for all.

TWO

WHAT ADVANCED MEDICAL CARE CAN DO FOR THE HIGH-RISK PREGNANCY

Years ago women who could get pregnant simply got pregnant. Those with certain health problems were either discouraged from getting pregnant or did so at all costs. Some used the limited methods of birth control available to them, fearful of the effects of pregnancy on themselves and potential children. Many got pregnant. Many babies died—before, during or soon after birth. Many women died, too. Great numbers of those who did not die suffered lifelong illnesses or disabilities as a result. Doctors could do little about such problems. It was heartbreaking and frustrating for loving mothers, fathers and family members as well as for dedicated physicians and other health professionals.

Many people remember one very moving story that touched a nation. In August 1963 president of the United States John F. Kennedy and his wife Jacqueline lost a son, Patrick Bouvier Kennedy—40 hours after birth. This same tragedy had happened to many, many couples over the years—prematurity resulting in a breathing difficulty known as hyaline membrane disease—and death. But this time an entire nation and the world watched and waited.

People wondered why nothing could be done. It was the first time the problems of pregnancy received worldwide public attention, although research had been going on for years to remedy many of them.

At Brooke Army Medical Center in Texas the day before his death, the young president watched a unique simulation in a specially designed oxygen tank, aimed at developing technology for space travel. President Kennedy surprised everyone when he asked if this kind of advanced technology being developed to sustain men in outer space might someday sustain premature babies. He would not live to see highly sophisticated space age technology modified for utilization in medicine—for the benefit of unborn and newborn babies, children and adults alike.

Then, premature babies with lung problems had little chance of survival. There was no way to stop premature labor and delivery. There was no way to help mature a fetus's lungs before delivery. There were only crude ways to determine if a fetus was in trouble inside the womb or at the time of delivery. There were few ways to manage or sustain the newborn who had problems. Doctors could do little—other than to keep the babies warm, sometimes give them oxygen—and hope for the best. Many couples suffered losses, and others all but gave up on ever having a family.

Today, it's an entirely different story. Doctors, specially trained, skilled and experienced in high-risk obstetrics, can take aggressive action in most cases, because the knowledge and technology are now available to help them assist the miracle of birth. Space age technology, then, has had a major impact on the care of mothers and babies. Yesterday's science fiction is in many ways today's reality. It has enabled great strides to be made in diagnosis, treatment and management of high-risk mothers and unborn/newborn infants.

Thirty years ago no one could have imagined we would actually be able to see a developing baby inside his or her mother's womb—long before birth—without making a single incision. No one dreamed special drugs would be developed to help a fetus's lungs mature before birth when premature labor occurred. No one could have guessed that the amniotic fluid surrounding the fetus would provide scientists and doctors with so much vital information, or that special imaging of the fetus would be used to evaluate and record the developmental changes during the nine months of pregnancy.

Who would have guessed that the technology used to monitor the condition of astronauts during space flights would be modified and perfected in order to record an unborn baby's heartbeat and fitness at the time of labor and delivery? This procedure, known as fetal monitoring, would detect problems so steps could be taken to lessen or alleviate them. And three or four decades ago, the study of genetics was still in its infancy. With the advent of the electron microscope, the development of many special techniques and the work of dedicated scientists, genetics came into its own, adding new dimensions to prenatal diagnosis.

"Man and his machines," it would later be called. But technology is more than just machines. It involves greater knowledge, better methods of care, new drugs, advanced surgical techniques and much, much more.

Suddenly women with such medical conditions as diabetes or serious heart disease had an excellent chance of having successful pregnancies. Those who developed toxemia (hypertension—high blood pressure—in pregnancy, along with other changes) were still in jeopardy for problems, but much more could be done, with more successful outcomes. Certain infectious diseases could now be managed during pregnancy and at the time of birth, with better results for both mother and child. Special tests could tell a couple if a child would be born with devastating chromosomal abnormalities. Rh disease could suddenly be prevented in most babies, and in those with the disease, special testing and treatment could prevent death.

People who could not otherwise have started a family could now consider the risks and make a choice—knowing that much more could be done than ever before.

Progress hasn't ended there. Those fearful that some inherited/ genetic disease might result if they had children have elected to undergo genetic counseling. Many find their fears have substance, while most find their fears were baseless—and are finally freed to have the children they always wanted. Others who could not become pregnant have been assisted through drugs or artificial insemination. The list goes on and on.

But there have been some criticisms. Medical science had become so sophisticated that many felt pregnancy and childbirth had become terribly impersonal—sterile and antiseptic. They had a right to be angry. But to be fair, many of the measures criticized were originally initiated out of concern for both mother and newborn baby.

Fear of infection led to specific policies about handling babies and about the importance of wearing masks and gowns. Women were kept in hospitals for days to recover from delivery, while babies were kept in nurseries far from their mothers—even when no problems were known or even suspected. Mothers were told that formula was as good as breast milk, or better, and were discouraged from nursing. Fathers were far removed from the entire birthing process and other "little" family members knew nothing about what was going on with mommy, who was suddenly away from home. In the late sixties and early seventies, high technology was the center of attention. People had temporarily been excluded—and the pendulum had swung to an extreme.

Dissatisfaction with the lack of personalism and warmth in prenatal care and delivery rose. People rightfully wanted to be a part of, not apart from, the birthing process. "Natural childbirth"—while not a new discovery—grew in popularity. Bonding became a key issue to parents and hospital personnel. Some even preached home birth, but specialists who feared potential hazards instead developed alternative birthing centers—with homelike atmospheres—in hospitals, thereby providing the best of both worlds. Today, most doctors and hospitals emphasize the value and importance of a warm, personal experience in childbirth.

This change in attitude needs to be put into some perspective. It wasn't until medical science knew more and could do more that procedures like natural childbirth were accepted as safe and even recommended.

Greater care is now taken to ensure warmth and personalism whenever possible—even when technology is vital for the safety of mother and baby. Health professionals, in general, want "giving birth" to be a very happy and beautiful experience for all. The various aspects of technology should enter the picture only when the safety or well-being of mother and child are potentially jeopardized.

With the many great strides in research and technology have come some other apprehensions—many questions and concerns about where all of this technology is leading. Technological advances and greater knowledge in medicine and science have yielded obvious good—and some bad. Questions have been raised about the rightness of "tampering with birth" and "tampering with life."

Some people feel that, even with the changes toward a more personal experience in giving birth, technology itself is imposing and has no place in the nature of birth. Others raise some very basic moral and ethical questions about the path of technological advances—those which could lead to misuse and abuse. There are concerns about genetic engineering and abortion and even fears of a plot to develop a superior race, thereby eliminating all the unique and fascinating little quirks and nuances that make every single human being special—one of a kind.

Is there a chance the Earth will be inhabited by little automatons—looking, thinking and acting alike? Only if this technology,
like other scientific advances, is not carefully scrutinized and monitored. Only if the current goals in perinatology—safer pregnancy
and identification and alleviation of both maternal and fetal problems, in order that children may lead healthier and happier lives—
are changed.

The "rightness" or "wrongness" of current fetal technology is
very much a matter of personal interpretation, morals and ethics.
For some people artificial insemination has no place in the world.
For those who could not otherwise have children, it is a welcomed
advance. For some the use of fetal monitoring infringes on the
beauty and intimacy of childbirth. But for those whose baby has
been saved because fetal monitoring alerted the doctor to fetal distress and enabled corrective measures to be taken, that technological
advance was a blessing. The issues are real, and the answers, in
many cases, can only come from the individuals involved—from
their needs, desires and personal feelings.

Regardless of your enthusiasm or skepticism about technology,
you should realize that advances in perinatal care have given new
hope to many who, in the past, had no hope. Many more mothers
and babies are doing better than ever before. Serious or fatal problems are becoming increasingly rare each year, and there is real
cause for even greater optimism in the near future.

The truth is—in many cases the mother who is diagnosed and
treated as high-risk can expect a better outcome than the mother
with no known risk factors, who stands a greater chance that problems will go unidentified and unattended. Careful, attentive management, early identification of problems and prompt intervention
are the keys to success.

TEN

A BIRD'S-EYE VIEW: ULTRASOUND

Hundreds of feet below the water's surface, the lurking submarine lies in wait for the slowly approaching battleship. Unknown to the submarine, the battleship beeps out high-frequency sound waves that travel well in water. As they reach the submarine, their "sonar" message bounces back to the battleship, is reflected into a special transducer and is then visualized as a pulsed "beep" pattern on a screen. From this message the distance, depth and size of the hiding giant are measured and calculated.

With the development of sonar, underwater vessels, mines and other types of weapons could easily be located and identified. The submarine no longer ruled the ocean and freely cruised the shores.

Because of sonar's military use, information on the technique was "classified" until after World War II. Once the war was over, researchers and scientists began utilizing the basic technology of sonar to develop highly sophisticated medical diagnostic equipment. First used for medical purposes in the 1950s, it now has broad applications in all areas of medicine, including high-risk obstetrics. It was a milestone in the development of non-invasive, highly reliable method of diagnosing fetal problems and development.

How Does Ultrasound Work?

Called "sonography," "pulse-echo sonography," "ultrasonography"—or simply, "ultrasound"—this technique is based on the principle of producing inaudible (high-frequency) cycles of sound vibrations (anywhere from 20,000 to millions of vibrations per second). These sound waves bounce off dense objects, like the unborn baby and back into a special transducer that directs them into sophisticated equipment for processing. The sound waves are converted so they can be projected onto a fluorescent screen as black-and-white images or in gray tones. Photographs and/or films can be made of these images to preserve them for later evaluation or review.

Since the speed of sound is known, the time it takes the pulsed sound waves to reach an object and bounce back into the transducer can be measured. From this information, the exact location of various structures can be calculated and "seen" on the fluorescent screen. Using physics, mathematics and biomedical instrumentation, the tissue densities, the size and shape of structures, and the distance between them can be determined.

Static Pulse-Echo Sonography

The earliest uses of ultrasound in medicine, including obstetrics, involved the technique called "static pulse-echo sonography," which allows structures to be located and their size and relationships to be measured. It does not measure or detect movement.

The "A-scan" pulse-echo allows us to look at a one-dimensional echo and measure distances. A "B-scan" records a two-dimensional cross section of the uterus and its contents—it allows us to look down into the lower abdomen and visualize its contents. One or both of these scans can be used to assess fetal growth (by measuring head size), the amount of amniotic fluid, multiple fetuses, the location of the placenta and abnormalities of the uterus.

Real-Time Ultrasonography

Real-time ultrasonography is a much more sophisticated, newer technique that shows movement. It uses a special transducer that sends out multiple sound waves in a specific sequence. When these serial transmissions are received back in the transducer, decoded, projected and constantly updated, they allow the monitoring of fetal movement and of many fetal structures.

This highly technical tool allows us to see the fetus move within the womb; watch the heart beat and even evaluate the function of the heart valves; determine fetal breathing movements, position and posture—or simply watch the fetus suck his or her thumb! Able to detect structures as small as two millimeters, this type of ultrasound equipment is so sophisticated it can visualize and count the pulsations in the umbilical vessels.

Will I Need Ultrasound?

Ultrasound, whether static or real-time, greatly helps our ability to evaluate fetal growth and well-being and is recommended for a variety of reasons. While it is not recommended in all pregnancies, whether high-risk or not, its use is becoming more and more prevalent. Each technique has its advantages and limitations. If recommended by your doctor, the type of procedure to be used will depend upon the kind of information needed, your stage in pregnancy, and the technical expertise and experience of those in the center in which you will have the study.

Monitoring Fetal Growth

One of the earliest uses for ultrasound in obstetrics was the determination of fetal head size. This remains its most common use. In fact, in some populations of women the use of ultrasound for this purposes is as high as 25 percent. While it is possible to locate the embryonal sac early as 6 weeks into the pregnancy and "see" the fetal head as early as 12 or 13 weeks, assessing fetal growth becomes practical and important in the middle trimester of pregnancy.

Normal growth has been well studied, and the general growth pattern and sizes at various stages of gestation are well-known. Fetuses grow at a very predictable rate early in pregnancy but with some degree of variation being normal later on. Additionally, most problems that cause deviation from normal fetal growth begin to show their effects during late pregnancy (the last trimester). These factors make ultrasound a useful tool in assessing fetal growth beginning around the 14th week of pregnancy, until approximately the 26th week.

During your pregnancy, your doctor will compare what he or she expects the size of your uterus to be based on your calculated dates with the actual growth that has taken place. If the size or growth pattern is unusual—either too large or too small—he or she might suggest ultrasound. Although this type of information can be obtained from either real-time or static-echo ultrasound, the static diagnostic technique is the one routinely used to evaluate fetal head size.

In assessing fetal growth, the most common measurement taken is of the size of the fetus's head. The biparietal diameter (the distance between the two sides of the skull) is compared to known standards of fetal growth. Additional information is obtained by comparing head size to chest and body size, as well.

If the size of the fetus's head correlates with your calculated dates before 28 weeks gestation, your doctor (and you) can feel comfortable that your expected delivery date is reasonably accurate. (Remember, a variation of two weeks or so is common and normal. The estimated delivery date is just that—an estimate—because of differences in fetal growth and development in later pregnancy.)

If on the other hand, the fetus is larger or smaller than expected, a second ultrasound scan may be done several weeks later to allow the doctor to compare the two measurements to evaluate any fetal growth deviations and to improve the accuracy of the original prediction of gestational age of the fetus.

Many doctors request ultrasound scanning before the 26th week as a routine in indentified high-risk pregnancies, especially if the risk factor(s) is likely to alter fetal growth or lead to possible early delivery. This allows greater certainty about the gestational age of the fetus.

Using ultrasound to measure fetal growth during the *last* trimester of pregnancy is not accurate by itself in dating the fetus. Factors associated with increased growth (for example, maternal diabetes, obesity and familial or personal tendency to have large babies) as well as those causing decreased growth (like maternal smoking, placental insufficiency and many other high-risk factors) have their greatest impact late in pregnancy. Comparison of an earlier scan with a late one can, however, help to assess the growth of the older fetus.

When ultrasound was first introduced to obstetrics, it was hoped it would allow doctors to determine if a baby was at term (mature and ready for delivery) and help with decisions about delivery—especially the timing of cesarean section, if deemed necessary, or induction of labor. While it was obvious most babies *were* "at term" if their heads were a certain size (as long as infants of diabetic mothers were excluded), a significant number still had immature lungs. In fact, as many as 15 percent of babies throught to be at term by estimated dates plus ultrasound late in pregnancy still had problems (usually respiratory) because of early delivery. As will be discussed in Chapter 11, it became clear that a combination of diagnostic ultrasound and a way to assure fetal lung maturity would be most beneficial in reducing fetal problems.

Assessing Unusual Uterine Size

Other factors besides fetal growth affect the size of the uterus during pregnancy. Many of these can be identified by ultrasound, often eliminating the need for other studies that might be more invasive and/or potentially more risky.

Ultrasound can identify abnormalities of the uterus itself—fibroids, cysts, unusual shapes—as well as identify a very rare condition—called "hydatidiform mole"—that is associated with very early pregnancy. (A hydatiduform mole is technically considered a tumor of the the placental cells—trophoblasts—and is derived as a product of conception. It often causes toxemia, rapid uterine growth, vaginal bleeding and inevitably aborts. It is usually a non-malignant process, but on occasion it may invade the mother's tissues and become malignant.) Some uterine problems may affect fetal development later, because of crowding, for example, and may present difficulties at the time of delivery.

Multiple gestations—twins, triplets or more—can be detected by ultrasound performed early in the middle trimester, often long before the doctor or mother is aware of the existence of more than one baby. In this case the uterus grows larger than with a single fetus. Larger uterine growth occurs in part because of the babies—but also because there is simply more amniotic fluid.

The amount of amniotic fluid produced during normal pregnancy is quite stable and contributes to normal uterine growth. Too much fluid ("polyhydramnios") or too little fluid ("oligohydramnios") may be associated with fetal and maternal problems. (For example, polyhydramnios is present in as many as 40 percent of pregnancies of diabetic mothers.) The amount of amniotic fluid can be determined during an ultrasound examination, and some fetal deformities that may be associated with polyhydramnios may also be detected by ultrasound.

Ultrasound and the Placenta

The placenta can be visualized very early in pregnancy. Determining placental size and location later in pregnancy is an important use of ultrasound. Placental position is vital in several situations.

"Placenta previa"—a condition in which the placenta is located low in the uterus, extending completely or partially over the cervix—can be associated with abnormal bleeding early in pregnancy and with serious bleeding and potential disaster during labor and delivery. While about 20 percent of women appear to have placenta previa as shown by ultrasound examination at 20 weeks, fewer have this condition persist throughout pregnancy. Those who do, however, require cesarean delivery for the safety of both themselves and their babies. Knowing the location of the placenta is also important to ensure greater safety in performing other diagnostic tests, such as amniocentesis and/or fetoscopy and placental aspiration. Ultrasound is used as a compliment to these procedures.

Unusual size of the placenta—too large or too small—can be associated with fetal problems or with maternal conditions that put mother or baby or both at high risk. For example, a small placenta can be associated with fetal growth retardation and may be caused by such problems as maternal hypertension.

Ultrasound before Amniocentesis and/or Fetoscopy

Since its introduction to obstetrics, ultrasound has played an increasingly important role in helping reduce the risk associated with diagnostic amniocentesis. By helping medical personnel locate the placenta, the umbilical cord and the various parts of the fetus, the best site for inserting the amniocentesis needle or fetoscope can be determined. Either static pulse-echo (non-motion) or real-time echo (motion) can be used. The ultrasound scan is done immediately before the other diagnostic procedures.

Detection and Diagnosis of Fetal Abnormalities

As experience increases and technology improves, it is increasingly possible to diagnose fetal malformations prior to birth with real-time ultrasound. While it is not yet possible to identify many malformations, ultrasonic techniques have identified certain obvious abnormalities in fetuses.

Occasionally such an abnormality is found unexpectedly at the time ultrasound is being done for another reason. When polyhydramnios or oligohydramnios is present, fetal deformity may be among the causes. For example, ultrasound studies may detect blockages of the fetal intestine as a cause for polyhydramnios. In some situations medical intervention is necessary.

One of the most common uses for ultrasound in detecting fetal abnormalities relates to defects of the central nervous system—so-called neural tube defects. Such conditions as spina bifida (open spine) or anencephaly (a serious defect in which there is little brain development) can be associated with abnormally high levels of a substance called alpha-fetoprotein (AFP) in the mother's blood and/or amniotic fluid. Ultrasound may detect some of these defects if used in conjunction with alpha-fetoprotein determinations in pregnancies at risk for neural tube defects. (There will be more information about alpha-fetoprotein in Chapter 11.)

Quite a few fetal abnormalities have been detected by ultrasound, and further study continues. However, ultrasound's use in the identification of most fetal deformities is still limited almost exclusively to major perinatal centers.

The Ultrasound Procedure

If your physician recommends a diagnostic ultrasound test for you, the procedure would be somewhat as follows.

You will be asked to drink four to six glasses of water before the test begins and will need to "hold" a full bladder throughout the procedure. The water distends the bladder so other organs can be seen easily and is used as a marker. This is a little uncomfortable for most women, but it is the only discomfort of the entire ultrasound procedure.

Once your bladder is sufficiently full, you will be asked to lie flat on your back on an examination table. Your abdomen will be "greased" with an oil that allows the ultrasound transducer to slide easily over your skin and helps with the conduction of the sound waves.

The transducer, which looks very much like a broadcast microphone, is attached to the ultrasound machine by means of a long, somewhat flexible arm. The technician (or physician in some centers) will place the transducer on your abdomen and, using slight pressure, crisscross the abdominal surface in a gridlike pattern— back and forth, back and forth, up and down, up and down— sliding across the oil. You may be able to watch the picture being produced.

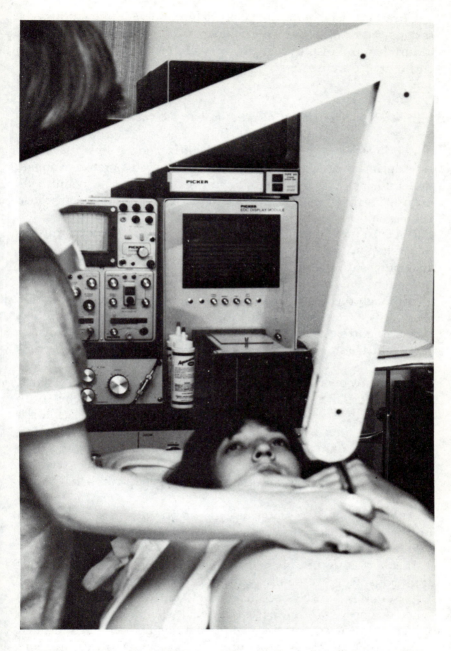

ULSTRASOUND: The technician slides the ultrasound transducer (similar to a broadcast microphone) across the mother's abdomen in a grid-like pattern. The information is relayed through the transducer, up the movable arm and into the sophisticated equipment visible in the background.

Ultrasound itself is a painless procedure. Some women, however, say it's rather difficult not to empty the bladder during the procedure because of the feeling of pressure on the full bladder. The entire procedure is usually completed in less than 30 minutes.

The Safety of Obstetrical Diagnostic Ultrasound

A non-invasive procedure, diagnostic ultrasound seems reasonably safe during pregnancy. However, research in laboratory animals (not humans) has shown that high-energy waves and continuous exposure can produce heat—a thermal effect—which can cause cellular and tissue damage or destruction.

It seems, then, that the safety of diagnostic ultrasound is probably dependent upon the intensity, frequency and duration of exposure. Like other rather new procedures, it may have risks that are as yet unknown, and its risk-benefit ratio must be considered.

Although there is still some question about what possible subtle long-term effects the low energy diagnostic levels of ultrasound waves might have on the fetus or the mother, there are presently no conclusive studies showing that the diagnostic levels cause problems.

One study worth noting was done by NICHD (the National Institute of Child Health and Human Development). The study followed 1,952 pregnancies and continued to follow the children for one year after birth. The results showed that, of the 303 pregnancies where ultrasonography was used as an adjunct procedure to amniocentesis, there were no increased developmental or physical differences in the children of the exposed group compared to the control group.

Although long-term studies are now in progress, it appears, based on short-term data, that the use of diagnostic ultrasonography is safe during pregnancy.

In addition to the apparent lack of risk, there seem to be significant advantages to the use of diagnostic ultrasound in pregnancy. Ultrasound is an excellent alternative to radiation exposure (X ray) when diagnostic work is necessary. And when used in conjunction with amniocentesis, fetoscopy or placental aspiration, it has resulted in safer procedures, since locating the placenta and the fetus and its various anatomic structures is possible.

It appears, then, that ultrasound is a very valuable diagnostic tool. It also appears to be quite safe, especially in light of presently available information and other alternatives.

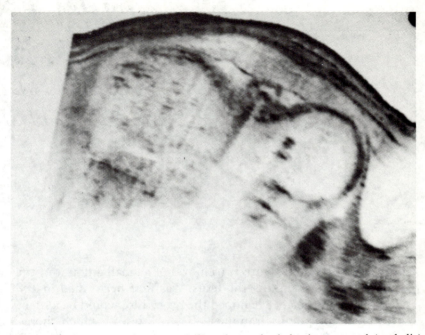

ULTRASOUND: The ultrasound film shows the baby in a normal (cephalic) presentation—head down into the pelvis.

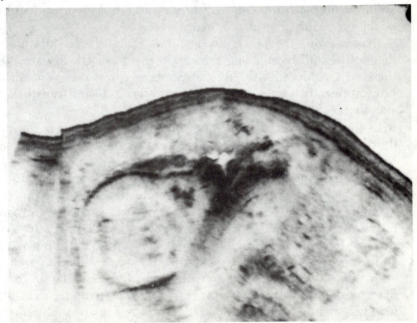

ULTRASOUND: In this ultrasound film we can see that the baby is in a breech presentation (buttocks first into the pelvis).

ELEVEN

DIAGNOSING THE UNBORN BABY: AMNIOCENTESIS

Surprisingly, amniocentesis (removal of a small amount of the amniotic fluid surrounding the fetus) was first performed in 1882 by a German physician. He hoped the procedure would be a successful treatment for polyhydramnios—a condition in which there is an abnormally large amount of amniotic fluid. It was probably believed that polyhydramnios was the cause rather than the result of fetal and/or maternal problems. Little was accomplished, and the use of the procedure was abandoned.

In the 1950s the procedure again came into use, this time for diagnosing and monitoring fetuses at risk from Rh disease. Over the next two decades the diagnostic techniques were refined, and intrauterine treatment—through intrauterine blood transfusion—was successfully begun.

In the 1960s further progress in the ability to analyze amniotic fluid, coupled with new methods of growing fetal cells in the laboratory, led to a unique and exciting use for the procedure. The first intrauterine diagnosis of a chromosomal abnormality was accomplished in 1967, and one year later the detection of an inherited metabolic disorder prior to birth was reported. Since then, progress in intrauterine diagnosis has been rapid and substantial. It is now possible to diagnose virtually all known chromosomal abnormalities and many inherited biochemical (metabolic) disorders, as well.

In the 1970s advances in knowledge made it possible to use amniocentesis to determine fetal maturity. A better understanding of fetal lung maturity and the cause of respiratory distress in premature infants has resulted in the refinement of tests of fetal maturity.

What Is Amniocentesis?

It is important to remember that amniocentesis is a procedure. It is the vehicle—the tool—used to obtain a sample of the amniotic fluid for fetal diagnosis. Derived from Greek, the word comes from "amnion," meaning caul (referring to fetal membranes) and "kentesis," meaning puncture. In other words, puncturing the fetal membranes—the amniotic sac. The procedure involves withdrawing a small amount of amniotic fluid from the uterus by inserting a needle through the woman's abdomen into the amniotic sac. The fluid obtained can be analyzed in many ways.

Interestingly, the amniotic fluid was once believed to be simply a stagnant pool of fluid surrounding the fetus. Actually, the fluid is rich in chemicals that are the source of much valuable information about the fetus and its well-being. Fetal cells found in the fluid can be studied in detail.

Amniotic fluid is produced throughout pregnancy, and its composition changes somewhat as pregnancy progresses. The fluid is initially produced by the placenta, but the fetus as it matures contributes to the fluid, as well (cells from the fetus's developing surface, urine produced by its tiny kidneys and fetal lung products). Since amniotic fluid is in part derived from the fetus, doctors and scientists can learn a great deal about the fetus from careful analysis of the fluid and its cells.

The Amniocentesis Procedure

Ultrasound is performed just before the amniocentesis procedure, in order to visualize the exact position of the placenta, the fetus and the umbilical cord. This makes amniocentesis safer and the procedure more efficient.

As soon as the ultrasound examination has been completed, and with the patient remaining unmoved, the amniocentesis begins. The abdomen is carefully washed with an antiseptic (often red or brown in color). Based on the information received from the ultrasound, the place where the needle will be inserted is determined and is marked on the abdomen, often with the blunt end of a cotton applicator or with a marker-type pen. Surgical drapes are placed across the legs and upper abdomen, leaving only the working surface exposed.

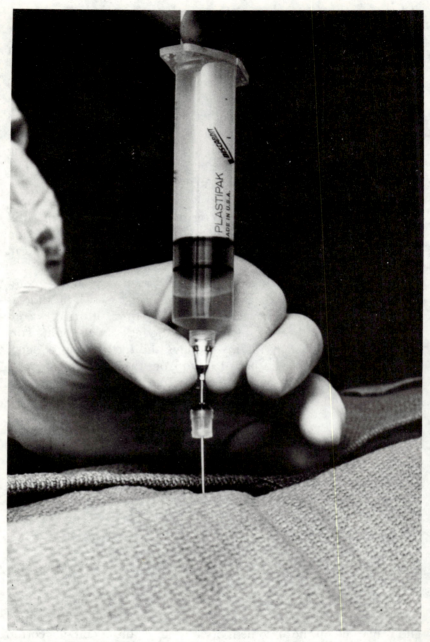

AMNIOCENTESIS: Amniotic fluid is withdrawn from the amniotic sac. The thin, hollow needle is placed through the mother's abdomen and into the amniotic sac after ultrasound determines the fetal position. Most women say that amniocentesis causes minimal to no discomfort or pain.

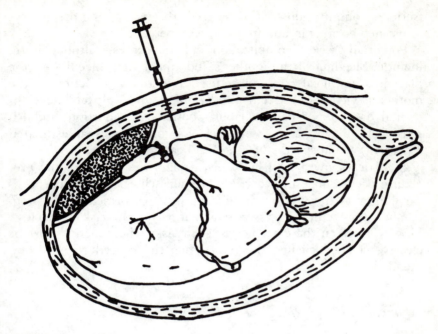

AMNIOCENTESIS: The drawing shows one of many possible needle placements for performing amniocentesis. The needle placement is determined by the fetal position (which is identified by ultrasound).

A special hollow needle is then carefully inserted through the abdomen and into the amniotic sac. Between 5 and 40 milliliters of the amniotic fluid are drawn through the needle into a syringe. The needle is removed, and a small sterile bandage is placed over the insertion point.

The entire procedure usually takes less than an hour, from the start of the ultrasound until the needle is removed after the fluid sample has been obtained. The actual duration of the amniocentesis itself if a matter of only a few minutes.

Risks of Amniocentesis

Amniocentesis appears to be relatively safe. A report prepared by the U.S. Department of Health, Education and Welfare (now the Department of Health and Human Services), Public Health Service and the National Institutes of Health, after compiling current data from the United States and Canada, stated that "when all significant (serious) complications are considered, the risks to the pregnancy, fetus, newborn or infant are below 0.5 percent."

Potentially serious complications of amniocentesis, although rare, include: bleeding of the mother's abdominal wall; bleeding of the placenta, umbilical cord, or fetus if punctured; infection of the mother as well as of the fetus (in the uterus); possible fetal developmental damage; premature labor; spontaneous abortion; and Rh sensitization. Only a small number of amniocenteses (an estimated 2 percent) are unsuccessful—no fluid can be obtained.

Statistics show a fetal loss (miscarriage) as a result of the procedure occurs once in every 200 women who have amniocentesis early in pregnancy. When amniocentesis is performed late in pregnancy—for example, to assess fetal maturity—this risk is even less. However, given the existence of such risks, the benefits must be clearly weighed against the risks when the procedure is recommended.

Amniocentesis and Rh Disease

Today, a blood test for Rh antibodies can easily determine Rh sensitization of a mother and is done routinely during the pregnancy of an Rh-negative woman. When the mother's Rh antibodies appear during pregnancy, indicating the fetus is at risk for problems, amniocentesis is usually recommended. Analyzing the amniotic fluid, (first around the 22nd to 25th week of pregnancy, then repeated at one- to three-week intervals), allows the doctor to assess the fetus's well-being as the disease progresses.

With serious Rh disease, the fetus's blood is rapidly destroyed. When this occurs, blood products are found in the amniotic fluid. With amniocentesis the amniotic fluid is withdrawn and these chemicals analyzed. The chemical levels are used as an indicator of how at-risk the fetus is for problems.

With moderate Rh disease, early delivery of the fetus may be necessary. When this is possible, examination of the amniotic fluid for indications of fetal lung maturity is an aid in optimal timing of the delivery. Maturity is routinely assessed when amniocentesis is done for Rh disease in the last six to eight weeks of pregnancy.

Amniocentesis and Fetal Lung Maturity

During the 1950s and 1960s when amniocentesis was used for monitoring Rh disease, researchers were studying amniotic fluid for clues to fetal lung maturity. A breakthrough in this area would lead to increasing certainty about the safest time to deliver a very sick infant—early enough to prevent death from Rh disease, but late enough for the fetus to survive outside the womb.

The earliest tests of fetal maturity using amniotic fluid analysis were not precise. The principle was based on the observation that the types and numbers of fetal cells in the fluid change during pregnancy. While not exact, analysis of these cells offered some clues to fetal maturity. Similarly, it was found that the measurement of various chemicals in the amniotic fluid could be useful. For example, the amount of creatinine (a chemical waste product of muscle breakdown excreted in fetal urine) is increased in the amniotic fluid in late pregnancy due to increased fetal muscle mass and fetal kidney maturation. The levels of creatinine can be measured, and this information can be used as a rough predictor of fetal maturity.

Although the earlier information was important, the greatest breakthrough came in the late 1960s. It was discovered that respiratory distress syndrome (also called "hyaline membrane disease"), the greatest risk for premature infants, was due to a deficiency of a lung substance called "surfactant." Surfactant develops in the last part of gestation, and its levels are directly correlated with the risk for respiratory distress syndrome.

Based on the knowledge that fetal lung fluid makes up part of the amniotic fluid in the last trimester of pregnancy, Dr. Louis Gluck and others began searching—successfully—for a chemical test of the amniotic fluid that would indicate the presence of surfactant. From this research emerged what is called the "L/S ratio"—the lecithin/sphingomyelin ratio—as a predictor of fetal maturity.

The L/S ratio—the relationship between the amounts of these two fatlike compounds in the amniotic fluid—rises in late pregnancy. Its rise is associated with a diminishing risk of lung immaturity and respiratory distress syndrome. When this ratio is over two (by special measurements), fetal lung maturity is almost certain. Although rare, problems may occur in infants of diabetic mothers, even with high L/S ratios.

A test developed relatively recently is also a possibility in determining fetal lung maturity. A chemical called "phosphatidyl glycerol" may prove to be an even better indicator of lung maturity and is also found in the amniotic fluid. This analysis appears to accurately predict lung maturity, even in diabetic mothers. Phosphatidyl glycerol levels can be determined in some laboratories today.

Amniocentesis for Diagnosis of Fetal Defects

By far the most common reason to perform amniocentesis is for the diagnosis of possible hereditary or chromosomal abnormalities. In fact, it is estimated that 85 percent of amniocenteses are performed to evaluate chromosomal abnormalities, and three-fourths of these are done in women 35 years of age or older.

Of the more than 3 million births each year in the United States alone, 3 percent to 5 percent of babies will have serious congenital malformation, chromosomal abnormality or another genetic disorder. Additionally, at least one-fifth of infant deaths in the United States are due to congenital defects and hereditary disease. Diagnosis of many of these problems is now possible, in large part because of advances in analyzing the fetus's amniotic fluid.

While "genetic" amniocentesis—performed to detect fetal abnormalities—is usually done because a woman or a couple has a known increased risk for a problem, it is reassuring to know that 99 percent of the time no abnormality is found. That means the majority of fetuses are free of a chromosomal defect or presently detectable hereditary metabolic congenital defect. Although this does not guarantee fetal health or the absence of other congenital anomalies or developmental defects not detectable by amniocentesis, it can tell us some of the abnormalities the fetus *does not* have.

In those situations where the results of testing identify a seriously abnormal fetus, many parents face a difficult and delicate decision. Some may choose to terminate the pregnancy. Often, however, parents simply wish to know if a defect is present, so they can better prepare for the care of their child. In the vast majority of cases, amniocentesis reassures prospective parents who feared that a possible chromosomal or genetic abnormality would be inherited by their child because of increased risk that no such problem is present. In fact, reassuring parents may well be the greatest contribution of amniocentesis.

Amniocentesis for fetal diagnosis is ideally done between the 16th and 18th weeks of pregnancy. At this time the procedure is relatively safe, and enough fluid can be withdrawn for diagnosis. Since several weeks may be required to complete the analysis of the fluid, this allows enough time for results to be obtained, so decisions, if any, can be made about the pregnancy.

Amniotic fluid obtained by amniocentesis can be analyzed in several ways. The cells that originate from the fetus's developing skin covering can first be grown—"cultured"—then analyzed to determine their chromosomal makeup. The chemical content of these cells can also be determined, so abnormal chemicals can be detected. Additionally, the fluid itself can be analyzed for abnormal products that result from metabolic defects.

Alpha-fetoprotein Levels

Abnormally high levels of a fetal blood substance called alpha-fetoprotein (AFP) in the amniotic fluid are associated with several serious congenital abnormalities called "neural tube defects." Measurement of amniotic fluid AFP is a very useful diagnostic test in pregnancies where the risk for these nervous system defects (anencephaly, spina bifida, encephalocele) is high.

While its function is not known, alpha-fetoprotein is produced by the fetus in very large amounts during the first 12 weeks of pregnancy and is found in very high concentrations in both amniotic fluid and in the mother's blood. The ideal time to look for abnormally high levels of alpha-fetoprotein is at about 15 to 17 weeks of pregnancy. Accurate estimation of the fetus's gestational age is extremely important in interpreting the laboratory information.

While neural tube defects account for the largest number of fetal abnormalities seen, there are other causes for abnormally high AFP levels in the amniotic fluid. Other less common causes include: fetal death or threatened spontaneous abortion, congenital nephrosis (a hereditary type of kidney disorder), omphalocele (a rare birth defect in which the contents of the abdomen protrude out of the umbilical cord), failure of the upper part of the intestine to develop (esophageal and duodenal atresia) and, rarely, hydrocephaly ("water on the brain"). Rh disease causes high AFP levels in the *last* trimester but not usually in the second trimester. Fetal death and anencephaly are usually the causes when extremely high levels of AFP are found.

It may be advantageous to measure the level of AFP in the blood of all pregnant women as a screening device for neural tube defects and other problems. This possibility is now being studied. While this technique looks promising and would be more practical than amniocentesis as a screening mechanism for larger numbers of pregnancies, it is presently not available in many areas.

Elevated maternal blood AFP requires further investigation and is more likely to be false-positive than amniotic fluid AFP. In any case, elevated levels must be interpreted with caution at this time. Serum (blood) AFP determinations will only detect 80 percent of fetuses with neural tube defects, so while it is appropriate for screening a low-risk population, it is not adequate for a high-risk group, where amniocentesis is indicated.

When Amniocentesis Should Be Considered

Amniocentesis is not recommended or necessary in all pregnancies. The fact is, it is not even recommended for all high-risk pregnancies. Its use depends on the reason the woman is considered high-risk.

Amniocentesis may be recommended if:

- Rh incompatibility has been determined, and the fetus must be assessed, so intervention can take place if he or she is in jeopardy.
- Fetal lung maturity needs to be determined because early delivery must be or is being considered.

Amniocentesis for fetal diagnosis of possible chromosomal or metabolic defects should be considered if:

- You are 35 years of age or older.
- You already have a child with Down's Syndrome, or another person in your or your partner's family has Down's Syndrome.
- You have already had a child with multiple congenital anomalies of unknown cause.
- You have already had a child with a chromosomal abnormality.
- You have experienced multiple spontaneous abortions.
- There is a sex-linked disorder in your or your partner's family.
- There is a possibility of Tay-Sachs disease (Ashkenazi Jews), sickle cell disease (American blacks) or beta thalassemia (those of Mediterranean extraction).

Amniocentesis to measure alpha-fetoprotein levels may be recommended in the following situations:

- Whenever amniocentesis is being done for another purpose.
- If either you or your partner has had a previous child with a neural tube defect.
- When there is congenital nephrosis in either your or your partner's family.
- If there is elevated maternal blood AFP on two occasions, and an ultrasound has not made a definitive diagnosis.
- Occasionally, when you or your partner have had a previous child with hydrocephaly.

Diagnostic Accuracy of Amniotic Fluid Analysis

While accuracy varies to some extent depending on the type of analysis performed, amniotic fluid studies are extremely accurate. The usefulness and accuracy of amniotic fluid analysis and monitoring in Rh disease is well established and is the key to successful treatment of the affected fetus.

Similarly, estimations of fetal lung maturity by determination of the L/S ratio are accurate in most pregnancies. The added ability to measure phosphatidyl glycerol may make this examination even more reliable.

With genetic amniocentesis—that done to detect fetal abnormalities—cultures of fetal cells can be achieved successfully in 98 percent of procedures. Statistics show that diagnostic accuracy for chromosomal abnormalities exceeds 99.5 percent when the work is performed in a major center with obstetrical experience as well as in-depth diagnostic laboratory experience and expertise. Additionally, detection of other genetic disease by amniocentesis is increasingly reliable and accurate.

Amniotic fluid AFP (alpha-fetoprotein) measurement appears to be effective in identifying at least 90 percent of the major neural tube defects, and the certainty of diagnosis is increased if ultrasound is used to further investigate abnormal results.

What's the Bottom Line?

While not recommended or indicated in all high-risk pregnancies, the procedure can be tremendously reassuring to the majority of those at risk for specific hereditary or chromosomal problems. It is also rather reassuring when it determines sufficient fetal lung maturity in situations where the infant is at risk unless delivery is accomplished as soon as possible.

Anyone considering amniocentesis for the detection of chromosomal abnormalities should undergo genetic counseling first and weigh the risks and potential benefits of the procedure. Anytime amniocentesis is recommended, no matter what the reason, you should have a discussion with your doctor about the risk-benefit ratio.

TWELVE

IDENTIFYING PROBLEMS EARLY: FETAL MONITORING

Like takeoff and landing in an airplane, labor and delivery are considered the most potentially dangerous and stressful times of a pregnancy for both mother and baby. In fact, without modern detection of problems and appropriate intervention, you would have a greater risk of dying on the day of your birth than you would for the next 40 years of your life. Although many risks to the unborn child can be identified before labor, four out of five problems that threaten the fetus's life arise unexpectedly during labor and delivery.

Considering this, doctors needed and wanted to find a safe and efficient means of evaluating the fetus at risk for problems during labor, so they could take appropriate action when necessary.

"Electronic fetal heart rate monitoring" (usually called simply "fetal monitoring") was developed as a means of evaluating the child during labor in hopes of recognizing fetal distress. (Essentially, the procedure assesses the baby's heart rate pattern as it responds to uterine contractions and the stresses of labor.) If fetal distress could be recognized early, then steps could be taken to avoid death or damage.

Early recognition of problems, new management techniques and sophisticated intervention have been the key to saving lives, ensuring better outcomes for others and increasing the quality of life for many newborns. Because of this, most (if not all) high-risk pregnancies will have fetal monitoring recommended during labor and delivery.

It wasn't until 1818 that a Swiss surgeon (Francois Mayor) noted that he could hear fetal heart sounds by placing his ear on the abdomen of a pregnant patient. In 1848 a noted physician made the proposal that the fetal heart rate might be useful in diagnosing fetal distress so intervention could take place. The fetoscope (a stethoscope that attaches to the doctor's head) was developed in 1917, allowing the physician to listen to the fetal heartbeat.

Yet it is not easy to identify subtle changes in the baby's heart rate just by listening through a fetoscope. Because muscle contractions of the uterus muffle the heartbeat, constant listening would be required to detect all the changes displayed by an electronic monitor. Additionally, the human ear is not able to detect subtle changes in rate very well or identify mild irregularities in rhythm.

While working at Yale University School of Medicine, Dr. Edward Hon was the first to report on fetal heart rate monitoring using an EKG monitor attached to a woman's abdomen. Although the technology utilized was primitive in comparison to that available today, Dr. Hon and others were able to compile data showing that certain heart rate patterns, variances and increases/decreases in rates were associated with fetal distress.

This work was a milestone in obstetrical care. As methods became increasingly refined, with better and more precise equipment available, more information could be gathered. Dr. Hon, again a forerunner in the field, introduced a special electrode that could be attached to the presenting part of the fetus (usually the scalp). This allowed for direct and much more precise information gathering. From there, more advances have been made in hardware, knowledge and interpretation of data. Presently, fetal heart rate monitoring is the best means available to evaluate the baby at risk during labor.

What Is Fetal Distress?

In order to appreciate the reasons for fetal monitoring, it is first necessary to better understand fetal distress. What the doctor or nurse needs to know during labor is if the fetus is receiving an adequate oxygen supply. If it is not, the fetus will experience distress. The purpose of fetal monitoring, then, is to identify the fetus who is experiencing hypoxia (inadequate oxygenation.)

When the fetus's oxygen supply is reduced—for any reason—there are changes in its bodily functions. These changes are interpreted as fetal distress. The heart rate changes—in several possible ways—in an attempt to deliver more oxygen to the tissues. As the oxygen supply gets lower and lower, the tissues show more and more of the adverse effect. Acid builds up, and the body cells don't function well. If the oxygen supply is not improved, permanent damage to the child can occur.

Prolonged or severe fetal hypoxia can potentially lead to mental retardation, cerebral palsy and other neurologic damage; and fetal acidosis (due to hypoxia) can result in kidney, lung, gastrointestinal, central nervous system and other damage. Ultimately, severe and prolonged hypoxia will lead to death.

The Task Force on Predictors of Fetal Distress (NICHD Consensus Development Conference on Antenatal Diagnosis) noted that "currently available data suggests that approximately 30 percent of stillbirths and early neonatal deaths are attributable to intrapartum events." ("Intrapartum" is the medical term for the time of labor and delivery.) The same report also pointed out that "approximately 20–40 percent of cerebral palsy, and 10 percent of severe mental retardation are currently attributable to intrapartum factors."

The placenta, a unique structure that develops on the uterine wall and is attached to the embryo/fetus by the umbilical cord, plays a major role in fetal well-being. This organ provides oxygen (and nutrients) to the fetus, acts as a heat-exchange mechanism and is a protective barrier against various harmful substances. It also eliminates waste products and produces estrogen, progesterone and protein hormones. During labor, however, the fetal oxygen supply is the most critical placental function and for this reason electronic fetal heart rate monitoring is used to detect mild hypoxia and to prevent potentially damaging severe hypoxia.

Uterine arteries and other smaller blood vessels supply enriched blood to the placenta. If these arteries are somehow occluded (compressed or blocked), blood flow to the placenta is either lessened or cut off. If the placenta itself is not functioning properly (for a variety of reasons), again blood flow is reduced or stopped.

There can be many reasons for decreased uterine blood flow and therefore decreased oxygenation of the fetus: excessive thickness of the placental membrane, reduced surface area of the placenta, placental abruption (separation of the placenta before delivery), placenta previa (placenta that is attached over the cervix), umbilical cord occlusion, prolapsed umbilical cord (cord that slips out of the uterus before the baby is delivered), hypertension, uterine rupture, some drugs and anesthetics, vigorous exercise (which shunts blood away from the uterus to the muscles) and uterine contractions. Some of these causes of reduced blood flow to or from the placenta are reversible, while others are not.

Other problems that can lead to fetal distress (inadequate oxygenation of the fetus) are: difficult or prolonged labor, prematurity, multiple fetuses, toxemia, pre-existing inadequate fetal growth, premature rupture of the membranes, congenital abnormalities and abnormal position and presentation of the fetus.

The Principles behind Fetal Monitoring

As noted previously, fetal distress can result from a variety of factors. When the uterus contracts during labor, blood flow to the placenta, and therefore to the fetus, is momentarily decreased. It's somewhat like forcing the baby to hold his or her breath—for as long as 60 seconds. A healthy fetus with a healthy placenta usually has no problem with this stress and suffers no apparent ill effects from the labor. Although the infant's heart may slow during the contraction, it quickly resumes its normal steady rate as the contraction subsides.

In some situations (and for the many reasons already mentioned), the child cannot tolerate the stress of labor. In particular, if the placenta's functioning has been only marginal at the end of pregnancy (called "placental insufficiency"), or if the fetus is receiving less than optimal oxygenation, he or she may not recover as well from the uterine contractions. The result is a change in the fetal heart rate, characterized by slowing that is delayed until the contraction has peaked and lasts after the end of the contraction.

These changes may be subtle. There may be a variation in rate or pattern, or there may be a time delay before the heart rate pattern returns to normal after a contraction. Certain patterns, rates and variations have been associated (through clinical study and observation) with fetal distress or certain specific problems. For example, pressure on the umbilical cord (umbilical cord occlusion) produces a particular heart pattern that can be recognized easily (and the problem eliminated by simply repositioning the mother, in most cases).

There is solid evidence that fetal heart rate monitoring can reflect fetal distress—that is, fetal hypoxia. Because of this association of fetal heart rate patterns and physiological changes in the fetus, it is estimated that about 60 percent to 70 percent of pregnant women in the United States are monitored during labor.

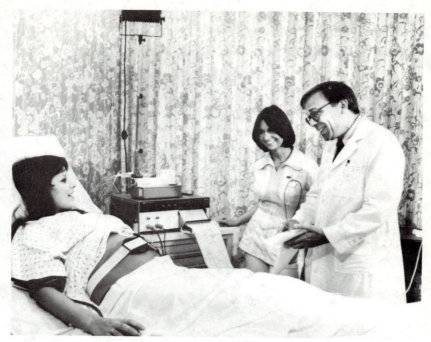

EXTERNAL ELECTRONIC FETAL HEART RATE MONITORING: Dr. Roger Freeman talks to a woman in labor as her contractions and her baby's responses to those contractions are monitored. The belts around her abdomen relay the information to the equipment in the background, which records the information on graph paper as two line tracings (seen coming out of the monitoring machine).

Two Types of Electronic Fetal Monitoring

"External fetal monitoring" is a method in which continuous information is gathered through two lightweight belts loosely placed around the woman's abdomen during labor. One of the belts contains an ultrasonic transducer (a Doppler), which detects the fetal heartbeat. This device works like sonar, detecting fetal heart movement through the use of sound waves. The other belt contains a tokodynamometer, which records each uterine contraction. Information from each of these belts is transmitted to a specially designed electronic fetal monitoring machine, which converts it into a series of line graphs and records the information on a strip of paper.

A non-invasive technique, external fetal monitoring has advantages and disadvantages. For one, the frequency of contractions is fairly accurately recorded through external fetal monitoring, but

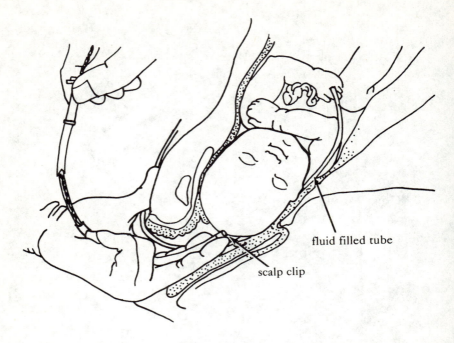

fluid filled tube

scalp clip

INTERNAL ELECTRONIC FETAL HEART RATE MONITORING: The physician is shown carefully attaching the scalp clip to the baby so that his or her heart rate and pattern can be more precisely monitored. The fluid-filled tube which measures the intensity and the length of uterine contractions is seen extending under the baby's head and over the right arm to the left hand. Reproduced with permission from Freeman, Roger K., M.D., and Garite, Thomas J., M.D. Fetal Heart Rate Monitoring, Baltimore: Williams & Wilkins, 1981.

recording of the duration and intensity of contractions is much less accurate than with "internal fetal monitoring" (discussed below). Since the position of the patient and that of the belts has a great deal to do with the accuracy of the recording, external fetal monitoring is less comfortable for the patient, since her movement has to be more restricted to maintain a good tracing.

In many situations, external monitoring is adequate. However, because it is an indirect technique—that is, nothing is directly attached to the fetus or uterus—the information will be less precise. In some pregnancies (particularly some high-risk pregnancies) where more accurate information is needed for serious decision making, the second method of fetal monitoring—internal fetal monitoring—may be recommended.

Internal fetal monitoring works on exactly the same principles as external monitoring but provides a much more accurate record of the baby's response to the stresses of labor. The procedure requires that the membranes be ruptured (the water broken), either naturally or artificially. In this procedure a very thin, fluid-filled plastic tube is inserted through the vagina into the uterine cavity alongside the fetus. This tube detects changes in pressure inside the uterus with each contraction. The pressure changes are transmitted through the fluid in the tube and recorded on a strip of paper as a line graph, just as the external belt did. However, this method produces a much more reliable and accurate record of uterine contraction strength, duration and frequency, by recording the actual pressure within the uterus.

Insertion of the fluid-filled tube is mildly uncomfortable, much like the discomfort experienced during detailed manual examination. Once inserted, however, there is little or no discomfort, and the woman (unlike with the external belts) has a little more freedom of movement and position.

In order to record the fetal heartbeat, a tiny electrode is attached with a small spiral to the baby's presenting part (usually the scalp). This electrode (which barely breaks the skin) works like a small electrocardiogram lead, recording a tracing of the infant's heartbeat and its variations with uterine contractions.

Fetal scalp blood sampling allows the doctor to measure the acidity (pH) of the baby's blood. A minute amount of blood can be taken from the fetus's presenting part, similar to a simple pinprick, and blood gases (pH, a measure of acidity; pO_2, the level of oxygen; and pCO_2, the level of carbon dioxide) are analyzed to determine whether he or she is at serious risk because of inadequate oxygenation. This is rarely necessary and is only used to clarify the significance of certain fetal heart rate patterns.

If the placental oxygen transfer (through simple diffusion) of carbon dioxide and oxygen is insufficient, a buildup of waste chemicals occurs, and metabolic acidosis takes place. If the problem is umbilical cord occlusion, the result can be fetal respiratory acidosis—which can be more rapidly reversed. At certain levels, blood acidity can signify a degree of oxygen deprivation that can put the fetus at serious risk for damage or death if he or she is not delivered quickly.

The Risks of Electronic Fetal Monitoring

There appear to be no risks to either the mother or the fetus associated with the use of external fetal heart rate monitoring. Most women experience little or no discomfort from this non-invasive procedure, and the only disadvantage seems to be some restriction of motion in order to achieve a good tracing.

Internal fetal monitoring, on the other hand, carries with it a minimal risk of infection for both mother and baby. Because the vagina is not sterile, and a foreign object (the fluid-filled tube) is placed in the uterine cavity through the vagina, there is a slightly increased risk of infection of the lining of the uterus. It is difficult to determine an exact percentage of risk or even a percentage of occurrence of maternal infections. However, most reports seem to agree that the risk is minimal.

There seems to be some indication that infection is more prevalent in patients who were internally monitored then later delivered by cesarean section, than in those who later delivered vaginally. Available data, however, show that long labor, many vaginal examinations and prolonged rupture of membranes are far more significant causes of infection than fetal monitoring itself.

Likewise, attaching the electrode to the scalp (or buttock) of the fetus can be associated with infection of the newborn, because the skin has been broken. Most such infections are localized on the scalp, with little spread to the rest of the body, although in a few rare cases generalized infection (sepsis) has occurred. The risk for small scalp infection is about 1 percent or less, and serious infection is so extremely rare that a known percentage of occurrence cannot be given. Local medication is usually all that is required for scalp infections. And with newer and more powerful antibiotics, such infections of both mother and baby are usually successfully treated.

The Importance of Expertise in Interpreting Data

Those inexperienced in interpreting fetal monitoring data can, at times, over-react to the data, diagnose serious fetal distress and recommend cesarean birth to prevent potential complications or fetal death. Interpretation of data is neither easy nor clear-cut. It's not like a gauge on a car that flashes red when you're out of oil or beeps when you are low on gasoline. Instead, it takes a keen, skilled, well-trained and experienced eye.

Taking this analogy one step further, imagine what it would be like if there were no gauges on your car's dashboard. You wouldn't know how fast you were going, when you were about to run out of gas, whether the car was overheating or when the oil was becoming dangerously low. In such a situation you would learn to identify visual or auditory cues that could warn you of potential problems. With more understanding of your car, you would begin to sense the amount of driving you could do without running out of gas; you'd become attuned to abnormal sounds and warning signs and learn how to examine the engine to determine if it was overheating unduly after driving; and you'd learn the feel and sound of the car at different speeds in order not to break various speed limits. Without devices such as gauges, you would obviously be less than precise, however. Even with training and experience, you would still have to interpret the situation.

Exaggerated? Yes, but this situation is similar to that 20 years ago, when a doctor had little else but a stethoscope and experience as tools for identifying fetal problems during labor and delivery.

Fetal monitoring is one step up from this. There still isn't a red light or green light or a gauge that tells the doctor what to do next. Monitoring does not give more information, but the data must be interpreted very carefully. If we look at the car analogy again, this becomes clearer. Few people—even very experienced drivers—could get into a sophisticated race car for the first time and efficiently read and interpret the information given them. The numerous and complicated gauges and equipment require more knowledge and greater skills and expertise to interpret than those found in a regular car. In fact, there is simply no comparison between the two vehicles. Accurate assessment of how a race is performing, whether potential problems exist and how to manage difficulties is required of the driver to stay in the race—and learning these skills takes time as well as special training.

Fetal monitoring is really no different. It, too, requires special training, experience and attention to detail to carefully interpret data presented on the monitor graphs. As more and more professionals are trained not only in the mechanics of electronic monitoring but also in the careful interpretation of the data, we can expect more accurate decisions about the appropriateness of intervention and a potential reduction in the rate of cesarean deliveries.

The Conflict over Electronic Fetal Monitoring

The controversy surrounding electronic fetal monitoring has much less to do with the monitoring itself—and much more to do with its possible influence or association with the rising rate of cesarean births. (See Chapter 16 for details.) Although there has been a worldwide rise in the rate of cesarean delivery (removal of the baby from the uterus through a surgical incision in the woman's abdomen), the United States has experienced a greater rate of increase than other countries. (Scientists and physicians in the United States, it should be noted, have pioneered much of the work done in perinatal care and its resultant technology.) The worldwide increase in management of pregnancy by obstetrical specialists has resulted in a greater use of technology, with emphasis on avoiding fetal brain damage, reducing morbidity and mortality rates, increasing the quality of life of the infant, and protecting the health and well-being of the mother.

The real question is—are too many unnecessary cesarean deliveries being performed because of misinterpretation of fetal heart rate monitoring data or over-reaction to the data? Interestingly, the early studies done by Dr. Edward Hon showed that once fetal monitoring was introduced (in 1967), the rate of cesarean births to prevent or alleviate fetal distress was reduced by half, and the fetal death rate during labor decreased markedly, about 75 percent. At Los Angeles County-University of Southern California Medical Center, there were one-third fewer intrapartum deaths than usually expected once fetal monitoring was instituted. But even more striking was this: Only those patients who had been identified as "high-risk" were monitored, and they had an overall *better* outcome than the low-risk mothers who were not monitored.

Subsequent studies have supported the belief that electronic fetal monitoring is useful and effective. At Women's Hospital in Long Beach, California, a tertiary care center specializing in high-risk pregnancy, 17,000 patients, both high-risk and non-high-risk, have been monitored during labor and delivery. Only one viable-sized baby has been lost during labor. This is impressive when compared to worldwide statistics, in which 1.5 to 4.0 deaths are expected for each 1,000 patients in labor. Due to the success experienced at the hospital, all women in labor at Women's Hospital are monitored if they agree to the procedure.

Other studies have shown different results. Three randomized prospective studies of 2,000 women found that the outcome of pregnancy was no better for monitored women than for those who were not monitored. However, several studies involving about 140,000 patients studied retrospectively show a clear reduction in mortality for electronically monitored babies.

So the fact that the studies do not all agree is the basis for the continued controversy regarding the usefulness of routinely performing fetal monitoring for all pregnant women during labor and delivery. Practically speaking, what you find across the country is a difference in the use of and the reliance on fetal monitoring. Interpreting electronic fetal monitoring data and making decisions about intervention to protect both the fetus and the mother does require skill and experience with monitoring tools. There is therefore the potential for less experienced health professionals to misinterpret the fetal heart rate tracings, which could result in the over-diagnosis of fetal distress—and consequent unnecessary cesarean sections.

However, the increase in the rate of cesarean section to prevent or alleviate fetal distress may be due to three things: better identification of fetal distress, difficulty in accurately interpreting some monitoring data, and the greatly increased safety, for both the mother and baby, of the cesarean birth procedure.

The recent consensus report from the National Institutes of Health concluded that electronic fetal monitoring offers benefits to high-risk pregnancies, but the benefits to normal pregnancies are questionable.

Therefore, if you were identified as high-risk, it would be important for you to be monitored during labor in an institution where electronic fetal monitoring is well established and properly utilized. You should not hesitate to inquire about this when selecting your hospital and physician.

THIRTEEN

TESTS TO DETERMINE FETAL FITNESS AND FETAL LUNG
MATURITY

When you consider the great complexity of fetal growth and development—from conception until delivery into the outside world—it is a wonder that things go so well the majority of the time. However, the possibility for fetal damage or death is not insignificant. Between 15 percent and 25 percent of pregnancies end in miscarriage during the first three months of gestation. This is usually due to abnormal fetal formation and may really be regarded as nature's way of eliminating (early in pregnancy) very serious defects incompatible with life. In other words survival is impossible. There is very little that could or should be done to interfere with this process.

During the last half of pregnancy, however, a condition called *uteroplacental insufficiency (UPI)* is responsible for the majority of fetal deaths and probably causes a significant number of babies to be born with brain damage. UPI is caused by various maternal disease processes that result in decreased uterine blood flow which in turn reduces the supply of oxygen to the fetus. Some of the maternal conditions that cause UPI are chronic hypertension (high blood pressure), diabetes, pre-eclampsia and eclampsia, prolonged pregnancy and chronic kidney disease. At times there is no known maternal process which predisposes the fetus for UPI. We do know, however, that unrecognized UPI can cause a lack of fetal growth (called fetal growth retardation) or even fetal death. Therefore, a history of a previous (or current) growth retarded fetus or a history of a previous stillbirth are also considered risk factors for possible UPI in current or future pregnancies.

After the 26th week of pregnancy the possibility of fetal survival is a reality. If it suddenly becomes necessary to rescue the fetus from its uterine environment because of inadequate oxygenation due to UPI, then delivery after the 26th week is a reasonable alternative. In other words, the chance for survival outside the uterus may be greater than continued intrauterine fetal existence when UPI (which progressively worsens) is recognized.

Because it is always important to balance the potential risks associated with prematurity against the risks for UPI, it was vital to develop both tests for UPI and others for fetal maturity. Therefore, if UPI is identified and a decision for early delivery becomes necessary, tests for fetal maturity may also play an important role in this decision making process.

The *contraction stress test (CST)* and the *non-stress test (NST)* discussed next are used to diagnose uteroplacental insufficiency, hopefully before the fetus is compromised (experiences damage). These tests essentially measure the oxygen transferring capacity from the mother's blood to the fetus via the placenta.

What Is the Contraction Stress Test (CST)?

Until a decade ago, doctors had a limited number of biochemical tests that could assist in evaluating the fetus. Although helpful, all of the available tests were limited in their usefulness. What doctors needed was a reliable test to determine fetal fitness (or lack of it) at the time when fetal survival outside the womb was possible. *Contraction stress testing* was begun systematically in the early 1970s following a report from the University of Southern California (by Dr. Michael Ray and Dr. Roger K. Freeman—one of the authors of this book). This first pilot study in the United States showed this test (then called the oxytocin challenge test) to be potentially able to prevent fetal death from UPI in high risk mothers if they were delivered when the test was clearly abnormal. Further study has showed that when the test results were normal the chance of fetal death (caused by UPI within a one week period) was extremely small—less than 2 per 1,000.

The *contraction stress test* (CST) is based on the same principles as fetal heart rate monitoring performed during labor. This test is based on two important principles. The first principle is that when the uterus contracts, the uterine blood flow and oxygen transfer is momentarily diminished to the placenta and thereby to the fetus. The second principle was learned from previous experience with fetal heart rate monitoring, as we discussed in Chapter 12: We know

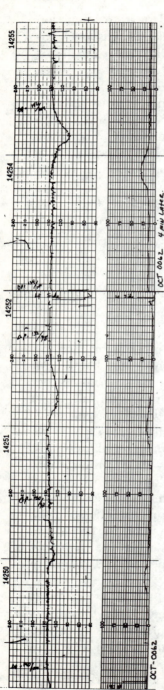

CONTRACTION STRESS TEST: Note in this test that the fetal heart rate (top line tracing) slows after each contraction (called late decelerations). The fetal heart rate also shows no accelerations. This then is a "positive" (non-reactive) contraction stress test. What this means is uteroplacental insufficiency (UPI) and delivery would be indicated.

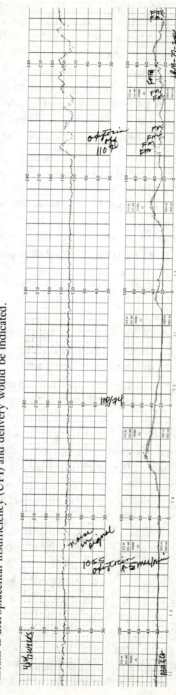

CONTRACTION STRESS TEST: The *bottom line tracing* shows the expectant mother's contractions. Note how the tracing goes up with each contraction and goes back down as the contraction subsides. The *top line tracing* shows the fetal heart rate. The heart rate doesn't slow after contractions and at the end of the tracing the heart rate accelerates. This would then be a "negative" contraction stress test—meaning the fetus is doing well at this time.

The test would be repeated weekly until delivery to make sure the fetus was continuing to do well and intervention wasn't necessary.

that the fetal heart rate will slow in a characteristic fashion during a uterine contraction—when the oxygen supply to the fetus falls below a critical level. Therefore, by observing the fetal heart rate response to uterine contractions, the doctor can determine if there is fetal fitness or if UPI exists. A characteristic slowing of the fetal heart rate which begins halfway through a uterine contraction and lasts until after the contraction is over is called "late deceleration." Late deceleration is a sign of UPI. When the uteroplacental reserve is normal, there is no late deceleration observed with contractions.

All women normally have uterine contractions which occur irregularly throughout pregnancy. The expectant mother herself may or may not even be aware of these spontaneously occurring contractions. When the contraction stress test is performed, two loosely fitting belts are placed around the woman's abdomen. One belt contains a tokodynamometer (the same as is used during labor with fetal heart rate monitoring) which records any uterine contractions which may occur spontaneously. If there are fewer than three contractions measured during a ten minute interval, uterine contractions will be stimulated either by administering oxytocin (a naturally occurring hormone) or by having the mother massage her breasts/nipples in the same way as when she prepares her nipples for breast feeding. In our hospital (Women's Hospital in Long Beach, California) we only recently discovered this breast stimulation technique and it has largely eliminated the necessity to administer oxytocin in the majority of women having a contraction stress test.

The other device which is also placed around the woman's abdomen is called a Doppler ultrasound transducer. High frequency sound waves (ultrasound) are transmitted through the mother's abdominal tissues and the Doppler device basically searches for the motion of the fetal heart (which is detectable when the reflected waves change their frequency). This is called the "Doppler principle" and allows the fetal heart rate to be recorded from the mother's abdominal wall.

What Is the Non-Stress Test?

In the last few years it has been reported that accelerations of the fetal heart rate in association with fetal movement are signs of well-being. Because of this fact, simply observing the fetal heart rate for accelerations appears to be a reliable measure of fetal condition.

This method of evaluation is called a *non-stress test (NST)* and is commonly used today as a simple screening test, with the contraction stress test used as an effective backup.

When the fetus has heart rate accelerations during an NST, the test is called a "reactive NST," which means that the test is reassuring. If there are very few or no accelerations during the NST, the test is then called a "non-reactive NST" and a contraction stress test (CST) is indicated to determine the significance of the NST results.

How the NST and CST are Performed

The *non-stress test* involves simply placing the two belts containing the tokodynamometer and Doppler ultrasound transducer around your abdomen. Fetal movement and fetal heart rate acceleration are then noted. Of course, this same information is always available when a contraction stress test is performed, so in reality an NST is a CST minus the contractions. However, if you have sufficient spontaneous contractions while the NST is being performed, then a spontaneous CST has been accomplished. The NST takes 30 to 60 minutes to complete and causes you no discomfort or pain.

The *contraction stress test* is performed in a similar manner as the non-stress test. You will usually be taken to a quiet room near the hospital's labor and delivery area and asked to lie on a bed or reclining chair. The special electronic belts will be carefully placed around your abdomen and a baseline reading of the fetal heart rate and your uterine contractions will be recorded.

Your blood pressure will be taken frequently, as often as every ten minutes throughout the test, to make sure hypotension (lowering of the blood pressure) does not occur. A lowering of blood pressure can take place when you lie on your back, because your enlarged uterus blocks off some of the blood flow from your legs back to your heart. This can ultimately lead to less blood flow to the placenta and reduced oxygenation to the fetus. Hypotension then could cause a misleading test result.

Since all women experience contractions throughout late pregnancy, baseline contractions and the fetal heart rate are generally recorded for 20 minutes or so. During this time if three contractions occur in a span of ten minutes, and the recording of the heart rate is deemed adequate—the test is considered completed. (There is enough information to assess the fetus.)

If, however, three contractions do not occur within a ten minute period, or the fetal heart rate recording is inadequate, uterine contractions will be stimulated either by breast massage or by the administration of oxytocin. When the breast or nipple stimulation method is chosen to induce uterine contractions, the nurse will give you a warm, moist washcloth to put on your breasts. Often this is sufficient to stimulate uterine contractions. If this is not sufficient, the nurse will ask you to massage the nipple area with the warm cloth (usually one side at a time) for about five to ten minutes. Sometimes rolling the nipples will work well. If the nipple stimulation method does not produce sufficient uterine activity, an IV (intravenous line) will be started so oxytocin can be administered.

Oxytocin is a hormone which stimulates uterine contractions, and is administered with an infusion pump, a machine specially designed to pump a very precise amount of fluid (and medication) through an intravenous (IV) line. The oxytocin is continued until three contractions lasting 40 to 60 seconds each are recorded over a ten minute period.

Once the test is completed, you would be kept on the monitor until the contractions return to their baseline level. If your contractions continue after breast/nipple stimulation (or oxytocin) has been stopped, a small amount of oral alcohol may be given to halt the contractions. Usually the contraction stress test takes from one to two hours to complete and can be momentarily uncomfortable during the time of the contractions. Most women, however, find the test *minimally* uncomfortable at worst.

When Are NST or CST Recommended?

Depending on the severity of the problem identified—and its relative risk for causing UPI—testing could be recommended as early as the 26th week of pregnancy (the time of reasonable fetal viability) or any time thereafter. For example, if you had chronic hypertension with pre-eclampsia, or one of the more severe classes of diabetes mellitus, testing would probably begin no later than 30 or 32 weeks of pregnancy. Such things as a history of previous stillbirth or advanced maternal age, or other minimal to moderate risks would warrant testing at around the 34th week. It very much depends on the problem(s) identified and the risk it places on the fetus for uteroplacental insufficiency.

Of course, the best of circumstances would be to allow the fetus to mature to term (if at all possible), try to control the existing problem and retest weekly to follow the fetus closely. However, much of the time carrying the fetus to term is not possible when the CST has been positive (shows persistent late decelerations), since fetal loss may occur at any time. In reality, even with very high risk women, both the NST and/or CST are usually completely normal and provide reassurance that it is quite safe to continue the pregnancy (not have to deliver the baby early). Prior to the use of the NST and CST, certain high risk women were delivered prematurely in an attempt to avoid fetal death or damage from UPI just on a statistical basis (facts collected over a period of time which showed certain women to be at greater risk for UPI). With the development and availability of the NST and CST, we can now avoid unnecessary intervention (early delivery) when the tests show fetal fitness and rescue the fetus in need of premature delivery only when it is best to do so.

Situations in Which CST Would Not Be Recommended

There are situations, which by their nature, would make CST contraindicated (not recommended). Women with a history of premature labor, an incompetent cervix, placenta previa, premature rupture of the membranes, a previous classical cesarean section, those with multiple gestation (twins or more), or those at risk for uterine rupture would in general not have CST recommended and would be followed by NST and/or estriol levels.

However, it should be noted that when all other factors point to fetal distress in late pregnancy, then CST may be recommended anyway. The test would be recommended to substantiate fetal distress so intervention could appropriately occur.

Estriol Testing as a Compliment to CST and NST

Estriol is a hormone found in the plasma portion of a pregnant woman's blood. Research has shown that the plasma estriol level normally rises slowly early in pregnancy, then quickly rises beginning in the 24th week, continuing throughout the remainder of the pregnancy. Abnormal levels of estriol may signify that the fetus is in serious trouble and may die before birth.

Measurement of the mother's estriol levels, then, can be another very useful means of monitoring fetal fitness during late pregnancy. Laboratory testing can be done on either a sample of the mother's blood (called the plasma estriol level) or on urine collected for an entire 24-hour period.

Determination of estriol levels might be recommended two or three times weekly or even daily in some situations. Results are usually recorded on a graph, and compared to the known normal estriol values for the week of pregnancy the woman is in. (These values for a specific week of pregnancy have been studied extensively and are excellent determinants.) The goal in measuring estriol levels—like with CST and NST—is the early detection of uteroplacental insufficiency (UPI). Estriol levels herald a warning when they are chronically low, if they fall gradually, or when an abrupt fall is noted.

Estriol reflects the *nutritional portion* of placental function more than the oxygen supply function. Therefore, an abnormal pattern— low or falling levels—may be seen before the CST or NST is abnormal. However, this is not the case when the *oxygen supply* is affected more than the nutritional supply. For example, an abrupt fall in the estriol level in a woman with diabetes may be a "late finding" because nutritional UPI occurs much later than hypoxic UPI in diabetic mothers. This "late finding" may precede fetal death by only a matter of two days or less.

Determination of estriol levels though is an excellent compliment to the NST and CST because it helps to detect or verify fetal distress in late pregnancy. One or both of these tests might be used in different stages of pregnancy, depending on the particular risk factors for you.

Depending on the type of risk and its degree—mild, moderate or severe—NST or CST may be performed as initial diagnostic measurements for uteroplacental insufficiency, or in conjunction with estriol testing. With some problems, careful monitoring of estriols is used as a screening mechanism, and only when levels become abnormal is NST or CST performed. In other situations the opposite occurs: NST or CST begin as early as the 26th week of pregnancy and estriol levels are determined only if the NST or CST is abnormal. The protocol used depends on the problems which put the fetus at risk for uteroplacental insufficiency and decisions are generally made on a very individualized basis.

The L/S Ratio as a Compliment to NST and CST

As we discussed in detail in Chapter 11 (Amniocentesis), fetal lung maturity is dependent on the presence of surfactant which develops in late pregnancy. A deficiency of this lung substance often leads to respiratory distress syndrome (sometimes called hyaline membrane disease) in the newborn baby.

From extensive research it was discovered that the relationship between two fat-like compounds (lecithin and sphingomyelin) was an excellent predictor of fetal lung maturity. The measurement of these two compounds in the amniotic fluid can indicate the presence or deficiency of surfactant, and thereby determine fetal lung maturity or immaturity.

If the CST is positive at any point (indicating fetal danger) and delivery of the baby must be considered, it is important to know if the fetus' lungs are mature—if he or she could survive outside the womb. Although premature birth can involve a whole host of potential problems (discussed in more detail in Chapter 15), the major fear and the major risk for non-survival comes from respiratory distress syndrome.

When the L/S ratio is sufficient to expect fetal lung maturity, the risk of serious problems is greatly reduced when delivering a premature infant. Therefore, if time allows, amniocentesis would be recommended if a positive CST resulted. If, on the other hand, the CST is so severely abnormal to signify impending fetal death, there might not be time for other diagnostic measures and swift action would be mandatory.

Very recently a new substance found in the amniotic fluid called phosphatidyl glycerol (PG) has been found to be perhaps even more accurate than the L/S ratio in determining fetal lung maturity. This may be especially helpful for diabetic mothers, where the L/S ratio has been found in some (but not all) investigations to be less reliable. If promising results continue and methods for measuring PG become more simple, this test for fetal lung maturity may replace the L/S ratio.

The Use of Corticosteroids for Lung Maturity

Again, if time and the situation permit (low estriol levels, positive

CST but the fetus is still reactive—yet the fetus' lungs are still immature), corticosteroids may be administered to the mother to accelerate fetal lung maturity so the fetus can be delivered safely within 48 to 72 hours. Betamethasone (a corticosteroid) must be administered at least 24 hours before delivery to be at all effective and is markedly more effective if administered over a 48 to 72 hour period. It is thought that betamethasone speeds up the production of surfactant necessary for lung maturation. (More detailed information about corticosteroids can be found in Chapter 15.)

The Overall Impact of Testing for Fetal Fitness and Fetal Lung Maturity

At Women's Hospital in Long Beach, we have had a very active program of contraction stress testing and non-stress testing for the past seven years. Even with an ever increasing number of women with high risk pregnancies, we have been able to reduce the fetal death rate substantially. The fact is—high risk mothers who are followed by our CST protocol have no greater risk for fetal mortality than low risk mothers who are not monitored.

Essentially, there are two different philosophies with respect to the role of the CST and the NST. Some specialists advocate the NST as a screening test and use the CST if the NST is abnormal. We have found that another approach—using the CST on everyone who is high risk for uteroplacental insufficiency—seems to give slightly better information than using the NST as a screening test and using the CST only when the NST is non-reactive.

The advantages of NST screening include less time per test, less cost and less inconvenience for the woman. However, with the recent development of breast/nipple stimulation for inducing uterine contractions, the need to start an IV and administer oxytocin has been largely eliminated. Because of this, using contraction stress testing for primary fetal surveillance for UPI appears to be quite feasible and reasonable for all women who do not have any contraindications to inducing contractions.

Overall, the use of contraction stress testing, non-stress testing and estriol levels as means of determining fetal fitness have been very instrumental in saving the lives of countless babies. Coupled with tests to determine fetal lung maturity (measuring the L/S ratio and possibly PG in the amniotic fluid) have turned the odds in favor of the mother and baby for a better pregnancy outcome.

These tests have played a major role in the last few years in bringing new hope and greater optimism to mothers whose unborn babies are at risk for death or damage because of uteroplacental insufficiency. The point is—these tests have made a major difference in the outcome for a substantial number of babies.

FOURTEEN

WHAT YOU SHOULD KNOW ABOUT LABOR AND DELIVERY

The time of labor and delivery signifies the cumulative effort of nine months of growth and development and the readiness of the baby to leave the protective womb of his or her mother.

Years ago it was thought that the mother's hormones and various physical mechanisms were solely responsible for determining the readiness of the fetus and for initiating labor. The infant was viewed simply as a bystander in the entire process of pregnancy, labor and delivery. We now know the unborn child, in combination with the mother, plays a significant role in determining readiness for delivery. The entire procedure is a complex process of action, reaction and interaction.

Being Prepared

It's important for all women (high-risk or not) to be prepared for labor and delivery. The woman who doesn't know what's going on will usually be anxious, often stressed, uneasy about what to expect and what is expected of her, and feel she is apart from rather than a part of the birthing process.

Childbirth classes and prenatal courses have played a major role in preparing the expectant mother and her partner for all aspects of pregnancy, labor and delivery. Most courses cover the gamut of topics: from preparing the nipples and breasts for nursing to breathing exercises, from nutrition to what to take to the hospital, from fetal monitoring to cesarean birth, and all those aspects in between.

The best classes are probably those recommended by your doctor or (in many cases) those available at the hospital at which you will deliver. For the high-risk woman it is best to make sure the classes cover many of those aspects of diagnosis and medical intervention that may, if necessary, be recommended for you. Some perinatal centers (regional tertiary care centers) have special courses or programs for those women identified or potentially high-risk or those with specific high-risk problems. These are available in preparing the woman for both natural childbirth and cesarean birth in case intervention must occur. Many of these courses not only provide excellent information but emotional support, as well.

Many high-risk problems simply require watchfulness and careful evaluation during pregnancy, labor and delivery. The point is, the majority of women identified as potentially high-risk may well deliver naturally and at term. Therefore, prepared or natural childbirth classes are highly recommended. If the center where you will deliver has a special course for those identified as high-risk, so much the better.

Solid information—knowing the facts—will make you a better decision maker. And knowing the facts actually makes it a lot easier for you (both physically and emotionally) to deal with medical intervention if and when it is recommended. When you know about something ahead of time, you have a chance to adjust to the possibility and put it into perspective.

Most women who are at risk for problems have astonishing determination and commitment. They deal with high technology well when they really understand what is going on and why something is recommended and are actively involved in the decision making— rather than just being passive participants. They tend to do well partly because today the odds are in their favor—in most cases. And they want to know. They are bright, sharp, involved and committed. They ask questions and expect clear, honest answers. In fact, they are, in general, an amazing group of women to work with—and for. They are also proof that when it comes to pregnancy, labor and delivery, the more you know and the more prepared you are, the better you will do both physically and emotionally.

The Truth About Discomfort or Pain during Labor

Basically, one of the major purposes of prepared childbirth classes is to help the expectant mother enter labor as relaxed and as involved as possible and better manage discomfort or pain. In other words, she learns to work with rather than fight the labor. And because she knows what the process of birth is, the options, the possible complications and what doctors can do to intervene, she is more at ease and feels in control.

For many women total natural childbirth without pain relief works well. For others it is beneficial, but if discomfort or pain becomes severe, they feel they have somehow failed or are weaklings. This is far from the truth. Some women describe minimal pain—more like a tightening or cramping sensation. But the great majority of women during labor will experience varying degrees of significant discomfort to real—often severe pain.

No one really knows why women going through the similar experience of labor have differing degrees of discomfort or pain, just as no one really knows why people (male or female) undergoing such similar experiences as surgery, broken bone, headache, bruise, etc.), have differing degrees of discomfort or pain. It appears that the degree of pain experienced in any situation is dependent on a variety of complex factors: hereditary influences, sensitivity to any stimulus, chemical secretions, state of mind, or even preparedness or lack of it. The nerve pathways and the brain function are complex chemical and electrical networks. Unraveling those conduction, production and interpretation networks will take some time. What we do know is that people experience different degrees of pain and appreciate that fact.

And so it is with labor and delivery. Special exercises and a full explanation of what to expect and what to do can help manage the discomfort and pain of labor and are beneficial. However, you should be aware that there are situations where analgesics and anesthetics (pain relievers) are appropriately used for the management or relief of severe pain, if forceps delivery must be done or if cesarean delivery becomes necessary.

Honesty is the key. The fact is, most women can tolerate the discomfort of labor to a point—even if they experience moderate to severe pain. The key is "to a point." What tends to bother women more is not the degree of off-and-on discomfort or the physical effort involved in labor but the duration of labor if it becomes extensive. Even without severe pain, prolonged labor can wear down anyone, and this can lead to problems for both mother and baby—in terms of physical well-being.

Doctors, too, understand how desirable it may be for many women to have a natural birth. If, however, a woman experiences severe pain, she should feel comfortable asking for pain relief and realize that there are many safe methods available. Occasionally anesthesia or analgesia may even be in the best interest of the baby. Why? Because severe pain can cause so much stress in the mother that she releases adrenalin. Adrenalin can cause constriction of the blood vessels which supply the uterus. This may result in poor blood supply and therefore inadequate oxygenation to the fetus. Fetal hypoxia may occur.

A few things you should try to remember are: Any discomfort or pain ceases as each contraction subsides; the process of labor is self-limiting—that is, you need only experience it for a certain period of time—until the baby is born and the placenta (afterbirth) has been expelled; and the discomfort or pain is not a warning signal that something is wrong with your body, as pain generally indicates. This is where preparing physically and psychologically helps so much. The more you understand the mechanisms of labor, the easier it is to cope with it.

While some women are able to go through labor without pain relief, the great majority of women experience significant pain and require some type of pain medication. If labor without medication is possible for you—that is good. However, if you require pain medication during labor, you are the rule—not the exception!

The Normal Process of Labor

Active labor itself averages about 12 hours in most first-time pregnancies (sometimes as little as only a few hours but occasionally as long as 18 to 24 hours) and usually a much shorter time in subsequent pregnancies. While labor itself normally lasts less than 24 hours, the process leading up to it begins in the four to six weeks preceding delivery.

Before the Start of Labor

During the first seven to eight months of gestation, the fetus floats freely in the amniotic fluid, moving in many directions. Most women are aware of this and only toward the last part of pregnancy become convinced the fetus stays in more or less the same position.

Before labor begins, the fetus must turn into the correct position for delivery. This is most commonly the "head down" (cephalic) presentation, but 3 to 5 percent of term babies establish themselves in other positions, such as breech (buttocks down). As the eighth month progresses, the fetus's head engages in the pelvis—it becomes wedged into the cervix and well down into the bony portion of the birth canal (the bony part of the pelvis and vagina). While "engagement" usually takes place before labor during a first pregnancy, it may not occur until during labor itself, especially in later pregnancies.

Preparation of the birth canal is also a gradual process and probably occurs in response to hormones secreted during the last months of gestation. The ligaments and structures of the pelvis become more flexible, allowing some stretching during labor and delivery.

"Braxton-Hicks contractions" are contractions of the uterus— tightening of the uterine muscles—that occur throughout late pregnancy, even if they are not felt or are not painful. These gradually become stronger in the last several weeks of pregnancy and may become bothersome enough to be misinterpreted as true labor. While not actually labor, this repeated tightening of the uterine muscles plays a role in preparing the birth canal for labor and perhaps in getting the fetus positioned correctly.

"Effacement" is the shortening and thinning of the cervix that occurs prior to active labor for most women pregnant for the first time (called "primiparas"). The cervix, usually firm and tightly closed, is about an inch or so long before effacement.

As the cervix thins and dilates, the mucus plug that has been in the cervix protecting (sealing) the entrance to the womb may become dislodged into the vagina and be expelled. A woman may notice this rather gelatinous piece of mucus after it has been expelled.

Rupture of the baby's amniotic sac—often called "breaking your water"—may occur before actual contractions are felt but means that labor will usually start within 24 hours. Sometimes "rupturing the membranes" (another term for the same event) is signaled by a very obvious gush of warm, clear liquid from the vagina. Other times the "rupture" is actually a gradual leak of the fluid and may not be as obvious to the woman. Most often, rupture of the membranes does not occur until labor has started or may even need to be done artificially during labor.

It's important to remember that there are many variations of these processes—based on individual differences. While preparation for actual labor at term is a gradual process for all women, it is usually much more prolonged for the woman delivering for the first time. For example, the first-time mother (primipara) will usually have completed cervical effacement (thinning) before active labor begins. The "experienced" mother (multipara), on the other hand, may start active labor without any prior effacement but may already be dilated.

The First Stage of Labor

The cervis (mouth of the uterus) is actually only 1 inch long (extending into the vagina) with an opening of about ⅛ of an inch. During the first stage of labor, this remarkably flexible structure must become paper thin and open to 10 centimeters (4 inches) in diameter in order to allow the baby's head to pass into the vaginal part of the birth canal. Uterine contractions, starting at the fundus (top) of the uterus then spreading out and down, cause dilatation of the cervix. Hormone secretions in the mother are responsible for softening the cervix and preparing it for thinning and dilation.

With each contraction the lower end of the uterus and the cervix itself stretch a little. Unlike other muscles of the body, which retract (go back to their original position), the uterus has special muscle fibers at its upper portion that stay shortened after a contraction, thereby allowing the lower portion to stay stretched—even after the contraction has subsided. Each labor contraction, then, widens the cervix and lower uterus. At the same time, the upper wall of the uterus gets thicker, slowly and methodically pushing the baby downward. These complimentary actions are the hallmarks of a successful first stage of labor.

The first stage of labor lasts different lengths of time for different pregnancies—it may be relatively long or short, depending on the efficiency and strength of the uterine contractions. Usually, though, cervical dilatation progresses at a rate averaging about one centimeter each hour.

The baby's head is turned sideways—parallel to the shoulders (almost like turning your head and pressing your chin down on your shoulder)—during this part of labor. Once the cervix is fully dilated to 10 centimeters, the crown of the baby's head passes the cervix with the help of contractions and the squeezing of the uterus from top to bottom. The first stage of labor has been fully achieved.

At some point during the first stage of labor (based on your doctor's determination), you will be admitted to the hospital to complete labor and delivery. Hospitals and doctors differ in some routines, so it's important that you ask ahead of time so you'll know the doctor's and hospital's routine. It is best not to eat or drink anything if you think your labor has started. Depending on your risk status, you may not be allowed to eat or drink while in labor in the hospital.

An intravenous solution (IV) may be started to give you liquids by vein. It is also important because it allows for the administration of any necessary medications. In some hospitals you may be required to have some laboratory tests (blood and urine). Some physicians recommend enemas and shaving of the genital area and require a shower, while others require only some or none of these.

Fetal monitoring—external or internal—will more than likely be started, since it is recommended for all high-risk pregnancies. Your progress in labor may be followed by frequent vaginal examinations as well as fetal monitoring.

A note about true labor: Women experience contractions off and on throughout the latter part of pregnancy. These are called "Braxton-Hicks contractions," as mentioned before. Sometimes indigestion also occurs and may seem like labor. True labor can mean a contraction here or there at the beginning, but the telltale sign of active labor is that the contractions become regular and can be timed. For example, 30 minutes apart, then 20 minutes apart, 16 minutes apart, and so on down to 2 minutes apart. As labor progresses, then, contractions are more regular and more frequent as well as more intense and longer lasting.

Standing up or walking around doesn't stop them, as is often the case with false labor or with indigestion. And much of the time, the beginning of labor feels more like back pain than abdominal pain. Active contractions also have a distinctly different sensation of starting up higher and moving toward the pelvis or lower abdomen.

Many women are confused about the term "false labor." While it may be used to mean other things, it most commonly refers to exaggerated Braxton-Hicks contractions. Particularly intense contractions may be interpreted as true labor and lead to a trip to the hospital. Although the contractions are real and may be quite regular, they are not efficient in dilating the cervix rapidly.

The Second Stage of Labor

The purpose of the second stage of labor is to advance the baby down the birth canal, through the pelvis and cervix, and into the vagina and out! This is where the mother's work really begins. The process of the baby's descent is greatly aided by the mother who bears down with each contraction. As you can imagine, it's a rather tight squeeze in there. But mucus, vernix (which coats the baby's skin like a cream) and other secretions help the baby slide over tissues and muscles as the uterus squeezes—closing down slowly from the top to push the baby downward. The mother assists by pushing down with each contraction. (It's almost the same pushing sensation as having a bowel movement.)

As the new little life is maneuvered through the birth canal, contractions are stronger. As the baby descends, the head begins to turn so it faces down and backward (somewhat like placing your chin on your chest).

For the first-time mother who is delivering in the "usual" hospital atmosphere, part of the second stage of labor will be completed while she is still in the labor room. She will spend 15 minutes to two or three hours "pushing the baby down" and will be taken to the delivery room when the baby's head has reached the outlet of the vagina. (This is called "crowning"—the crown, or top of the head, protrudes during a contraction.) The experienced mother, on the other hand, is usually moved to the delivery room for the entire second stage of labor, because this stage usually progresses quite rapidly for her.

Just prior to the baby's delivery, the doctor will perform an "episiotomy" (an incision in the perineum—the area between the anus and the opening of the vagina). This incision is performed under local anesthetic (an injection at the site where the cut will be made) and allows for a wider opening without unnecessary muscle and tissue tearing and stretching. An episiotomy is usually a good idea, especially during the first delivery of a term baby, because muscle ripping, tearing and stretching in this area are difficult to repair satisfactorily. In fact, irreparable damage may occur without an episiotomy.

As the baby's head reaches its destination, it is pushed through the vaginal opening by a contraction and the mother's assistance in bearing down. The baby automatically turns his or her head, so the head is facing sideways. The baby's shoulders wait at the vaginal opening and are delivered one at a time with the next contraction. Once the head and shoulders are delivered, the rest is easy. The baby's trunk is guided out, and the hips and legs follow by literally sliding out. Because the baby is so slippery, he or she is usually caught with a towel. The nose and mouth are either suctioned as soon as the head is delivered or as soon as the entire baby is out.

At this point, hospitals and doctors differ as to their procedures. Some doctors and hospitals place the baby on the mother's abdomen, clamp the umbilical cord, take the newborn to a small table under a warmer, wipe the baby off and check the baby's general condition. They may apply silver nitrate or antibiotic drops to the eyes to prevent serious eye infections due to gonorrhea, then return him or her to the mother and encourage the baby to suck at the breast, be cuddled and held for better mother-child bonding. Other hospitals and doctors place the newborn on the mother's abdomen, clamp and cut the umbilical cord, wipe the baby off, then immediately encourage the baby to suck on the breast for a period of time before attending to the other aspects of care.

The goals of baby care in the delivery room are to be sure that the baby is breathing well and getting enough oxygen and stays warm. While the exact sequence of events may differ, most babies are dried off and placed under a heater for some time and observed. The baby's "Apgar score" is counted twice—at one minute after delivery and again at five minutes. (The Apgar score is a way to look at the baby's condition—color, breathing, heart rate, muscle tone and activity. The best possible score is 10, but scores above 7 are quite good. Babies who need some help to start breathing tend to have low Apgar scores. Low scores usually mean the baby needs to be watched carefully for at least a short time after labor.) Only after the baby is stable—breathing well and vigorous—are the other things done, such as eye care and nursing.

The order of all of these events can vary from hospital to hospital and doctor to doctor. Make sure you check with your doctor about the steps he or she follows as well as ask about the hospital policies at the prepared childbirth classes. If you have any special requests or certain preferences, make sure you discuss them with your doctor early in the pregnancy to make sure you are aware of the policies and procedures and can agree with them. This also applies to your feelings about the use of analgesics and anesthetics for pain relief during labor and delivery. Don't wait until the latter part of pregnancy to discuss your feelings and wants and hear what your doctor feels and thinks about these important issues.

It's vitally important that you understand the situation—particularly if you are high-risk. In many cases it is essential that the baby be evaluated immediately by a pediatrician or neonatologist, and at times the baby will be taken to the hospital's special care nursery for his or her safety and well-being (more detailed information will be provided in Chapter 19). Often mothers feel cheated if they only get a glimpse of the baby. It's a normal maternal instinct to want to cuddle and caress your baby. This can be a very difficult time for mother and father, and health professionals should be sensitive and understanding about this. No one likes to have to take a newborn from his or her mother right away—but at times it must be done for the newborn's well-being.

In some situations the mother and father are prepared for this and realize, even in their disappointment, that it is best for the baby. At other times the couple are not prepared, because no one is quite sure if intervention or careful management or immediate evaluation and treatment will be necessary. A frank discussion with your doctor often helps.

The Third Stage of Labor

The purpose of the third stage of labor is the separation of the placenta from the wall of the uterus and its delivery. Often mothers don't even remember this part of labor, because they're so involved with the joy of the new baby. Actually, it's usually a simple matter of another contraction or two, which pushes the now-detached placenta out with a little help from the physician as well as a small amount of intravenous oxytocin hormone. If the baby has been suckling, this stimulates contractions, or the uterus contracts on its own.

Once the placenta is out, the doctor will examine it closely to make sure all of the placenta has been removed from the uterus. He or she may need to examine the inside of the uterus (through the vagina), an uncomfortable procedure. Then the episiotomy incision is carefully sutured (stitched) with an absorbable type of suture material, and the area is cleaned of blood and tissue.

If the baby is sucking, contractions (sometimes relatively uncomfortable ones) will occur. This helps tighten the uterus and prevent excessive bleeding. The action of nursing (even though there is little milk present) stimulates oxytocin, which in turn stimulates uterine contraction. As the uterus contracts and tightens, pressure is placed on the blood vessels, and this controls bleeding. If the baby does not get the hang of sucking (and many do not at first), the uterus will usually contract some on its own.

The Fourth Stage of Labor

Although heretofore there have only been three stages of labor identified, many more physicians and health professionals are now recognizing a fourth stage. The first one to two hours after delivery are important to the mother's recovery, particularly in terms of the control of bleeding.

During this time observation and monitoring of the woman's vital signs (temperature, pulse and respiration) as well as careful measurement of blood pressure every 10 to 15 minutes are vital. Blood pressure is important, since post-delivery high blood pressure can occur and require medication. On the other hand, if blood pressure drops, it may indicate more than the usual blood loss or the need for more careful control of bleeding.

As a means to control and eventually stop bleeding, the uterus is externally massaged and pressed to stimulate contractions. Rubbing and pushing on the uterus cause it to contract, constricting blood vessels naturally. Any blood left in the uterine cavity is also expelled. This process can be uncomfortable. The uterus has been through a lot and is sensitive. Some women describe this as feeling like someone is pushing on a bruise. Often, too, the new mother is weary and just wants to rest. This can therefore be very irritating. It's important to remember this procedure is done for your safety and well-being. The nurses are really not trying to be mean—as is often perceived. They know this is uncomfortable and irritating and even painful for some women. They also know it needs to be done to control and stop bleeding. Excessive blood loss can lead to shock—and this is precisely what it is hoped this procedure will prevent.

If the uterus does not respond well to manipulation, and bleeding continues, oxytocin may be administered intravenously to stimulate uterine contraction. This usually takes care of the problem. The average blood loss that occurs due to normal delivery is around 500 milliliters (about two cups, or a pint). To the layperson the blood loss often seems considerable, but in actuality it is not.

Assisted Vaginal Delivery

In some situations vaginal delivery may need to be assisted during the second stage of labor, so the infant can be promptly delivered. This stage of labor may not progress well in several types of situations: Fetal distress toward the end of the second stage may make speedy delivery imperative; medication or anesthetic may be given to the mother and make it difficult or impossible for her to help push the baby out; the second stage may be prolonged, and the mother may be tiring; or the baby may be somewhat larger than expected and the force of contractions not great enough because of a "tight fit."

Intervention at the time of delivery can be invaluable in these situations. Forceps delivery and vacuum extraction are the most common types of assistance used to speed delivery in the second stage of labor.

Forceps Delivery

Forceps are carefully designed and constructed instruments used to help deliver the head of the baby. They are used as a pair. One is carefully inserted into the vagina along each side of the fetus's head, and then the two forceps are attached together. The doctor pulls steadily on the forceps with each contraction, in order to help the fetus's head advance through the birth canal (much as the mother's pushing would do).

Forceps can only be safely applied when the baby's head is sufficiently low in the vagina. Most forceps deliveries are performed to shorten the second stage of labor—only after the head is on the perineum (visible during a contraction) and are called low-forceps or outlet force deliveries. Sometimes the baby has temporary forceps marks or bruises near the cheeks and ears, and the mother may suffer discomfort and small tears of the sides of the vagina. However, this type of assistance is useful and generally safe for both mother and baby.

Some forceps deliveries are more difficult because the baby's head is higher in the birth canal or the baby's head needs to be rotated to continue vaginal delivery. These types of forceps deliveries are called "mid-forceps maneuvers." While they are clearly indicated in certain situations, most obstetricians have abandoned the more difficult mid-forceps deliveries and are utilizing cesarean delivery more liberally in such situations (because of the higher risk of injury to mother and baby in mid-forceps maneuvers).

Vacuum Extraction

Vacuum extraction is a relatively new technique for helping vaginal delivery along during the second stage of labor. With this procedure a special suction cup is attached to the presenting part of the fetus (almost always the head), and careful suction is applied, which holds the cup to the head. The doctor can assist the descent of the baby by pulling on the tubing attached to the cup. Pulling is done with each uterine contraction, and the extractor is held firmly between contractions. In this way, the fetus can be helped to advance through the birth canal.

Vacuum extraction is a safe way to assist delivery and is usually less uncomfortable for the mother than forceps delivery. However, it may be difficult to get the vacuum cup to stay attached to the fetal head in some situations. If the cup repeatedly releases, a cesarean delivery may then be necessary. Use of vacuum extraction leads to a very characteristic circular bruise on the top of the baby's head.

Pain Control during Labor and Vaginal Delivery

Labor and delivery are accompanied by varying degrees of discomfort or pain (as discussed previously). While some women are able to labor many hours and deliver their infants without pain relief, many will want or need some type of medication. In certain situations the stress associated with severe pain may be potentially harmful enough for the mother and child that both would benefit from some form of relief.

Natural childbirth—childbirth without medication—involves preparation of the mother and her mate for the birthing process as well as use of various techniques to deal with fear and pain or discomfort of labor and delivery. Such measures as education about the process of labor and delivery, physical and breathing exercises, relaxation techniques and specific distraction routines to use during contractions are helpful in coping with the stress of giving birth. While there are claims of shorter, less complicated labors, fewer cesarean births, and fewer newborn and postpartum problems, scientific proof is lacking. Nonetheless, natural childbirth preparation has distinct advantages in reducing the amount of medication needed during labor and in increasing the mother's ability to cope with the stresses of labor.

Better preparation for the birth process as well as more concern about the effects of anesthetics and analgesics have led to the use of less medication during labor where possible. On the other hand, greater knowledge of the process of labor and the effects of the various pain-relieving medications on both mother and fetus have resulted in safer pain relief methods when needed during the birth process. With professional expertise and proper monitoring, obstetrical pain relief can be effective for the mother and safe for both mother and fetus.

Pain relief can be partial or complete—and provided in a variety of ways. All have advantages and disadvantages. Most pain control during labor and vaginal delivery is *analgesia*—relief of pain without complete loss of all sensation. *Anesthesia*, on the other hand, involves complete absence of all sensation, including pain, and is required for cesarean birth and some difficult vaginal deliveries. (The use of anesthesia for cesarean births is discussed in Chapter 16.)

Pain during early labor originates from contractions of the uterus and dilation of the cervix. This pain is felt in the lower abdomen and the lower back. As the baby moves down the birth canal during the second stage of labor, pain is caused by stretching of the vagina and perineum (the area between the anal opening and the vulva and vagina), as well as pressure on the rectum. Because these areas are supplied by different nerves, more than one type of pain control may be needed for the best possible results, depending on the stage of labor and the special requirements of the mother and fetus.

Narcotics, Sedatives and Tranquilizers

One of the most common ways to provide pain relief in labor is with the use of various medications given by injection or IV (intravenously). Narcotics, tranquilizers and sedatives are most often used during the end of the first stage of labor, and their effects usually last through the second stage. They are often given in conjunction with local or regional analgesia.

Narcotics such as meperidine (Demerol® and others) are effective in relieving pain and decreasing anxiety in the laboring mother. These medications can be used in established active labor and are effective in all stages of labor. However, meperidine and other narcotics do cross the placenta easily and can have some effect on the newborn's breathing and behavior. Their effect on the fetus depends on the dose given, the way it is given (by injection or IV) and how close to the time of delivery the drug is administered. When given intravenously, meperidine provides very rapid pain relief for the mother (in 5 to 15 minutes). Its maximum effect on the fetus takes about one hour. If given as an injection into the muscle, on the other hand, it produces maternal pain relief more gradually. When administered this way, it has its peak depression on the baby's breathing in two to four hours.

Therefore, the doctor determines how to give the medication based on when he or she expects the baby to be born, trying to minimize its effect on the baby at the anticipated time of birth. Nalorphine (Narcan®) can be given to the newborn at the time of delivery to counteract meperidine's effects immediately if the baby's breathing is severely depressed.) Meperidine can also cause "sleepiness" and poor feeding in the newborn for up to several hours depending on the total dose given to the mother.

Other sedatives and tranquilizers are sometimes used instead of or with narcotics. Most commonly used are hydroxycine (Vistaril®), promethazine (Phenergan®) and propiomazine (Largon®).

All of these are effective in reducing anxiety and cause little or no depression of the mother's breathing. Each has relative advantages and disadvantages. All cross the placenta and may cause varying effects on the fetus, such as floppiness, poor feeding and low body temperature. Some can cause a fall in the maternal blood pressure (and therefore in fetal oxygenation) and possible slowing of labor. Barbiturate drugs, although used in the past (especially in very early or false labor), are administered infrequently today.

Epidural Anesthesia

A very effective means of providing pain relief is to inject a local anesthetic (one of the "caine" drugs, such as chloroprocaine or bupivicaine) in the vicinity of a nerve or nerves that supply the painful area. An "epidural" very commonly used is one method of doing this. Epidural anesthesia involves inserting a needle into the back and injecting a "caine" drug into the area outside of the spinal canal called the "epidural space." Often a small plastic catheter is left in place so that, if the effect of the anesthetic wears off at some point during labor and delivery, more can be administered.

An epidural can be given when labor is well established and progressing and provides very good pain relief during labor and delivery, while having few effects on the fetus. Because it occasionally interferes with muscle function, limiting the mother's ability to bear down and help in pushing the baby out without assistance, the use of forceps may be indicated. Epidural anesthesia, also called "epidural block," may cause hypotension in the mother (low blood pressure) which is easily treated. Rarely, spinal headache may occur because of inadvertent puncture of the spinal canal.

Other Nerve Blocks

Paracervical block is a technique that can be used in the first stage of labor to relieve the pain caused by dilation of the cervix. It involves the injection of a local anesthetic into the area of the dilating cervix. Since the anesthetic may slow early labor, it is not used until labor is active and progressive.

Paracervical block does not produce good pain control during the second stage of labor, so another type of analgesia (pudendal or local block) may be used then. Also, this method is associated with temporary bradycardia (slowing of the fetal heart rate) for reasons that are not totally clear. Because of this, it is usually not used in complicated labors.

Pudendal block is a "nerve block" of the nerves involved in relaying pain in the second stage of labor due to the stretching of the vagina and perineum. Local anesthetic (a "caine") is injected through each side of the vagina into the area of the pudendal nerves. This type of block produces enough pain control for episiotomy and low-forceps delivery. There seem to be no ill-effects on the fetus from its use.

Local infiltration of the lower vagina and perineal area with a "caine" anesthetic just before delivery is often done as an analgesia for episiotomy, even though another type of pain control (narcotic, epidural) or natural childbirth was effective throughout earlier labor. This has virtually no fetal effect and allows both the episiotomy incision and repair to be performed with good pain control.

Spinal Anesthesia

Spinal anesthesia provides excellent and complete pain relief for vaginal delivery as well as cesarean birth. It involves injection of a local anesthetic (a "caine") into the spinal canal through the lower back. The mother is tilted to keep the anesthetic from flowing too far up the spine and just to the level needed for necessary pain relief. While total pain relief during labor as well as vaginal delivery is possible, the mother's muscles are also very weak or paralyzed, so assistance by forceps or vacuum extraction may be necessary.

The advantages are that the mother is awake and alert but free of pain. However, she may be at risk for hypotension, but this is usually easily remedied. A small number of women have "spinal headache" for a day or two afterward, although this occurs in much fewer than 10 percent when very small spinal needles are used. (The use of spinal anesthetic for cesarean delivery is discussed in Chapter 16.)

General Anesthesia

True general anesthesia, that is, anesthesia by injection or gas to produce unconsciousness, is uncommon for vaginal delivery today. It does, however, in very specific situations, have some usefulness. An IV is usually placed and a short-acting anesthetic administered. Once unconscious, the woman is immediately intubated (that is, an anesthetist inserts a tube into her windpipe) to prevent her from aspirating (inhaling) stomach contents and to maintain an open airway for delivery of oxygen and anesthetic gases.

Although general anesthesia can cause the newborn to be less alert and less vigorous at birth (often called "depressed" or "depression") this type of anesthesia may be necessary in certain situations. For example, if mid-forceps delivery needed to be done quickly because of fetal problems, and nerve block or another method was not possible, general anesthesia might be the best option. General anesthesia is also sometimes used to relax the uterus and allow for indicated manipulation of the fetus—such as with a second twin that needs to be turned or for relaxation of the cervix during vaginal breech delivery. It is also valuable in totally unmanageable patients (mentally retarded or hysterical).

Various methods of general anesthesia have been used in the past and still continue to have benefits in some situations. Certain gases can be inhaled by the mother to dull pain during a contraction, but these do not produce unconsciousness. This type of temporary pain relief might be used in very rapidly progressing labor along with local anesthetic for episiotomy. While relatively safe, occasionally this method will result in some neonatal depression (less vigor and activity) and more anesthesia than is usually desired in the mother.

The Risks and Benefits

While it might be possible and desirable for many women to avoid medication for pain during labor, analgesia and anesthesia can be safe and effective. With careful attention to timing, dosage and method, pain relief can make labor and delivery safely comfortable for the mother, even if high-risk. Studies show that both short- and long-term harmful effects on the fetus can be avoided by careful attention to the details of administration and monitoring as well as by prompt and efficient intervention if the infant is depressed at birth.

It is always best to discuss the use (or nonuse of analgesics and anesthetics with your doctor long before your due date (preferably early in pregnancy), to make sure both agree to the possible method(s) to be employed if deemed necessary or desirable during labor and delivery. You should have a frank discussion of the risks and benefits of each method, so you can make an informed judgment.

Complications of Labor

The best thing about almost all problems experienced during labor today is that medical intervention is possible, and results are for the most part excellent. In this section we will be discussing general categories of problems (not covered in earlier chapters) that can cause complications during labor.

As mentioned, the potential complications of labor can fairly easily be placed in general categories. These include complications due to: dystocia (the function or performance of the uterus or the size and shape of the pelvis); placental problems; position of the fetus; multiple births (twins, triplets, etc.); fetal problems due to such factors as abnormality, growth retardation, prematurity or disease; and the health status of the mother as well as the effect of any specific condition (diabetes, heart disease, etc.) on her well-being and that of the fetus.

Dystocia Due to Abnormal Function and Performance of the Uterus

The uterus obviously plays a major role during pregnancy, labor and delivery. In fact, this strong, specially designed precision muscle/organ is the mechanical driving force in labor. It is the uterus, its contractions and function during labor, that pushes the baby out into the new world (with the help of the mother, of course!). During labor, contractions must be strong enough to do their job but not too strong, and the uterus must be able to perform efficiently and effectively.

If the uterus is not performing properly and efficiently, labor can be unreasonably prolonged, endangering the health and well-being of both mother and baby. Since for most high-risk pregnancies electronic fetal heart rate monitoring is recommended, the fetal response throughout labor will be recorded and the mother closely monitored. If fetal distress or maternal problems develop and the labor has not progressed to the second stage, then an emergency cesarean birth would be recommended. If labor had progressed to the second stage, forceps delivery (with pain medication) would probably be the course of action recommended.

If the problem is due to contractions that are too weak, intervention would again be based on the stage of labor and how well the fetus and mother were tolerating labor so far. If contractions are quite weak, the cervix may not even dilate sufficiently to allow completion of the first stage of labor. Even if contractions are sufficient to completely dilate the cervix, they may not be adequate to push the baby down the birth canal and out.

If labor does not progress for any reason, it is simply called "failure to progress," and this always requires some form of intervention. If contractions are too weak, but the fetus and mother are tolerating labor well, the doctor may want to let the woman continue to labor (as long as baby and mother are well) with the assistance of oxytocin administration. (This is a hormone that stimulates contractions and increases their force and frequency.) In many cases this is all that is needed for labor to progress without further incident.

When oxytocin is used to stimulate labor, over-stimulation can be detected and corrected with continuous electronic fetal monitoring. It may be necessary to stop the oxytocin, give oxygen to the mother and change her position if over-stimulation is detected.

Rarely, contractions may be excessive even without oxytocin. Sometimes this is caused by premature separation of the placenta. If this is the case, and fetal distress occurs, it may be necessary to do a cesarean delivery in order to prevent the fetus's suffering from oxygen deprivation.

A general rule of obstetrics is not to allow the second stage of labor to exceed two to three hours and to intervene appropriately at any time in labor when fetal distress or maternal problems occur.

Dystocia Due to Abnormal Size and Shape of the Pelvis

If the shape of the pelvis is unusual or simply too small, complications of labor can occur. If the space (birth canal) between the pelvic bones is too small for the baby to fit through, the bony prominences of the pelvis intrude or the tailbone is in the way, for example, labor will not progress normally. These are called "outlet obstruction," and depending on the problem, the course of action will vary.

If progress in labor stops, and the bony prominences of the pelvis are involved, or the pelvis is too small in proportion to the baby's head (called "cephalopelvic disproportion," abbreviated CPD), the only course of action possible would be cesarean birth.

Ultrasound can be used to predict very large babies, because the chest size can be seen to exceed the head size by a significant amount. Especially in diabetic mothers, this can lead to "shoulder dystocia," where the head delivers but the shoulders get stuck. This is a very serious and often unpredictable complication. Because this potential problem is well-known for diabetic mothers ultrasound is usually performed before labor to determine if vaginal delivery would be safe or if cesarean delivery is necessary for the safety of both mother and baby. X ray measurements of pelvic size (called "x ray pelvimetry") is rarely used anymore, because it seldom helps in management and involves exposure of the fetus to small amounts of radiation.

Position of the Fetus

The normal delivery position of the baby is head down toward the pelvis. Called "cephalic presentation," this is the most advantageous position in terms of greater ease of delivery. About 85 percent of cephalic deliveries occur with the "occiput anterior" position. This means the back of the baby's head points to the front of the mother's pelvis, and the baby's face looks at the back of the vagina. About 10 to 15 percent of the time, the cephalic presentation occurs with the "occiput posterior." This is where the fetal face looks at the front of the mother's pelvis. This "posterior" position is often associated with a prolonged second stage of labor and may even require manual or forceps rotation and sometimes a cesarean delivery.

Basically, the fetus is free-floating in the uterus: He or she has enormous mobility due to the space and the protection of the amniotic fluid—and changes positions often. Many fetuses are found in unusual positions—including breech—until the last few weeks of pregnancy. Up until the 32nd week of gestation (around the 8th month), the doctor will usually not be too concerned, since the greatest number of those in a breech position or another unusual position will move to the cephalic presentation before delivery.

If your doctor suspects a breech or other unusual position (through physical examination), he or she may order an ultrasound for verification. One approach to patients with breech presentation after 37 weeks is to consider a "version." This is a procedure in which the fetus is turned by the physician by direct manipulation of the fetus abdominally. The procedure carries the risk of umbilical cord entanglement and, rarely, placental abruption. For this reason, all obstetricians don't agree that the benefit exceeds the risk. At the Women's Hospital in Long Beach, California, we have been using real-time ultrasound to monitor the fetus during the procedure and ritodrine (a uterine relaxant drug) to permit easier manipulation. We do the procedure in the hospital so that, if a complication occurs, we can do an immediate cesarean delivery. With this approach we can safely convert most breeches to cephalic presentations and allow a normal labor and delivery.

Breech and Other Unusual Presentations

In a "frank" breech presentation, the fetal buttocks are the presenting part (in the pelvis), and the legs extend straight out and up over the fetus's shoulders in the womb. A "double footling" breech is where both feet are the presenting parts, and the fetus "sits" on his or her haunches in the uterus. A "single footling" breech means that only one foot is down through the cervix, but the buttocks are downward.

In a frank breech presentation the buttocks are delivered first, with the legs, trunk, shoulders and head following. In a footling breech presentation the feet will be delivered first, followed by the legs, buttocks, trunk, shoulders and head.

In all breech deliveries the concern lies with delivering the baby's head—it's the largest part—safely and quickly. While most often term breech babies could be safely delivered vaginally, it is nearly impossible to determine for sure which ones would have problems prior to the actual delivery. Therefore, cesarean birth is commonly recommended, especially for first-time mothers.

A face presentation means that the face is the presenting part, with the fetus's neck extended back. The greatest problem with this is that the face doesn't mold well to the birth canal, as the crown of the head does. (This helps make the fetus's descent more efficient.) The extension of the neck makes the delivery more difficult and can possibly lead to fetal injury.

Another unusual problem is shoulder presentation, a type of transverse lie in which the shoulder is in the pelvis and is therefore the presenting part. The only course of action in this situation is scheduled cesarean birth if the condition is identified prior to labor or emergency cesarean delivery if it is recognized during labor. In effect, in a transverse lie the fetus is lying lengthwise in the lower portion of the uterus across the cervical opening. Nothing, then, is really in the pelvis. In some cases an arm or leg may "prolapse"—slip out—into the opening. With a transverse lie there is no way to deliver the fetus vaginally, and there is danger of uterine rupture if labor is allowed to continue. If an arm or foot has prolapsed into the birth canal, the umbilical cord may also slip out and place the fetus in jeopardy. Again, cesarean birth is the only answer. As the fetus is removed through the abdominal incision, the prolapsed part is carefully pulled back into the uterus and out through the incision.

More premature babies are born breech (as many as 25 percent at 30 weeks) than term babies (3.5 percent), since the fetus usually turns into the cephalic presentation as full-term approaches. Because the fetal head is relatively larger than the body in a premature baby, the risk of vaginal delivery is even greater than for a term breech. In addition more problems arise due to the complications associated with prematurity.

While prematurity is the most common factor associated with breech presentation, other causes may be implicated for babies' presenting as breech at term. If the fetus's head does not "fit" into the pelvis correctly (if it is too large), the fetus may accomodate by not changing into the cephalic presentation. If the umbilical cord is too short, the fetus may stay higher or in a different position in the uterus. Such conditions as fibroids, a two-horned uterus and other uterine abnormalities may prevent the fetus from moving easily into a cephalic presentation. If there is upper or midbirth canal obstruction—for some unknown reason—the fetus may adapt itself to the situation.

Breech presentation is also common for infants who have congenital malformations, especially of the head. For example, hydrocephalus ("water on the brain") or anencephaly (lack of brain development) often result in breech presentation. Hydrocephalus has this effect because the head is too large and anencephaly because the head is too small. Additionally, other congenital abnormalities (such as congenital hip dislocation) are associated with breech presentation but are probably the result rather than the cause of unusual position.

Years ago many babies in a breech or unusual position died, and many others experienced varying degrees of damage due to hypoxia and birth injury. Today, so much more is known about the various unusual positions and how and when to intervene (with refined instrumentation and much safer procedures) that the vast majority of babies do quite well.

With sophisticated diagnostic tools available to detect potential problems, some obstetricians argue that most of the time the delivery procedure can be pre-planned: Allow the mother to labor if all indications point to an uncomplicated breech delivery; if delivery becomes complicated (without warning), perform an emergency cesarean birth immediately; or schedule a cesarean birth as close to term as possible for the safety of mother and/or baby. There is a growing consensus among many obstetricians that, even with careful selection, one cannot guarantee a non-traumatic vaginal delivery.

It is usually recommended that all breeches over 26 weeks gestation be delivered by cesarean section (if delivery is necessary or the mother goes into labor). See chapter 16.

Placental Problems

As discussed in Chapter 13, when the blood flow to the uterus is decreased, a condition known as "uteroplacental insufficiency" may result. Certain patients are at much higher risk for this complication than others (for example, women with hypertension or diabetes and those with prolonged pregnancies); therefore, testing would be started long before labor. Since uterine contractions further decrease uterine blood flow, these patients need careful electronic fetal monitoring during labor.

Should a contraction stress test indicate uteroplacental insufficiency, and the baby is sufficiently mature, delivery may be indicated. In this situation labor can sometimes be induced, but continuous fetal monitoring is a must. In any patient being monitored during labor, if uteroplacental insufficiency develops and can't be corrected, cesarean delivery is indicated, because more uterine contractions would only make the situation worse.

Even patients without known risk factors may develop unexpected signs of uteroplacental insufficiency during labor. One can therefore make a case for monitoring all laboring patients, as we do at Women's Hospital in Long Beach. Patients who require oxytocin during labor can benefit from electronic monitoring, because sometimes the labor produced by oxytocin exceeds the uteroplacental reserve of that patient.

If placenta previa occurs (meaning that a portion or all of the placenta covers the cervix or is lying in the lower portion of the uterus near the cervix), safe vaginal delivery is not possible. In this position the placenta not only blocks the fetus's mode of exit but usually partially separates from the uterus as the cervix dilates. This may result in massive hemorrhage that can threaten both mother and child. In this situation Cesarean delivery is necessary.

With placenta previa there is usually no pain with the bleeding, and it may either appear as simple spotting or be quite heavy. Any time bleeding or spotting occurs, you should contact your doctor immediately. If bleeding is severe, it is imperative that you seek appropriate medical care at once.

Sometimes the normally located placenta may separate prematurely. This is called "placental abruption." As the placenta separates, blood accumulates between the placenta and the uterine wall.

With massive abruption, the baby often dies, and the mother may suffer from a condition called "disseminated intravascular coagulation" caused by substances released by the separated placenta. This condition is very serious, because patients lose their ability to clot, and hemorrhage is further aggravated. Cesarean delivery and blood transfusion are often necessary when managing this very serious complication. Fetal death may be due to either uteroplacental insufficiency or prematurity.

The Bottom Line on Labor and Delivery

The most important thing for you to remember about labor and delivery is that *you* are in control. By learning all you can about the process and events of labor and delivery, the potential problems and the corresponding modes of intervention for your safety and that of your baby, you can better prepare yourself and be in control of the big event.

FIFTEEN

DRUGS USED TO STOP PREMATURE LABOR AND THOSE USED TO PROMOTE FETAL LUNG MATURITY

Prematurity (with all its potential problems) has always been a major cause of fetal and neonatal death and disability. Also, infants whose birth weight is low, because of either prematurity or fetal growth retardation, have been shown to have a greater incidence of neurological problems and intellectual deficiencies. Although great strides have been made in saving many premature babies and increasing the quality of life for countless others, the real answer to the problem of prematurity is the prevention of preterm labor. ("Premature" and "preterm" labor are synonymous.) Although more is known about labor today than ever before, the exact physiological and biochemical mechanisms of premature (and term) labor as well as their timing and order are not completely understood.

It appears that many endocrine (hormone-related) and physical changes in both the mother and the fetus play a significant role in the onset of labor. In the vast majority of pregnancies, these physical and biochemical events occur once the fetus has reached maturity (term). If not, we would be seeing a greater number of premature births.

Part of the reason for premature labor may be that the set of circumstances that leads to term labor may be quite different from that which is responsible for prematurity. No one quite knows yet. When it comes to premature labor, then, the real questions are: "What" triggers preterm labor? and "What" can be done to block this triggering mechanism or prevent this set of circumstances? Finding the answers to these questions will require further research to identify the exact mechanisms of labor (their order and timing), to detect labor's onset early, and to develop an effective form of intervention to countermand the various forces and events at work in the process of abnormally early labor. Until more is known and all the questions are answered, doctors are now using certain drugs (with some success) to halt premature labor as much as possible. As more research continues, it may someday be possible to identify the earliest warning signs of premature labor and effectively and safely stop this process entirely.

Obviously, the best answer to the many problems of prematurity is stopping preterm labor so the fetus can mature in the most natural and beneficial environment—his or her mother's womb—until full gestation is reached. But what if premature labor cannot be stopped for an extended period of time? The second part of the puzzle: Is there a means by which fetal lung maturity can be rapidly promoted when premature labor and delivery are inevitable? There has been some progress in this area and research continues. Although the drug now in clinical trials in the United States may not be *the* answer for all mothers in premature labor (and their babies)—its discovery seems to be a giant step in the right direction.

Drugs to Stop Premature Labor (Tocolytic Agents)

As discussed in detail in Chapter 2, there are certain factors that tend to predispose a pregnancy to premature labor. These include placental abruption, placenta previa, multiple gestation (twins, triplets, etc.), eclampsia (hypertension of pregnancy), liver disease, kidney disease, heart disease, a history of two or more previous premature births, incompetent cervix, fetal malformations, premature rupture of the membranes, cigarette smoking and even socioeconomic conditions (poor nutrition and lack of proper prenatal care). Some studies have shown an association between premature labor and alcohol consumption, genital infections, small stature in the woman, poor physical condition, physical and psychological stress, fetal hypoxia and possibly even genetic makeup.

Some of these predisposing factors can be alleviated, and some others can be managed successfully. With a few, little can be done to prevent and/or control them. The risk of premature delivery with placenta previa, multiple gestation, eclampsia, some maternal conditions (liver disease, kidney diseases, etc.), incompetent cervix, infections and some causes of fetal hypoxia may be modified or prevented with proper perinatal care and management. Those that can be eliminated by the woman herself include cigarette smoking, alcohol consumption, repetitive elective abortions, poor nutrition, neglectful prenatal care and poor physical condition. Those factors that women can do little or nothing about include their genetic makeup, some fetal malformations, placental abruption and their physical stature.

Nonetheless, even with careful management and the alleviation of some predisposing factors, premature labor still occurs. Doctors needed a means of stopping preterm labor (if at all possible) to allow greater fetal maturity. Although research continues on the mechanisms of labor (which, once they are completely identified, can tell us more about how to stop labor), early observations made it clear that a few classes of drugs appeared to have some ability to suppress uterine activity. When premature labor occurs, administration of medication, along with bed rest when indicated, is presently the favored means of intervention.

Drugs used for halting labor are called "tocolytic agents" ("toko" means labor or childbirth, and "lytic" means stop)—therefore, agents to stop labor. The classes of drugs employed for this purpose act differently and have varying degrees of success.

Ethanol (Intravenous Alcohol)

In 1965 the first report was published regarding the use of ethanol (intravenous alcohol) as an agent to stop premature labor. Although studies vary in their findings regarding the effect of ethanol on premature labor, most agree that it inhibits the secretion of oxytocin (a hormone that stimulates uterine contractions), is a central nervous system suppressant and probably has a specific effect on the uterine muscle itself.

What is seen during alcohol administration is a gradual but definite decrease in the intensity and frequency of uterine activity. In the majority of patients, uterine activity ceases soon after the administration of ethanol. However, this drug does not appear to be as effective as other agents and produces troublesome side effects, such as headache, nausea, vomiting and the unpleasant feeling of intoxication. With the present availability of better drugs, ethanol is less frequently used as a measure to stop premature labor.

Prostaglandin Inhibitors

Basically, prostaglandin inhibitors are anti-inflammatory agents used to prevent or slow down the synthesis or production of prostaglandins, which are a group of body hormones. Although no one is quite sure what role prostaglandins play in labor, they seem to be synthesized more during labor and have been found in the mother's blood as well as in the amniotic fluid.

Aspirin is a prostaglandin inhibitor. One study on the long-term effects of aspirin use in pregnancy showed that the drug prolonged gestation, as well as slowed labor when it occurred. The results were confirmed in another study, but chronic aspirin intake was also found to be associated with other potential maternal and fetal problems. Animal studies show that indomethacin, another prostaglandin inhibitor used in the treatment of arthritis, can also inhibit uterine contractions with few maternal side effects but has been associated with potentially serious fetal problems. Since there appears to be a potential for serious side effects and complications, prostaglandin inhibitors should not be used as a means to prevent or control premature labor until more research is performed. There are other agents available that appear to be both safer and more effective.

Progestins (Progesterone-Like Compounds)

It is interesting that a predominantly male hormone (progesterone) would be considered the "pregnancy-maintaining hormone," described as such in 1929. The relationship of progesterone and labor is as follows: Animal studies show that the level of progesterone in the mother's blood decreases before spontaneous labor occurs. This theory, which suggests that premature labor would occur if progesterone were to fall too early in pregnancy, is based on the previously mentioned studies but has not been confirmed with any consistency in initial human studies.

Nevertheless, some studies have now shown that the administration of 17-hydroxyprogesterone (17αOHP-C) to patients at high risk for premature labor may decrease that risk. However, there is concern that certain progestins (compounds chemically related to the naturally secreted progesterone hormone) may be teratogenic if given in the first three months of pregnancy. Therefore, when 17αOHP-C is used, administration should not begin until the fourth month of pregnancy or later.

Betasympathomimetics (Beta-adrenergic Agents)

When adrenalin—an adrenal gland secretion that acts on the sympathetic nervous system—is released, it has a specific effect on cell and organ activity. Research has shown that adrenalin has a great deal to do with uterine activity. While adrenalin is usually regarded as a stimulant—it acts as a relaxant for the uterus. That may seem like a contradiction—but it's not. Here's why.

Over the years two types of cellular receptors—places where adrenalin acts—have been identified. These are called "alpha receptors" (α receptors) and "beta receptors" (β receptors). In the uterus stimulation of α receptors results in excitement, and stimulation of the β receptors leads to relaxation. Beta receptors can be further subdivided into α_1 and β_2 receptors, based on the organs in which they are found. β_1 receptors are found in the heart, and β_2 receptors are found in the uterine muscle as well as in other organs, such as the lungs.

What was needed to control premature labor was an agent that stimulated the β_2 receptors without exciting the β_1 or α receptors. The drugs developed that have this characteristic are called "betasympathomimetic" or "beta-adrenergic" agents—or simply "betamimetic"—in other words, agents that "mimic" the β_2 activity of adrenalin and relax the uterus.

Ritodrine, isoxsuprine, terbutaline, fenoterol, salbutamol and orciprenaline are some of the beta-sympathomimetic drugs that are available. These drugs have been selected for tocolysis because they have relatively more β_2 than β_1 activity—that is, they relax the uterus but still have some effect on cardiovascular function. Isoxsuprine was the first betamimetic agent available in the United States, but some other newer agents appear to be more suitable.

Ritodrine is actually the only drug that has undergone extensive evaluation by the FDA (Food and Drug Administration) leading to its approval as a uterine relaxant in the United States. The use of ritodrine was approved in Austria in 1972, and approval followed in 1973 in the Netherlands, Switzerland, Spain and Belgium. Seventeen other countries approved the use of the drug between 1974 and 1978 because of the results of a 1971 seven-hospital collaborative study in four European countries, as well as many earlier studies performed internationally. Even with such excellent results, the drug was not approved by the FDA until 1979, when a 10-year study was completed. (Ritodrine was approved in the USSR in 1979, as well.)

Usually the administration of ritodrine intravenously decreases uterine contractions rather quickly. Once all contractions have ceased, the IV infusion is continued for 12 to 24 hours. Administration of the drug by mouth is begun 30 minutes before the IV administration is concluded, and if this oral treatment continues to be effective, the woman will take the ritodrine every 4 to 6 hours until she reaches term.

Therapy may be stopped if a maternal or fetal problem occurs (usually not associated with the drug's use) that requires immediate delivery when identified. If premature labor recurs during oral administration of ritodrine, IV infusion can be started again if there are no maternal or fetal problems that would make it unwise to postpone labor.

Although there are some side effects with ritodrine's use, for the majority of women these are minor and tolerable. Women have experienced one or more mild cardiovascular effects (increased heart rate, palpitations, nervousness, tremor, higher pulse pressure and/or an increase in cardiac output) and similarly mild bronchial effects. One or more of these side effects may occur during IV administration, but they are less prominent when a woman is on the oral maintenance stage of therapy. A temporary rise in maternal blood glucose and plasma insulin may also be seen during IV administration. This means that ritodrine must be used with care and with cautious monitoring in diabetic mothers. (In most situations ritodrine is not used at all in diabetic mothers.)

The greatest concern about the use of ritodrine is the problem of pulmonary edema (fluid accumulation in the lungs, usually in association with heart failure). Although pulmonary edema is an infrequent complication of ritodrine use, it can be a serious one. Pulmonary edema due to ritodrine administration can usually be reversed rapidly by stopping the drug and administering diuretics (medications that cause the body to eliminate excess water).

One plus is that the fetus appears to do very well with ritodrine. While the drug may mildly increase the fetal heart rate (by up to nine beats per minute, on the average), this is basically insignificant and has no adverse effects on fetal well-being. Some of the clinical studies carried out with ritodrine involved the followup of babies born to mothers who received the drug. No serious adverse effects could be attributed to the drug.

Women who would not be candidates for ritodrine intervention are those with hyperthyroidism, obvious heart disease, eclampsia or severe pre-eclampsia, intrauterine infection, severe vaginal bleeding, often women with diabetes or any other medical problem in which labor and delivery should not be postponed.

Currently many obstetricians believe ritodrine to be the drug of choice for women who experience premature labor and for whom intervention to stop labor would be beneficial. Effective in approximately 70 percent of premature labors, it is relatively safe for both the mother and her fetus. Other betamimetics (terbutaline, fenoterol, salbutamol and orciprenaline) are available but have not been as extensively studied as ritodrine and need further investigation.

Magnesium Sulfate

Magnesium sulfate has long been used as a treatment for toxemia (hypertension) during labor and delivery. Doctors also noticed that uterine contractions slowed when intravenous magnesium sulfate was administered at that time. They found that it acts on the uterine muscle itself and has fewer side effects than betamimetic drugs (but magnesium sulfate can cause pulmonary edema). As is the case with ritodrine, pulmonary edema due to the administration of magnesium sulfate can be reversed.

Magnesium sulfate is administered first in a large dose over five to ten minutes intravenously. The woman usually feels very warm and flushed at this point. The treatment is then continued by intravenous infusion. Often the patient is somewhat sedated by the effect of the drug. The fetus is not adversely affected by magnesium sulfate and the newborn, while occasionally a little limp at birth, does not show any serious side effects.

Magnesium sulfate appears to be approximately equal to ritodrine in its effectiveness but has fewer side effects. Also, it is not contraindicated in women with heart disease, toxemia or diabetes. For these reasons we prefer magnesium sulfate as our drug of choice to stop premature labor.

The Pros and Cons of Drugs to Control Premature Labor

It is often difficult for anyone not in medicine to sort out the pros and cons of one drug as opposed to another. For those involved in health care, this choice is at times very clear-cut. At other times these decisions are not so simple and are based on many factors— research results, the woman's medical history, her present condition and needs, the risks and benefits for this specific situation, the physician's experience with a drug or drugs, and personal preference when available drugs are similar.

However, for the reasons stated previously, we consider magnesium sulfate to be the drug of choice, but may use ritodrine if magnesium sulfate fails. Others prefer ritodrine. Terbutaline is much cheaper than ritodrine and appears to be very similar in efficacy and side effects. It is not approved by the FDA for tocolysis, but is available for the treatment of asthma. It is commonly prescribed because of its low cost, however, for the treatment of premature labor. The other betamimetics are seldom if ever used in this country.

Drugs to Promote Fetal Lung Maturity

In the majority of cases, inhibiting premature labor and allowing the fetus to reach term (as near as possible) are important in reducing fetal and neonatal death or serious disability. It is estimated that 8 percent of deliveries will occur prematurely—that represents approximately 240,000 neonates per year in the United States. Around 75 percent of perinatal deaths (fetal and neonatal) are due to a long list of problems resulting from or associated with prematurity. Therefore, it would be quite advantageous for a pregnancy to be prolonged to term, unless there were specific reasons why the risks of prematurity were less than those of trying to prolong pregnancy.

Obviously, our goal is to be able to avoid prematurity by preventing or stopping premature labor, but often tocolytic agents like ritodrine or magnesium sulfate will only work for a few hours or days. For this reason it is desirable to have some method available which can help accelerate fetal maturity in order to better prepare the fetus for survival outside the protection of the womb.

Many premature babies suffer from respiratory distress syndrome. We know that the fetus' lungs mature in the last few weeks of pregnancy, so infants born prematurely will often have immature lungs. The more premature the infant, the more likely that it will have lungs that are not sufficiently developed to support it outside the mother's womb. Other organs are immature, as well. The result: Many premature infants die, and those that do not, often experience serious lifelong disabilities. While newborn intensive care units and advances in neonatal medicine have made a difference in these rates, other strategies were needed to better ensure the newborn's safety and well-being.

A major breakthrough came from Graham C. Liggins, MD, a professor of obstetrics and gynecology at National Women's Hospital in Auckland, New Zealand. Dr. Liggins has been instrumental in studying the use of glucocorticoids—in particular the drug betamethasone—to speed up the process of lung maturation in the fetus. What's really amazing is that in 24 to 72 hours (72 hours is ideal), betamethasone can actually accelerate fetal lung development to a degree that usually takes several weeks in the womb.

Interestingly, Dr. Liggins discovered betamethasone's life-saving ability by accident. He was studying the mechanisms that control labor when he and his colleagues stumbled on the mechanism that controls fetal organ development. Using sheep, he found that the fetal lamb produced increasing amounts of a hormone called "cortisone" secreted by the adrenal glands as it came closer to term. It was noted that the increasing secretion of this hormone accelerated the development of major fetal organs required for the lamb's survival outside the womb, particularly the lungs. It seemed that this hormone also determines (in part) the time of the onset of labor.

Cortisone, then, appeared to play a significant role in organ development and the beginning of labor. Dr. Liggins found that if the adrenal gland of the fetal lamb was removed or the secretion of cortisone suppressed, labor would not begin, and the pregnancy would continue far beyond the time of full term. He also discovered that by stimulating the adrenal gland or injecting cortisone or betamethasone (a synthetic drug similar to cortisone) into the mother, labor could be initiated at any stage in the pregnancy. But most impressive was the fact that very tiny premature lambs who probably should not have lived did indeed survive because the drug had stimulated the maturation of their organs—most importantly the lungs.

In 1970 human studies of betamethasone began in New Zealand. Unlike fetal lambs, who had to be directly injected with the synthetic hormone, human fetuses could receive the drug through the placenta after it was administered to the mother. In this way there was no disruption of the fetus. Dr. Liggins' preliminary and long-term results, as well as results obtained internationally, have been promising. Even the very smallest of babies—1,000 grams or less (just a little over two pounds or less) at birth appear to benefit.

Betamethasone has not as yet been approved by the Food and Drug Administration in the United States. However, certain investigators (including our hospital) have been involved in clinical trials of this drug. So far, what this major breakthrough has meant is our ability to administer betamethasone to stimulate fetal lung development when premature labor has begun. The drug is administered over 24 to 72 hours while labor is temporarily stopped. This approach might be indicated in situations where prolonging the pregnancy over an extended period of time would not be advisable (for maternal or fetal reasons) or would not be possible, or in borderline situations where fetal viability is possible but prematurity is inevitable. Essentially, betamethasone administration may give the baby a jump on the problems of prematurity by maturing the lungs more quickly. Thus, the premature infant has a better chance of survival.

However, since corticosteroids appear to have such a profound effect on fetal lung development, the question of other effects (possibly adverse) is raised. Some animal studies have suggested adverse effects on the central nervous system, the immune system and overall fetal-neonatal growth. The long-term followup studies completed to date on human fetuses do not show any adverse effects. However, DES (another hormone used twenty to thirty years ago during pregnancy with no apparent adverse effects at the time) does not show its complications until after puberty in young women who were exposed to this drug during their gestation. While the proven beneficial effects appear to outweigh the risk of possible developmental abnormalities, we always have women sign a special consent indicating that they understand that the long-term effects of corticosteroids are not yet fully known. The clinical trials are continuing and follow-up studies are being performed to see if betamethasone is part of the answer to fetal lung maturity.

The Bottom Line

Tocolytic drugs and betamethasone (in particular) have been instrumental in reducing the devastating effects of prematurity. Tocolytic drugs with their ability to inhibit premature labor, and betamethasone with its ability to accelerate fetal lung maturity, have increased the likelihood of survival for many infants who would heretofore have died because of the devastating problems of prematurity or been crippled by serious lifelong disabilities. Although these drugs are not cure-alls for every problem of prematurity and are not 100 percent effective, they do represent great progress and promise for more successful intervention in premature birth.

SIXTEEN

AN IMPORTANT ANSWER TO SOME PROBLEMS: CESAREAN BIRTH

For thousands of years, cesarean delivery was deemed the last resort—the ultimate and only means of intervention possible to save the baby when there was no way to save the mother, or when the mother had died from illness or injury.

In fact, this was such a well-accepted set of circumstances that when a Virginia doctor performed a cesarean on his wife in 1794, he did not report it because he feared no one would believe his wife and the baby had actually lived! In the late 1800s one American medical historian noted that a woman had a mere 10 percent chance of surviving if cesarean birth was performed. The odds were not good for the mother and only slightly better for the baby. The procedure was rightfully feared.

As medical knowledge increased and more sophisticated technology was developed, the surgery became progressively safer. As is true of all surgery, greater safety came with the discovery of the importance of antiseptic (sterile) conditions, better anesthetics, antibiotics, improvements in surgical instrumentation and techniques, methods to control bleeding, postoperative observation and management, and pain control.

By the 1960s maternal mortality (death) due to cesarean birth was an extremely rare occurrence (as was maternal mortality in general). The emphasis began to shift from the primary protection of the mother to the increasing attempts to protect the fetus from death or damage, as well—a change from a one-patient strategy (protection of the mother) to a two-patient strategy (protection of both mother and fetus). This milestone in obstetrical care was made possible because of enormous technological advances, extensive research and greater knowledge.

People began asking why more could not be done to prevent fetal death and reduce permanent damage when death did not occur. Public pressure demanded answers and solutions. Due in great part to these public demands and encouragement, much of today's technology was developed.

Why Cesarean Birth?

Where does cesarean birth fit into all this technology and the emphasis on protecting both mother and fetus? As much more was understood about fetal growth and development, the causes for intrauterine problems and the ability to better diagnose problems early—various means of intervention were developed. An answer to some problems was cesarean birth (often called "cesarean section" or "C-section").

The premise was this: If intervention could occur early—then the outcome might well be markedly improved. Since a multitude of advances had made cesarean delivery a much safer alternative when problems occurred, the rate of cesarean delivery increased fairly rapidly.

Cesarean birth is considered a potential alternative in the following situations:

- Dystocia (abnormal labor) due to a variety of causes, such as cephalopelvic disproportion, unusual or abnormal presentation (for example, breech position), obstruction in the birth canal or inadequate contractions of the uterus
- Placental problems
- Various maternal illnesses, chronic illnesses or problems, such as hypertension, diabetes, kidney disease and others
- Fetal distress
- Fetal illness or abnormalities, such as Rh disease or some congenital defects
- Previous cesarean delivery—"repeat cesarean"

In all these situations the well-being of both the mother and the child must be taken into account. The reason(s) for and potential benefit(s) of the cesarean delivery must always be carefully weighed against the known or potential risk(s). When the health and well-being of the baby are involved, the procedure is performed in an attempt to prevent fetal death, avoid brain and other damage or disability, and improve the quality of life as much as possible. There are also situations where the mother's life and/or well-being may be jeopardized due to a known problem or suddenly compromised due to an unforseen problem.

Often cesarean birth simply cannot be avoided since maternal and/or fetal death would be inevitable or imminent without it. At other times the decision to perform cesarean delivery is not based on such "absolutes," in which scheduled or emergency cesarean is the only answer. Rather, the obstetrician's recommendation for cesarean must be based on his or her judgment with respect to the information at hand—it may be judged to be the safest alternative, given the individual circumstances in this pregnancy.

In some situations the need for cesarean delivery is known in advance of the start of labor. When this is the case, the timing of the operation will be based on the reason(s) for the cesarean as well as the maturity of the fetus. This allows the woman and her mate to psychologically prepare themselves in advance for the cesarean birth.

In other situations there is little or no warning that a cesarean will be necessary. Labor may not progress well for mother or baby, or a serious problem may develop, necessitating immediate intervention. Such an emergency cesarean—often called a "crash" cesarean—may be lifesaving for the mother, baby or both.

Dystocia (Abnormal Labor)

Dystocia is a term that simply means abnormal labor (from the Greek "dys," meaning abnormal, and "toko," meaning labor or childbirth). Dystocia, which can have a variety of causes, accounts for about one-fourth of cesareans done in the United States. This broad category of problems is also responsible for much of the rise in the cesarean birth rate seen over the past decade.

Progress of labor can be poor because of mechanical problems, such as abnormalities of the mother's pelvis, a baby that is too large for vaginal delivery, or an abnormal or unusual fetal position. In other cases uterine function is poor, and contractions are not effective in dilating the cervix and moving the baby down the birth canal. In either situation "failure to progress" in labor may lead to a recommendation for cesarean delivery.

Fetal presentation other than the cephalic, or "head down," position is often associated with abnormal progress of labor. Breech presentation, which occurs in about 3 percent to 5 percent of all deliveries, accounts for a large number of recommended cesarean deliveries, and there is an increasing trend in this direction. We know that breech babies have more problems than cephalic presentation babies regardless of whether they are delivered vaginally or by cesarean. (Breech is more common with prematurity, fetal malformations and multiple gestation.) Most obstetricians feel cesarean birth is safer because those problems due to birth trauma (especially with very large or premature babies) can be avoided completely. Term breech babies delivered by cesarean do not have greater morbidity or mortality.

The greatest problem with vaginal delivery of a baby in the breech position is usually the uncertainty about whether the baby's head can be delivered easily and safely. The breech (buttocks and hips) is smaller than the head and therefore presents little difficulty in delivery. However, there is danger that the head will not be able to be delivered easily and will require difficult, prolonged manipulation. Furthermore, there is some suggestion that the overextension (extreme bending backward) of the baby's head that occurs during vaginal delivery of a breech baby may lead to decreased blood flow through the arteries that supply the brain or may cause injury to the spinal cord in the baby's neck. The result in either case may be permanent neurologic damage to the baby.

While most women could probably successfully deliver a normal-sized term breech baby vaginally, it is impossible to accurately predict before the baby's head is stuck which ones will not be successful. Unfortunately, once the head is stuck, cesarean delivery is impossible, because the baby's body has already been delivered and cannot be pulled back up through the birth canal. Often special forceps are successful in safely delivering the difficult aftercoming-head. But once the head is trapped either by the cervix or the bony pelvis, the risk for fetal injury increases markedly.

Because of this potentially serious problem, many doctors feel that if the baby cannot be rotated (through external manipulation) to the cephalic presentation, a scheduled cesarean delivery is the best alternative, especially in a first pregnancy. (In a first pregnancy the pelvis has not been tested.) On the other hand, with those women who have already had one or more children vaginally without any problems, the doctor may be more likely to consider a trial of labor.

Premature or very small babies who are in breech position at the time of labor present a special concern. Breech presentation is more common in premature labor (25 percent at 30 weeks) than at term—

and as many as 15 percent (on the average) of all prematures are breech. The problem arises because the premature fetus's head is proportionately *much* larger than the breech and the shoulders. Consequently, the head may become stuck, because the much smaller buttocks and body can slip through a cervix that is incompletely dilated, but the head cannot pass. The only alternative at this point is a potentially life-threatening extraction and potentially serious trauma to the cervix and birth canal. For this reason most obstetricians opt for cesarean delivery when premature delivery of a breech baby is inevitable.

In some abnormal presentations (for example, transverse lie), vaginal delivery is impossible, and the forces of labor may put the mother at risk for rupture of the uterus. In others potential complications like prolapse of the umbilical cord are very common. In still others the mechanical difficulties caused by the fetal position require some sort of intervention. In all of these situations cesarean birth may be the safest (or only) way to preserve the fetus and prevent unusually difficult, prolonged labors.

While some causes of dystocia (abnormal labor) may be identified prior to the start of labor, others are not detected until labor has begun. In a typical situation of dystocia, labor proceeds for some time and the cervix begins to dilate, but then progress slows down or stops altogether. Two common causes of this failure to progress are cephalopelvic disproportion (CPD) and ineffective uterine muscle contraction (both discussed previously).

Failure to progress may occur at any time (depending on the cause) during the dilatation of the cervix or the descent of the fetus. Unless it is obvious or suspected that a baby is very large, the doctor may try to stimulate effective labor once again, as long as the fetus shows no sign of distress.

Such measures as resting the mother, increasing her fluid intake, walking or administering mild sedation may be enough for effective contractions to resume. Artificial rupture of the membranes, if still intact, often causes labor to continue actively. Oxytocin may be administered, with monitoring of the fetal heart rate and uterine contractions, in order to stimulate more effective contractions. If active labor resumes again, such measures would continue until delivery, as long as fetal distress did not occur and labor was not dangerously prolonged. (Prolonged active labor is associated with increases risks to the mother and child. With prolonged rupture of the membranes and poor labor progress, the risk of infection increases significantly. Damage to the fetus is unlikely if fetal hypoxia has not occurred and if no manipulation of the fetus is necessary.)

If oxytocin and other measures fail, if the mother tires significantly or if fetal distress occurs at any time, the doctor may feel cesarean delivery is necessary in order to preserve both mother and baby. This requires a judgment based on all available data: At what point is intervention necessary for the well-being and safety of the mother, the baby or both?

Placental Problems

Placenta previa, in which the placenta is positioned completely over the cervical opening, is a situation in which cesarean birth is absolutely necessary. Cesarean birth is planned at about 37 to 38 weeks gestation if fetal maturity is documented, unless massive bleeding or the start of labor occurs requiring earlier delivery.

Placenta previa presents two distinct obstacles to vaginal delivery. First, the placenta itself prevents the delivery of the baby by obstructing the cervix. In addition, if labor begins, it is likely that part of the placenta would be torn away from the wall of the uterus as the cervix dilates. With each contraction, the blood vessels near the cervix are pulled or torn, causing hemorrhage. An emergency cesarean would be necessary to save the endangered mother and fetus.

Placental abruption is another situation that requires emergency cesarean delivery. There is usually no warning when placental abruption occurs—the placenta suddenly tears off the wall of the uterus, either partially or completely. The woman experiences severe, sudden pain and perhaps a sudden gush of blood from the vagina. Without intervention she may progress into severe shock because of the blood loss.

With profuse bleeding comes collapse of the mother and a serious reduction of the oxygen supply to her fetus. The fetus itself is not usually bleeding, because blood loss comes from the mother's side of the placenta. But with its mother's blood loss and shock, the fetus experiences degrees of hypoxia. Both mother and fetus are in imminent danger of death or permanent damage. Vaginal delivery is possible with placental abruption if the fetal monitor indicates no fetal distress, and the mother is stable and laboring satisfactorily.

Maternal Conditions

Some *maternal conditions and illnesses* lead to the recommendation of cesarean section for the safety of the mother, the fetus or both.

Conditions that limit the mother's ability to withstand the stress of labor—for example, *severe heart or lung disease*—are best managed by scheduled cesarean birth at the time of the fetus is mature.

Scheduled cesarean delivery is an important part of the management of the problems experienced by the *diabetic mother* and her fetus. As many as 25 percent of babies of diabetic mothers may die after the 38th week of pregnancy. In order to reduce this risk, at least in part, the diabetes must be tightly controlled before pregnancy occurs and throughout the pregnancy. Additionally, testing of the fetus takes place as early as the 26th week of the pregnancy. Amniocentesis is performed to determine fetal lung maturity, a Contraction Stress Test (CST) is done weekly to evaluate fetal fitness and plasma estriol is evaluated—often daily—to further determine fetal well-being.

The baby is then delivered by scheduled cesarean at about the 38th week. The precise time of delivery is based on a determination of fetal lung maturity and on an assessment of fetal well-being. Because of early delivery and because fetuses of diabetic mothers are often very large, cesarean delivery rates usually run high in diabetics.

Active infection of the mother with *genital herpes (herpes simplex type 2)* puts the fetus at risk for serious infection if delivered vaginally. Such risk can be significantly reduced by well-timed cesarean delivery. In fact, the use of cesarean delivery to reduce this risk is increasing each year with the rise in herpes simples 2 genital infections.

Prolonged rupture of the membranes—for over 24 hours, or so—is associated with an increased risk of infection within the amniotic sac (called "amnionitis")—a risk for both mother and fetus. The mother is at risk for uterine infection and the baby for pneumonia, sepsis (generalized infection) and other serious, life-threatening infections. When the threat to either becomes great, especially if labor has not progressed enough to allow prompt vaginal delivery, cesarean delivery is recommended.

Another example where judgment may be needed is in severe *hypertension with toxemia.* In some situations labor may be progressing in its first stage, but there is difficulty in controlling the woman's blood pressure (even with medication). Severe hypertension during labor can cause difficulties for both mother and fetus. Although both may survive the labor, the doctor must consider the potential risks for brain damage for the fetus and other complications for the mother. The placenta may be compromised by the high blood pressure, thereby affecting the fetal blood supply and oxygenation, and oxygenation of the fetus may become too marginal to risk a continuation of labor. The potential risks to the mother include possible seizures, impending kidney failure and increased intracranial pressure, ultimately even leading to cerebral hemorrhage because of the severe hypertension.

Obviously, these extreme complications of toxemia are rare, but they can occur. The obstetrician must make judgments based on the situation at the time—the status of the mother and baby and the potential risks—and weigh these against the relatively low risks associated with cesarean delivery.

Fetal Distress

Since the advent of electronic fetal heart rate monitoring in the 1970s, the number of cesarean deliveries performed because of *fetal distress* has increased by about 10 to 15 percent. This increase is probably due to improved identification of fetal distress and the greatly increased safety of the cesarean birth procedure for both mother and baby. Also, since fetal heart rate monitoring is still relatively new, the increase may be due in part to some misinterpretation of the fetal monitoring data.

Before electronic fetal heart rate monitoring, fetal distress could not be as easily identified during labor. Identification of fetal problems was based on listening to the fetal heart through a stethoscope, usually between contractions. Because of the difficulty in interpreting what was heard, infants were often deprived of adequate oxygen for prolonged periods before this was detected. With increased utilization of fetal heart rate monitoring for both high-risk and low-risk pregnancies, as well as more experience in interpreting fetal heart rate patterns, fetal distress can be detected much earlier and its signs interpreted with more accuracy and assurance. Because of the improved safety of cesarean birth itself, prompt delivery of a distressed fetus is now favored and is a rational course of action.

The causes of fetal distress are many, as previously discussed. Often the causes of the distress lead to *gradual* fetal compromise, which gives the doctor time to try to correct the cause. If, however, the distress continues or worsens, prompt cesarean delivery would be required, especially during the first stage of labor (before complete cervical dilatation).

Some complications of labor may lead to a sudden, devastating decrease in the oxygen supply to the fetus—followed by severe fetal distress and impending fetal death. An example of such a situation in which there is no option but to perform a cesarean delivery immediately is worthy of a detailed discussion.

If at 35 weeks gestation a woman went into labor, the baby—although it would be premature—would be mature enough to survive, so attempts to stop labor might not be made. If the fetus had not engaged in the pelvis as yet, and the membranes had not ruptured, then the fetus would be floating freely in the uterus.

If the membranes were to rupture during a contraction and the umbilical cord suddenly slipped down (prolapsed) into the vagina, it would be compressed by the fetus. The fetus's blood supply (and therefore its oxygenation) would be decreased markedly, especially during the contraction. The fetal monitor would show a precipitous drop in the fetal heart rate, which would not return to the normal base line after the contraction ceased. An immediate vaginal examination would show that the cord had slipped out of the uterus.

The doctor or nurse who was attending the first stage of labor would immediately push the fetus up off the cord, holding the baby high up in the uterus. The mother would be quickly rushed into the delivery room and a "crash" (emergency) cesarean delivery would be performed.

Fetal Illness or Abnormality

Some fetal problems, by their nature, make cesarean delivery the preferred choice for the well-being of the fetus, when these have been identified prior to the start of labor. *Rh sensitization* of the baby is such a problem in which scheduled cesarean birth might be indicated. Because this disease leads to progressive anemia and can be a threat to the fetus as pregnancy progresses, very careful management is necessary. Amniocentesis would be used both to follow the disease's progress and to determine fetal lung maturity. Cesarean delivery would then be planned at the optimal time, taking into account both the threat of the Rh disease and the risks of prematurity. A CST may or may not be performed, depending on the degree of stress the fetus is already experiencing. Most Rh sensitized pregnancies do not require cesarean birth. If the baby is in serious jeopardy, however, due to the anemia, it would not have adequate oxygenation to withstand the stresses of labor. C-section is then the safest recourse.

Congenital abnormalities of the fetus often lead to cesarean delivery, because this is the only possible course of action. For example, a baby with hydrocephalus (an abnormality in which the baby's head is very large—too large to pass through the birth canal) could not be delivered vaginally. This and many other types of congenital defects may be associated with unusual presentations and dystocia.

Cesarean delivery may be recommended for a different reason in some other kinds of birth defects—to allow for safer, more immediate treatment of the defect itself or to preserve a sterile environment for the baby. This may increase the chances of survival of a baby with some forms of neural tube defects and abdominal wall problems, who could acquire serious infection during vaginal delivery.

Multiple gestation (twins, triplets, etc.) is another reason a cesarean delivery might be performed for greater fetal safety. Multiple births commonly are complicated by abnormal presentations as well as by some entanglement of the fetuses. Very small or premature twins are at increased risk for abnormal positions and cord problems in particular. Cesarean birth allows for prompt and safe delivery of *both* fetuses with few or no "surprises." Regardless of size, if either twin is in anything but a cephalic presentation, the risks for them from vaginal delivery are greater than from cesarean birth. For term babies who are both in cephalic position, on the other hand, there appears to be no demonstrable advantage to cesarean birth.

"Repeat Cesarean"

One of the most common reasons for cesarean delivery is called "repeat cesarean"—in which the procedure is performed because the woman had previously delivered by cesarean. This reason accounts for a large part of the increase in the cesarean birth rate noted in the past 10 years. While the belief that "once a cesarean, always a cesarean" is still valid for the most part, a growing question among obstetricians is whether there are situations in which vaginal delivery can safely follow a cesarean delivery.

The basic reason for recommending repeat cesarean is that the healed scar on the uterus is not as strong as the rest of the uterus, and the woman would be at risk for uterine rupture due to the forces of labor. Improved surgical techniques—in particular the use of the low transverse incision—reduce but do not totally eliminate this risk.

Currently, some obstetricians will allow a trial of labor for a limited number of carefully selected women who have had previous cesarean section. Such trials of labor should be done only with very careful monitoring and only in hospitals in which it would be possible to do an immediate cesarean delivery if a problem arose.

How Is Cesarean Delivery Performed?

A cesarean delivery is a major surgical procedure in which a fetus is removed from the uterus through an incision in the abdomen. It is performed under sterile conditions in an operating room and in the manner that is safest for both mother and baby.

If the surgical delivery has been planned in advance, you may be admitted to the hospital either the night before the surgery or early in the morning on the day surgery is scheduled. You may be given an enema the night before to empty your lower bowel. You will usually not be allowed to eat or drink anything for at least eight hours before the scheduled delivery. Your lower abdomen and pubic area will be scrubbed, and you will probably be shaved. Just before the scheduled cesarean, an intravenous (IV) infusion will be started, so you can receive fluids and any necessary medications, as well. You will usually have a small catheter inserted into your bladder, either before or after you have been taken to the operating room. (Some of these steps are omitted when emergency cesarean is necessary.)

After you arrive in the operating (cesarean delivery) room, the next step will depend on the type of anesthesia to be used. If a spinal or epidural anesthetic is to be administered, you will be asked to sit up or lie on one side so the anesthetic can be given. You will then lie on your back but tilted to one side (usually the left), so the uterus is not resting directly on the large blood vessels that supply the lower body. You may also be positioned and moved in order to allow the anesthetic to take optimal effect.

Devices for monitoring your heartbeat and blood pressure will be readied. Your abdomen will be "prepped" (washed) with an antiseptic solution and sterile drapes placed to leave only the operating field exposed. If your spouse or mate will be in attendance, he will usually sit near your head with the anesthesiologist. You may be asked to breathe extra oxygen through a mask or small nasal prongs when the surgery is ready to begin.

If general anesthesia is to be administered, the preparation of your abdomen will take place as indicated. Your spouse or mate will not usually be in the delivery room with you.

The Delivery Itself

Whether you have a general anesthetic or regional anesthesia (spinal or epidural), the steps of the surgery itself remain the same. With regional anesthesia you will be awake and aware of the steps of the procedure, because the doctor or anesthesiologist will talk with you about what takes place, and you can ask questions if you wish. Usually your field of vision is blocked, so you are unable to see the procedure itself. On the other hand, if general anesthesia is planned, it would be administered now and you would be unaware of the steps involved.

The first step in the surgery itself is an incision in the skin. Most commonly, the doctor will make a five- to seven-inch incision across your lower abdomen, just above the pubic bone. Called a *"bikini cut" low transverse incision)*, this type of incision seems to heal well and leaves a less noticeable scar than other types of incisions. However, the bikini cut is not always possible in situations where the baby is unusually large or other problems are anticipated. When deemed necessary, *a vertical cut* from the umbilical area (belly button) down to the pubic bone is performed. In either case, the doctor will then separate the muscles and other tissues and work his or her way down to the bladder and uterus. The bladder and nearby tissues are identified and their attachments to the uterus carefully separated. The uterus is then visible and ready to be opened.

There are two basic locations for incisions in the uterus itself. The most commonly used is called a *"lower cervical transverse incision" of the uterus*, made in a manner similar to the bikini cut on the skin. This incision is made across the uterus from side to side, in the lower segment of the uterus—the cervical area. If at all possible, this type of incision is preferred, because the lower portion of the uterus usually bleeds less and is associated with a somewhat lower risk of uterine rupture with subsequent pregnancies (because of the way it can be repaired).

The *classical incision* is a vertical cut made in the larger, more vascular body of the uterus. It allows more space for delivery and intrauterine manipulation, and provides some advantages with unusually located placentas. With very premature deliveries, especially if no labor has occurred, the lower segment of the uterus is insufficiently developed and a classical incision is necessary. There is more likelihood of uterine hemorrhage with classical incisions than with the lower segment cuts, and the scar is more likely to rupture with later pregnancies.

After the initial cut is made in the uterus (regardless of which type of incision is used), your doctor will carefully widen the opening to allow enough space for the baby to be delivered. The fetal membranes are ruptured (if they have not already ruptured), and the amniotic fluid is suctioned out of the uterus as much as possible.

The moment of delivery has arrived. The obstetrician reaches into the uterus and slips his or her hand under the baby's head, then carefully guides it through the uterine opening. The baby's nose and mouth are suctioned, and the rest of the delivery is started. First one shoulder then the other are guided out of the uterine opening, usually with help from the nurse or assistant surgeon pushing down on top of the uterus. (You may feel this as pressure, but not as pain.) After the shoulders are out, the rest of the body slips out of the uterus easily. The cord is clamped, and the infant is handed to a special neonatal nurse or the pediatrician or neonatologist present to tend to the baby's needs.

After delivery of the baby, the placenta is removed by hand. The doctor then carefully examines the placenta to make sure all of it has been removed. Oxytocin is administered intravenously to cause contractions of the uterus and reduce the risk of bleeding. The inside of the uterus is examined carefully, then the incision in the uterus is sutured (stitched up) and covered by the protective tissue near the bladder if possible. Next the muscles and tissues of the abdomen are sutured, then the layers of skin until the work is complete. The procedure usually takes less than 10 minutes from the first incision until the baby is delivered and about 45 minutes for the entire procedure.

After the surgery is finished, you will be taken to a recovery area for careful observation. Your blood pressure, pulse and breathing pattern as well as your temperature will be monitored carefully. You will be closely evaluated, both to make sure excessive bleeding from the uterus (vagina) does not occur and to allow for prompt intervention if such bleeding does occur. After the effects of the anesthetic wear off, you will be returned to your room for further care and rest. The IV will be removed, and you will be allowed to eat and move around as soon as it is safe for you to do so. The urinary catheter is usually removed in a day or so. Some doctors might prescribe IV antibiotics for several days, especially if you had been in labor or the membranes had already ruptured before the cesarean birth (since those factors are associated with a higher incidence of infection).

Some doctors and hospitals encourage fathers to attend cesarean births and allow considerable contact between mother, baby and father, if possible. After an initial "get acquainted" period, the baby is taken to the nursery for several hours of observation. If the baby is healthy, he or she will be taken to the mother as soon as the mother's condition permits. If the baby requires more treatment or evaluation, then the mother will be able to visit the baby in the special care nursery as soon as she is able to be up and about.

Anesthesia for Cesarean Birth

Because cesarean birth requires surgical cutting of the abdomen, complete anesthesia (elimination of all pain and sensation) of the abdomen is required. Relaxation of the abdominal wall muscles is also essential during the operation. There are several possible ways that a mother can be anesthetized for a cesarean birth. Each has benefits and risks. The choice of anesthetic depends upon the condition of both mother and baby, as well as the preferences of the mother.

With *general anesthetic* the mother is not conscious during delivery. This is undesirable for many women but may be preferred by others concerned about being awake during surgery. This kind of anesthesia can be extremely safe for both mother and fetus but requires an experienced anesthesiologist or anesthetist. The main disadvantage is that the baby may be less vigorous at birth due to the effect of the drug—but this is unusual.

General anesthesia involves the mother first being very quickly made unconscious by a short-acting IV medication then having a plastic tube (an endotracheal tube) inserted into the windpipe so the anesthetist can assure a good oxygen supply.

The anesthetic gas itself is mixed with oxygen and inhaled through the tube. Sometimes additional drugs to relax or paralyze the muscles are needed and used, especially after the baby has already been delivered.

General anesthesia is most commonly used in an emergency situation when speed is the primary consideration, or when spinal or epidural anesthesia is not successful. Its major drawback for the mother is the risk of aspiration (inhalation) of stomach contents into the lungs. This can usually be prevented by use of the endotracheal tube.

Spinal anesthesia is a commonly used type of anesthesia for cesarean birth. A lumbar puncture ("spinal tap") is done with a very small diameter needle, and a small amount of a "caine" anesthetic is injected into the spinal fluid. This kind of anesthesia causes very quick, complete pain relief and numbness. The portion of the body that is anesthetized can be regulated by changing the mother's position. Spinal anesthesia allows the mother to be awake during the birth and reduces her risk of aspirating stomach contents into the lungs.

The major risk of spinal anesthesia is maternal hypotension—low blood pressure—caused by a reflex that dilates the blood vessels in the lower part of the body. This reduces blood flow (and hence oxygenation) to the fetus and mother. A small number of women also experience what is called "spinal headache" after this kind of anesthesia. (Spinal headache is a fairly unpleasant headache that may last several hours to several days after the administration of spinal anesthesia. Thought to result from a small leak of spinal fluid from the spinal tap site, it can largely be prevented by using a very fine needle for the procedure and by having the mother lie flat for several hours afterward.)

Lumbar epidural anesthesia is increasingly being used for cesarean birth as well as vaginal delivery. This procedure also requires a needle puncture in the lower back into the epidural space which surrounds the spinal cord and its membranes. At times a small plastic catheter is inserted so more "caine" anesthetic can be injected without making another needle prick. Although a very good type of anesthesia, it is more difficult to administer and requires greater experience on the part of the anesthesiologist than does spinal anesthesia. It is also slower to take effect and requires the administration of more anesthetic than a spinal does. The increase in the amount of anesthetic may potentially cause the baby to be slightly less active (basically a little groggy) as it is absorbed and transferred through the placenta. Lumbar epidural anesthesia is much less likely to cause hypotension, and there is no complication from spinal headache.

While *local anesthesia* injected into the abdominal wall is occasionally possible, this is not a common or desirable type of anesthesia for cesarean birth. To be at all effective, large amounts of sedatives must usually be given to the mother, as well, resulting in a potentially increased risk of a depressed (less vigorous, less active) baby.

The choice of anesthetic used for cesarean delivery is based on the recommendation of your obstetrician and the anesthesiologist or anesthetist, in concert with your personal preferences and consent. As mentioned, each type of anesthesia has benefits and risks to be considered, and much of the time the choice depends on each

woman's individual situation. If a cesarean delivery is recommended
for you, be sure you understand the type of anesthesia being considered and its risks and benefits based on your needs and those
of your unborn baby. Never hesitate to ask questions until you are
sure you understand all the risks and benefits to you and the baby.

The Risks and Complications of Cesarean Birth

Much of the concern about cesarean section comes from the increased risk associated with the procedure as compared to vaginal
delivery. Some of these risks to the mother are similar to those
associated with other types of major surgery. Other risks are pe-
culiar to the cesarean procedure itself, perhaps compounded by
complications of the condition(s) that led to the procedure's use in
the first place. Also, any risk to the fetus—the "other" patient—
must be taken into consideration.

Maternal Mortality

As previously noted, until recently, a high maternal mortality rate
following cesarean delivery was one of the very important reasons
why operative delivery was a "last resort," and used almost exclusively for "maternal" reasons—that is, as an attempt to improve
the mother's outcome. As the procedure became safer, it could be
and was considered for "fetal" reasons—to potentially improve the
outcome for the fetus.

   As mentioned earlier, maternal mortality needs to be put into
perspective. What most people do not realize is that there are only
slightly over 300 maternal deaths recorded each year in the United
States. Unfortunately, the designation of "maternal death" here is
rather misleading and broad. These statistics include death due to
any cause both during pregnancy and during the 90 days after the
termination of pregnancy, regardless of its duration. Maternal mortality statistics are not broken down into specific causes, such as:
illness or accident not related to pregnancy, maternal complications,
complications of labor, vaginal delivery and cesarean birth. Therefore, great care must be taken in distinguishing between maternal
deaths due to the actual cesarean procedure and its associated risks
and those due to totally different and unrelated problems.

   The point is—it is a very rare occurrence today in this country
for a mother to die due to the pregnancy itself or to labor and/or

delivery. There was approximately one maternal death for every 10,000 births in 1978—about the same rate as for vaginal delivery alone in the 1950s—and the rate may be even lower now. By comparison, in 1935 there were approximately 60 maternal deaths for every 10,000 births—about *60 times* more than today. If the actual numbers of births in 1935 had been over 3 million a year, as there are today, there would have been more than *18,000* maternal deaths—compared to the current 300 or so.

These impressive reductions in maternal deaths (even including the unknown numbers not directly related to pregnancy, labor and delivery) are due to major advances in all aspects of perinatal care.

It is very difficult to assess the overall rate of maternal mortality due to specific causes. However, a number of studies have been completed and statistics compiled for various hospitals, cities and states. Although there seems to be a wide variance in the studies and experiences, it appears that the risk of maternal mortality due to cesarean delivery is about four times greater than that associated with vaginal delivery. This is based on information compiled in 1980 by the Consensus Development Conference on Cesarean Childbirth, U.S. Department of Health and Human Services, Public Health Service, National Institutes of Health. The same report notes that the risk of maternal death from repeat cesarean delivery (cesarean performed due to a previous cesarean delivery) is two times greater than that of all vaginal deliveries.

The Professional Activities Study of the Commission on Professional and Hospital Activities recently collected data from a large cross section of the many hospitals in the United States. Data were gathered and statistics for maternal mortality for both cesarean and vaginal deliveries were compiled for the years 1970, 1974 and 1978. The results for these many hospitals were noteworthy. In 1970 there appeared to have been 20.4 maternal deaths for each 100,000 vaginal deliveries and 113.8 maternal deaths for each 100,000 cesarean deliveries. In 1974 there were 15.2 maternal deaths per 100,000 vaginal deliveries and 62.9 deaths per 100,000 cesarean deliveries. The year 1978 saw another major reduction in maternal mortality: 9.8 deaths per 100,000 vaginal deliveries and 40.9 deaths per 100,000 cesarean births.

Again, the experiences of different institutions, areas of a state and even different states vary. A great deal depends on the skill and experience of the physicians and other health professionals, the diagnostic and treatment capabilities, and the technical resources. Results also depend heavily on the patients themselves—their basic health, their pregnancy problems, their prenatal care and the reasons for cesarean delivery. All of these factors must be considered in looking at the risks associated with cesarean birth.

Other Maternal Complications

Complications of anesthesia account for the most significant maternal difficulties seen during the cesarean operation itself. These risks depend on the type of anesthesia used. With general anesthesia there is danger that the mother will aspirate (inhale) stomach contents—food and/or acid—at the start of administration of the anesthetic. This complication, while usually preventable, may lead to serious lack of oxygen to the mother (and hence to the fetus) at a critical time. The mother may also have pneumonia later because of the irritation caused by the material that got into her lungs.

The major risk of spinal and epidural anesthesia is hypotension—low blood pressure—which leads to reduced blood flow to the placenta and potential fetal hypoxia. Careful monitoring of the mother's blood pressure and prompt intervention when necessary are essential in reducing damage due to this complication.

Excessive bleeding is another risk of cesarean delivery. The wall of the uterus has an exceptional blood supply during pregnancy, and cutting through the engorged blood vessels can pose a problem, especially with the classical cesarean incision. Usual blood loss with a cesarean birth is about 1,000 cubic centimeters (one liter, or approximately a quart). When blood loss is greater than that because of difficulties in repairing the uterus and/or poor muscle contraction, the mother may need blood transfusion(s). Serious problems may result if blood loss cannot be controlled. In very rare instances, when hemorrhage cannot be controlled in any other way, emergency hysterectomy (removal of the uterus) may be the only possible course of action.

Infection of the mother is one of the most frequent complications of abdominal delivery. The infection may involve the uterine lining (called "endometritis"), the urinary tract or the surgical wound and may also be more generalized and potentially life threatening (called "sepsis").

The risk of infection is greater for women who had been in active labor before cesarean delivery was performed and whose membranes had been ruptured. And the longer the membranes were ruptured, the greater the risk for infection. Because of this known association, some obstetricians advocate giving the mother one or more antibiotics by IV for several days after abdominal delivery, even if she does not show signs of infection, in the hope of preventing it. Others do not prescribe antibiotics as a routine preventive measure but obtain cultures (samples of the amniotic fluid and swabs from the fetal side of the placenta during the operation) to try to identify any hidden infection. The mother is treated only if she shows signs of infection, or if the cultures suggest infection.

Such maternal complications as *thrombophlebitis* (blood clot with inflammation) of either the pelvic veins or those in the legs are less common and often preventable. *Pulmonary embolism* (migration of a blood clot to the lung from another area of the body), while potentially life threatening, is quite rare. *Complications from other maternal diseases*, such as hypertension—either chronic or due to pre-eclampsia—or diabetes, are also possible. The incidence of all of these is statistically low because of improvements in the ways to manage and intervene in these diseases. Improved anesthesia, modern surgical techniques, antibiotics and other drugs, and better means to control bleeding and replace blood loss have also made serious complications relatively rare today.

Fetal Complications

Many studies of fetal risks associated with cesarean delivery are difficult to interpret. The effects of the cesarean delivery itself are hard to separate from those due to the potentially serious conditions that led to the cesarean in the first place. Such factors as fetal distress, problems related to underlying fetal abnormality or prolonged labor take their toll on the fetus.

However, there are two types of fetal risks worth noting. An increased risk to the fetus can be related to the *effects of anesthetics* given to the mother. As previously mentioned, maternal hypotension can be a direct result of spinal anesthesia and may compromise the oxygen supply to the fetus. Hypoxia may be recognized as fetal distress around the time of delivery, and the baby may require more resuscitation than expected right after birth. Likewise, the direct effects of the anesthetic drugs themselves on the fetus (either the absorbed "caine" drugs or inhaled gases) may lead to depression of the baby's breathing and activity, low Apgar scores and a need for resuscitation.

Respiratory distress is a problem often seen more commonly in infants delivered by cesarean section. Therefore, a question asked is whether the method of delivery has anything to do with the breathing difficulties. A closer look at some of the types of respiratory distress is necessary before this concern can be understood.

"Respiratory distress syndrome" (also called "hyaline membrane disease") is a term usually reserved for the lung problem of premature infants that results from lack of lung surfactant. Prior to the mid-1970s the incidence of this problem was much higher than it should have been in cesarean babies, especially those delivered electively (that is, by planned cesarean birth). In fact, one obstetrician reviewing the data from that decade suggested that as many as one-third of the approximately 40,000 cases of respiratory distress syndrome (RDS) seen annually resulted from unnecessary (and unexpected) prematurity and could have been prevented.

The focus here, then, should be on *elective* cesarean births—repeat cesarean delivery for example and on prevention of the RDS due to prematurity among these babies. The key to solving this problem is assuring fetal lung maturity before cesarean delivery (and also before the elective induction of labor). A strong joint recommendation was issued in 1979 by the American College of Obstetric and Gynecology and the American Academy of Pediatrics that fetal gestational age be *accurately* determined to be term, or that amniocentesis be performed to determine fetal lung maturity prior to planned cesarean delivery. With improved methods of assessing fetal maturity, the risk of unexpected respiratory distress syndrome following elective cesarean delivery now approaches zero.

Other types of breathing difficulties also occur in cesarean babies. A problem called "transient tachypnea of the newborn" (abbreviated TTN), or "retained fetal lung fluid" is quite common in babies delivered by cesarean. Usually a temporary problem without serious complications, this difficulty is less common in babies delivered abdominally after active labor had begun. The theory is that the squeezing of the fetus in the birth canal during labor pushes out some of the lung fluid normally present in the fetus, preventing this problem. In cesarean birth without labor, there is no opportunity for this fluid to be expelled before delivery. Further study of the problem will hopefully be helpful in understanding this and other causes of respiratory distress in mature infants.

The Controversy Surrounding Cesarean Birth

In the past decade there has been a great increase in the number of cesarean deliveries in the United States and worldwide. This increase is the basis for the controversy surrounding the cesarean delivery procedure. Questions have been raised not only by the general public but also by those in the medical profession regarding whether cesarean delivery is warranted in all cases and whether its increased use in fact improves the outcome for mother, baby or both.

The most recent studies showed a threefold increase in the cesarean delivery rate in the United States between 1970 and 1978. In 1970 cesarean deliveries accounted for 5.5 percent of births, compared to 15.2 percent in 1978. While variations in the incidence of cesarean birth were seen from hospital to hospital, state to state and region to region, there was a general increase in abdominal delivery throughout the country. Increased cesarean deliveries have been seen in other countries as well, although to a lesser extent than in the United States. Large hospitals tended to have higher cesarean rates than small ones, and at some the rate was as high as 25 percent of all births. The National Center for Health Statistics notes that cesarean delivery is the 10th most common surgical procedure in the United States.

The increase in the cesarean birth rate cannot be denied. The real issue is not the numbers of surgical deliveries, but whether the procedure is necessary in every case.

Undoubtedly, part of the increase is due to the procedure's relative safety today, which has made it a reasonable means of intervention when problems arise or are identified. The fact is that while the cesarean delivery rate has increased, the maternal as well as perinatal mortality rates have continued to decrease. That in itself is encouraging, but what remains to be seen is whether the long-term outcome for the babies will be affected positively.

Studies have shown that 90 percent of the overall increase in the cesarean birth rate can be attributed to four major conditions:

- Dystocia (including prolonged labor, abnormal pelvis and cephalopelvic disproportion)
- Previous cesarean delivery
- Breech presentation
- Fetal distress

Premature labor, prolonged pregnancy, premature rupture of membranes and placental problems account for the remaining 10 percent of the increase in cesarean deliveries. A look at each of these problems as they relate to the controversy is helpful in better understanding the cause and effect.

The greatest contributor to the increase in cesarean birth is *dystocia*, which accounted for 29.2 percent of the eight-year rise in cesareans in the national statistics. (The statistics are from the 1980 Consensus Development Conference on Cesarean Birth.) While certain conditions that lead to cesarean birth for dystocia—pelvic abnormalities, very large babies, fetal abnormalities—are not in question, others are more controversial. Prolonged labor—thought to be due to poor uterine contraction, for example—might lead to cesarean, especially if there is also a concern over the baby's size or indications of fetal distress. However, when fetal distress is not identified, wide variations in physician judgments may be seen. Statistics show that approximately 90 percent of babies delivered abdominally for this reason are of normal size, and that the survival rate is not better than for vaginal delivery. This problem needs to be looked at more closely and possibly a better way to evaluate potential difficulties developed.

The so-called *repeat cesarean* accounts for 27 percent of the increase in the cesarean section rate. The "once a cesarean, always a cesarean" belief was based on information available early in this century. The rise in repeat cesareans logically parallels the rise in primary (first-time) cesarean delivery. However, data gathered in the National Maternity Hospital in Dublin, as well as several smaller studies done in the United States, suggest that some women (as many as 40 percent to 60 percent) may be safely delivered vaginally. While guidelines are not completely defined as yet, there are some factors associated with safe vaginal delivery after a cesarean delivery:

- The woman has had only one cesarean delivery.
- In the previous cesarean, a low segment transverse incision was performed.
- Her cesarean delivery was uncomplicated and performed for reasons not present in this pregnancy.
- She experienced no complications immediately after cesarean delivery and no later problems.
- She is to deliver this baby in a hospital where an emergency cesarean can be safely performed if complications occur during the trial of labor.

While careful trials of labor in some women who have had cesarean delivery might be successful (thereby reducing the rates of cesarean births), this is *not* safe in many circumstances. It is important for women who wish to deliver vaginally after a previous cesarean to fully understand the potential risks of labor and work with their obstetricians in weighing the risk-benefit ratio for them.

Breech presentation accounts for about 15 percent of the rise in cesarean birth in the 1970–78 period. Whereas 11.6 percent of breech babies were delivered abdominally in 1970, 60.1 percent of them were delivered by cesarean in 1978. This increase has been an attempt to improve the outcome for breech babies. The upward trend of cesarean for breech presentation continues, especially with first pregnancies.

The greatest problem is that it is impossible to know which baby will be easily delivered and which is likely to require a difficult vaginal delivery, possibly resulting in serious damage or death. Analyzing the results in complicated, because breech babies have more problems, regardless of how they are delivered. (Breech is associated with fetal malformations and prematurity with its many potential problems.)

For term breech babies, the outcome is statistically much better when they are delivered by cesarean, according to a study done in New York City. Vaginal delivery is still a very important option to be considered in selected circumstances. However, the consensus of opinion today is to opt for the mode of delivery that is safest for both mother and baby—which appears to be cesarean birth in many pregnancies complicated by breech presentation.

The fourth most common reason for cesarean section, *fetal distress*, accounts for about 10 percent of the increase. This reflects, in part, the rise in electronic fetal monitoring, which allows for better detection of fetal distress. While early identification of fetal distress and intervention—including cesarean delivery, when appropriate—have led to improved outcome for babies, there is still room for greater precision in identifying fetal distress and determining at what point cesarean delivery is the only safe method of intervention.

Criticisms have not all been related to physiological considerations. Some critics have pointedly blamed *economics, convenience* and *legal considerations* as playing a major role in the rising rates. The fact is, doctors can earn more for operative delivery than for vaginal delivery, and cesarean birth results in longer, and hence more expensive, hospital stays for mothers and babies. If a complication occurs, (such as infection or hemorrhage) then the cost rises even more, due to necessary intervention. There are some studies that show a higher cesarean rate among women with insurance and other studies that show no difference between the insured and uninsured populations. Therefore, all studies have been inconclusive, since most results are contradictory.

Another consideration is the role of hospital review committees in monitoring cesarean rates. These committees review both the cesarean rate and the reasons for using this method of delivery in specific cases, to better ensure the appropriate use of cesarean birth in the hospital. Records are checked and any pertinent documentation (such as fetal heart rate monitoring strips) is reviewed. This type of peer review, particularly in perinatal networks (discussed in detail in Chapter 18), is effective in identifying physicians for questioning if there is a concern about their reason(s) for performing cesarean delivery. Although there are abuses found in every professional field, it would be difficult for any doctor delivering in a perinatal network where extensive peer review is performed to continue delivering by cesarean inappropriately.

These same principles hold true for cesarean as a convenience for the physician. Critics have charged that doctors opt for cesarean rather than be called in to deliver on days off or as a means to deliver quickly rather than waiting out a long labor. Again, doctors must be able to reasonably justify and document the need for cesarean delivery to a group of his or her peers. It is quite unlikely that anyone could fool not only the assisting physicians in the delivery room but the nurses and other technicians, time and time again, simply as a matter of personal convenience. And it is quite unlikely that a review committee in a reputable hospital or in a perinatal network would not question the appropriateness of the doctor's cesarean deliveries if there were no reasonable documentation of the need for such intervention.

As far as legal considerations go, it is felt by some that the fear of malpractice litigation due to poor outcome in vaginal delivery has played a role in the rising cesarean rate. In other words, cesarean delivery may be performed as a means of self-protection from potential lawsuits. Since in some situations a judgment must be made about whether to allow labor to continue or to deliver by cesarean, there have been some lawsuits that maintain that the poor outcome was the result of *not* performing a cesarean delivery. This trend in malpractice suits, some say, has led to more physicians' performing cesarean sections in self-defense. However, while there are abuses in every system, the Consensus Report on Cesarean Childbirth (1980) notes that economic, convenience or legal considerations as motivations for cesarean delivery are anything but common.

The Bottom Line on the Controversy

There are no clear-cut answers for the increased cesarean rate for all the indications discussed. The reasons for cesarean delivery and the results are under continued scrutiny and study by obstetricians and others concerned with the well-being of both mothers and infants. Only this continued analysis and careful monitoring by hospital review committees as well as by national organizations and perinatal networks will be able to answer the many questions now posed about the increased cesarean delivery rate.

As more studies are completed we will be better equipped to answer certain questions and determine if the increased safety of cesarean delivery is responsible for justifiable intervention and better outcomes (both short- and long-term) for mothers and babies. However, no one can dispute one simple fact—as the cesarean delivery rate has increased, the infant and maternal mortality rates have both decreased.

The Emotional Impact of Cesarean Birth

With the rising cesarean birth rate has come concern about the psychological impact of cesarean delivery—on the mother, on the father and even on the baby. There are many factors involved here, including whether the cesarean was planned or unexpected; how much preparation, if any, the mother and/or father had before the delivery; and what the father's role was at the time of delivery and thereafter.

Few studies have been done on the psychological effects of cesarean birth on the family, and those available are based primarily on questionnaires parents answered after delivery. Mothers understandably felt disappointed following cesarean birth and often took longer to recover physically from the birth process. Consequently, the father often played a greater role with the baby than when vaginal delivery occurred.

While there is usually greater stress both physically and psychologically with cesarean birth, several things can make the experience more positive:

- Preparation of all pregnant women and their mates for pos-

sible cesarean birth by their doctors as well as in prepared
childbirth classes
- More active and informed participation in the decision making about cesarean delivery by the mother and her mate
- Participation by the father in the delivery room during cesarean delivery whenever possible
- Hospital care that is family-centered, allowing for greater
  participation by parents in the overall care of mother and
  baby

With attention to all of these factors, cesarean birth can be a
positive, rewarding experience for families. Most regional perinatal
centers have special programs and take care to involve the parents
as much as possible, not only in the decision-making process, but
in the cesarean birth itself. Fathers and mothers are encouraged to
be supportive of each other and to take an active role in the care
of the baby whenever possible. We will begin seeing increasing
sensitivity toward the parents' and baby's psychological needs as
time goes by and more hospitals and professionals become aware
of the ways to make cesarean delivery (when indicated) a less stressful and more fulfilling experience.

*T*HREE

PERINATAL CARE: AN IMPORTANT MEDICAL ADVANCE

In the last three decades there has been a significant decline in the number of babies who die prior to and during labor and delivery and in the first year of life. Figures from the National Center for Health Statistics show a 45 percent reduction in fetal deaths, a 47 percent reduction in neonatal deaths and a 48 percent reduction in infant deaths in the United States from 1950 to 1976.

And these statistics do not begin to show the unbelievable number of babies whose quality of life has been substantially improved or who had potentially damaging or devastating problems avoided or their impact lessened because of timely and sophisticated medical intervention.

Impressive reductions in maternal mortality have also occurred over the years, as previously mentioned. There were around 60 times more maternal deaths in 1935 than today. Although we cannot say that death due to pregnancy is unheard of, we can now say it is very, very rare. Considering the more than three million births each year in the United States and only slightly more than 300 maternal deaths, you can see what a rare occurrence it is today. And with more knowledge, continued advances and early management of problems during pregnancy, this number will more than likely be reduced even further.

Such impressive reduction is fatalities and increases in optimal outcomes can be directly attributed to major advances in high-risk obstetrics, neonatology and pediatrics; greater knowledge, excellent professional training and continuing education; and the development of space age technology. All of these have enabled doctors to more successfully teach prevention and the importance of prenatal care, as well as identify problems and intervene throughout pregnancy, labor, delivery and during the neonatal period or infancy.

From microscopic analysis of amniotic fluid to evaluating the fetus inside the womb—from identifying problems early in labor to determining fetal fitness before labor—from the development of drugs to halt premature labor to those that promote fetal lung maturity—from early intervention in potential problems to corrective fetal surgery—all are major achievements whose sole purpose is to assist the miracle of birth. These advances—sometimes dramatic—have played a major role in ensuring safer pregnancies and substantially better outcomes for those at risk for problems.

Along with these striking advances (as well as greater specialization in all areas of medicine) has come the establishment of the regional tertiary care center (major regional medical center). A tertiary care center provides a level of medical care involving skilled sub-specialists with the necessary compliment of sophisticated technology and laboratory backup 24 hours a day. These centers are capable of managing the most complicated medical problems—in both the mother and the fetus/neonate.

In general, a tertiary care center has a perinatology department (high-risk obstetrics and neonatology), a neonatal intensive care unit, and the ability to perform sophisticated pediatric surgery, plus all the expertise, continuing education, experience and technology necessary to monitor, manage and intervene in the high-risk pregnancy. These state-of-the-art medical centers are found in most metropolitan areas in the United States.

Often these tertiary care centers are the hub of a regionalized network of perinatal care. In this way hospitals in the network can be evaluated and "classified" based on the level of care they are qualified to provide. This cooperative relationship allows for a step-up approach to the care of the mother and fetus/newborn. High-risk mothers are referred to the appropriate facility based on the level of care required. "Perinatal outreach programs" are frequently a special part of the regionalized program. This allows for continuing education for the professional, nursing and technical staffs at the area institutions; review of existing cases; discussion of treatment plans; and an understanding of when patients need to be referred for more specialized management or intervention to obtain optimal results. This type of liaison is beneficial to the area hospitals and the regional perinatal center (tertiary care center) alike, and especially beneficial to the patients the facilities serve.

We know that for some high risk problems minimal management and little or no special intervention are necessary—when the course of the pregnancy is excellent. For others, women should be under the care of a specialist in high-risk obstetrics (maternal-fetal medicine or sometimes called perinatology), with the support of a tertiary care center throughout the pregnancy. Your level of care will depend on your needs and those of your unborn baby. The best policy is to ask your doctor. If he or she is not a specialist in high-risk obstetrics, the doctor may feel it best to refer you to a specialist—if the reason for your being high-risk warrants this. If your physician is not a specialist in high-risk obstetrics but the hospital in which he or she has staff privileges is part of a perinatal network, then you would automatically be referred to specialists at the facility which could best meet your needs and that of your unborn baby (if the situation warranted this at some time during the pregnancy).

Because there are so many components to perinatal care today—the various professionals involved and the different levels of care provided by hospitals and professionals—we have divided Section 3 into four chapters which cover the various aspects of perinatal care and conclude with a chapter which looks to the future in perinatal care. *Chapter 17* explains the roles of the many health professionals who may at some point be involved with your care or that of your baby. *Chapter 18* is an overview of regionalized perinatal care, what you can expect from each level of care and how you "fit" into this specialized network. *Chapter 19* is an overview of infant special care (intensive care), the professionals, equipment and treatment, and your role in your baby's care if he or she is admitted to an infant special care unit. *Chapter 20* takes you one step into the future of perinatal care—an exciting future filled with more very important answers to the problems faced by mothers and unborn/newborn babies.

SEVENTEEN

THE SPECIAL ROLE OF THE HEALTH CARE TEAM

Over the years we have seen more and more specialization in medicine—a trend caused by the explosion in technology, the enormous volumes of research and information, and the seemingly minute-to-minute advances in all areas of care. The general public has also played a major role in this move toward specialization by expecting the finest skills and most up-to-date knowledge from their doctors. No single physician would be capable of "specializing" in everything (a contradiction of terms) to the degree necessary to meet the often unique needs of all patients. Because of these factors, physicians began to study intensely in their fields of interest and develop special diagnostic, management and treatment skills.

To put this into perspective, specialization was particularly necessary because of the great renaissance medicine has experienced in the last 50 years. If you take a close look at medical history, you will realize that progress was a tedious process. Milestones in medicine were achieved over thousands of years by piecing together information. For example: The circulation of the blood was not even described until 1628; the study of tissues and cells began to evolve in the 1700s (but the knowledge that our bodies constantly make new cells and replace older ones was not confirmed until the 1940s); the first surgery using ether as an anesthetic was performed in 1837 by an American physician; the study of germs did not really begin until the 1800s; Roentgen accidentally discovered the X ray in 1896; and the Curies isolated radium from pitchblende in 1903.

The point is, although the origins of some advances and breakthroughs can be traced to the remote past (such as surgery, which was described as early as 5000 B.C.), from 5000 B.C. until 50 years ago, progress was achieved very slowly.

In comparison, astonishing medical progress has occurred in the condensed time span of the last 50 years. To name a few of these recent advances: a spectrum of anesthetics; knowledge of the value of sterile conditions (antisepsis); instrumentation and methods to control bleeding and shock; the development of uncountable medicines to prevent, control, treat or cure devastating diseases or conditions, including antibiotics, chemotherapeutic drugs, immunizations, synthetic hormones, pain relievers, etc.; sophisticated monitoring, diagnostic and treatment equipment, such as heart monitors, electroencephalography (EEG), CAT scanners, the electron microscope, lasers, ultrasound, refined radiological equipment, linear acclerators, renal dialysis, respirators, defibrillators for the heart, pacemakers, etc.; organ transplants; refinements in surgical instrumentation, such as operating microscopes, and in surgical procedures; great strides in genetics and cellular pathology, and...well...the list goes on and on!

Considering these major accomplishments and many, many others, as well as the amount of information being continuously collected in each field and the skill necessary to provide care in any one field—specialization was the only way to go. As medicine continued to become more and more complex, more areas were specialized, and this trend was followed by sub-specialization.

To put this into perspective, in 1929 there were only 5300 obstetricians in the United States. The American College of Obstetricians and Gynecologists was established only 30 years ago. Today there are more than 25,000 obstetricians in this country. Obstetricians sub-specializing in the care of high-risk pregnancy (maternal-fetal medicine/perinatology) number 200. In gynecology there is sub-specializations in infertility, gynecological urology, endocrinology, oncology and other areas.

A similar movement forward specialization can be seen in the field of pediatric medicine. In 1900 there were only 6 pediatricians in this country and less than 50 other physicians who took a special interest in the care of children. The American Academy of Pediatrics was established only 51 years ago. Today there are more than 20,000 pediatricians in the United States. Sub-specialization in pediatrics now includes the areas of neonatology, pediatric cardiology, pediatric endocrinology, allergy and immunology, pulmonary medicine, hematology, neurology, nephrology, genetics, ambulatory care and adolescent medicine.

The point is, nearly every health care professional today has some area of specialization and often sub-specialization, as well.

Doctors, nurses, technicians and auxiliary personnel can concentrate in their areas of particular interest or concern. Every health care professional, then, has a special role, and in this way, the public's need for both general health care and unique or special care can be met.

Although specialization was a necessary step, with it came a concern that too much attention would be focused on specific physical problems or isolated areas of the body and that the total care of the patient would suffer. It became clear that a problem with one system of the body could directly affect other body systems. Therefore, it was necessary to develop a comprehensive approach to care that would meet the total physiological and psychological needs of each patient. This led to the structured team approach to health care. Now called the "health care team," a group of professionals work together to provide and direct the total care of every patient. The members of each patient's health care team can number only a few or many—depending on the particular patient's unique problems or needs.

Obviously, with so many professionals potentially involved in both your care and that of your baby, it is easy for you, your husband or partner and other family members to become confused. Although the professionals know who does what, when and why, you may sometimes be left baffled and a little bewildered by all these people and their roles in providing your care or that of your baby. When things seem confusing, remember that each health care team has a team leader. The team leader for your care would more than likely be your obstetrician or the maternal-fetal specialist designated by your obstetrician. The pediatrician or neonatologist would be the team leader for your baby's care. These specialists would be responsible for directing and coordinating the care provided by the other professionals on the team, to make sure all of your needs and those of your baby are met.

If you are ever in doubt or confused about who can or should answer questions or talk with you regarding your care or that of your baby, or if at any point you do not understand the role of certain health professionals, make sure to ask so you feel as comfortable as possible.

How Doctors are Trained

The various levels of health care are more easily understood when you know how doctors are trained. This also allows you to under-stand what certain credentials mean in terms of training, experience and expertise. In this way you will be able to better understand the level of training of the doctor(s) involved in your care and your baby's care as well.

Medical school training consists of four years of intense study of the basic medical sciences, as well as supervised hospital training experiences in all areas of medicine. Graduation from medical school allows a doctor to use the "MD" title, but further training is necessary before he or she can actually *practice* medicine.

All states in this country require at least one year of supervised hospital training after medical school, as well as the passing of a special examination in order for the doctor to be licensed to practice medicine. Before 1950 or so this year of training—called an *"in-ternship"*—involved experience in several fields of medicine (for ex-ample, internal medicine, surgery, obstetrics and gynecology, pe-diatrics) for almost everyone. Since the early 1970s the requirements for this initial year of training needed for licensing have changed to allow the new doctor to concentrate in a specialty area of medicine during the first year after medical school.

A *residency* is an intense hospital experience and training program in one of the fields of medicine and can vary in length from three to six years. To receive *board certification* in a specialty of medicine, a doctor must complete all the requirements of a full residency program, as well as pass rigorous certifying examina-tion(s).

If the specialist decides to sub-specialize—concentrate in an even more limited field of care within a given specialty—he or she would need to complete another one or more years of *fellowship* training after the completion of the residency. Fellows, then, are MDs, fully trained in their specialty (for example, obstetrics), who are in the process of in-depth learning, training and research in a sub-specialty (such as maternal-fetal medicine—high-risk obstetrics). Some fel-lowships entitle the doctor to be further board-certified in the sub-specialty, but not all sub-specialties have certifying boards as yet.

Most people are confused by the often long list of initials after a physician's name. The purpose of these initials is to identify (in part) the physician's training, experience and expertise. They also may tell you that the doctor has been certified by a specialty board, by completing the necessary training and passing rigorous exami-nations. So John C. Smith, MD, FACOG—is John C. Smith, *Medical Doctor, Fellow* in the *American College* of

Obstetricians and Gynecologists. Dr. Smith, in other words, has completed medical school and a residency in obstetrics and gynecology and is therefore a fellow in the American College of Obstetricians and Gynecologists (membership in which requires that the specialist complete board certification).

Sub-specialists usually do not have special initials after their names to indicate their additional training, but will often indicate their sub-specialty on a business card or directory listing. And do not be confused by the use of "Fellow"— a "Fellow" in this case is *not* a doctor training in a sub-specialty—but a *board-certified specialist*!

After physicians have completed formal training, they are required to participate in *continuing medical education* in order to maintain their licenses to practice and to stay up-to-date in their fields. Continuing education can take the form of lectures, special postgraduate courses or supervised clinical programs.

If you are not sure about your doctor's training and expertise— whether he or she is or is not a specialist or sub-specialist—the best thing to do is to ask. If your physician is not a specialist and you are concerned that you may need a specialist, instead of worrying about this, simply ask the doctor if he or she feels you may need specialized management for your high-risk status. Remember, all high-risk problems do not need specialized management throughout pregnancy for optimal care. And only certain ones require that your primary physician be a sub-specialist in maternal-fetal medicine instead of a specialist in obstetrics.

Members of the Health Care Team

Although it is impossible to predict exactly which professionals would be involved in your care or that of your baby, it is helpful for you to understand the various roles of the different health care professionals you may encounter at some point in your pregnancy, during labor and delivery, and after delivery.

For the Mother

Basic health care during pregnancy can be supervised by doctors with several different kinds of training and interests. Your individual needs and preferences, as well as the availability of specialized care, will determine the members of your health care team.

Family doctor: If your physician is a family doctor, then his or her role is to provide for the health care needs of all members of your family. Before the 1970s family doctors were more often general practitioners, meaning they had completed an internship after medical school. Some, however, had spent extra years of training in a particular field of medicine, as well. Since the early 1970s training programs in *family medicine* have been developed. These programs consist of three years of residency, with the first year fulfilling the requirements for licensure (as the previously mentioned internship did). During residency the doctor learns about all fields of medicine—internal medicine, surgery, obstetrics and gynecology, pediatrics, etc.—in more depth than is possible during a one-year internship. He or she also learns about family medicine—the art and science of providing care for the entire family. Your family physician may follow you if your pregnancy is uncomplicated and you have no risk factors, or may refer all his or her pregnant patients to obstetricians. If you have known risk factors and have a family physician, he or she will more than likely refer you to an obstetrician *immediately* for consultation and care.

Obstetrician: If your doctor is an obstetrician, he or she has had three years of residency training (after medical school) in both obstetrics (the field of medicine dealing with pregnancy, childbirth and postpartum care) and gynecology (the field of medicine dealing with diseases and problems of women, in particular those of the female reproductive system). He or she has had the necessary training and experience to manage high- and low-risk pregnancies and their complications. However, your obstetrician may refer you to a maternal-fetal specialist/perinatologist (if available) for either consultation and recommendations or for the complete management of your pregnancy depending on the problem(s). The American Board of Obstetricians and Gynecologists certifies these specialists, who can then become Fellows in the American College of Obstetricians and Gynecologists (ACOG).

In a perinatal center or tertiary care hospital, you will usually meet doctors in various stages of specialty training:

Resident in obstetrics: A resident in obstetrics is a doctor who is in one of the three years of training required to specialize in obstetrics and gynecology. Residents in training hospitals care for patients under the supervision and direction of their "attending" faculty of board-certified obstetricians and gynecologists.

Fellow in maternal-fetal medicine: A fellow in maternal-fetal medicine is a fully trained obstetrician/gynecologist who is studying high-risk obstetrics under the direction of a maternal-fetal specialist in a perinatal center. He or she will be a sub-specialist in high-risk obstetrics after completion of the two-year fellowship.

Nursing care:Nurses are professionals who are trained and experienced in providing care for your day-to-day physical and emotional needs. Nurses receive varying kinds of basic and specialized nursing training:

- *RN*: A registered nurse is licensed to perform all general and some specialized nursing duties. He or she has had either three years of nursing training (a diploma nurse) or four years of training and a college degree (a baccalaureate or degree nurse). Each hospital can determine what additional training or experience is needed to have special expertise and privileges in patient care.
- *LVN or LPN*: A vocational or practical nurse is licenses after completion of a special one- to two-year program in nursing. He or she performs bedside nursing and a number of other duties under the supervision of an RN.
- *Obstetrical clinical nurse specialist*: An RN who has completed one or more special programs in obstetrical care, perhaps with additional university or college training, as well. He or she has special expertise and privileges in a given area of obstetrics (for example, CST or fetal monitoring).
- *Obstetrical nurse practitioner*: A nurse with special training beyond the basic nursing courses and often with an advanced university degree. His or her preparation consists of advanced science and clinical training. The nurse practitioner usually specializes in a given area (for example, obstetrics, gynecology, pediatrics or family medicine) and performs many duties under physician supervision previously carried out only by doctors. You will most often find nurse practitioners working with doctors in their offices and providing such services as routine prenatal care, post-delivery checks and the like. Other nurse practitioners work in hospitals with maternal-fetal specialists.
- *Nurse-midwife*: An RN with special training in providing prenatal care as well as caring for mothers during labor and delivery under the supervision of a physician. Nurse-midwives are not licensed in some states.

Other professionals: You may also come into contact with individuals with expertise and training in special areas, who often play a special role in your care.

For the Baby

Your baby's health care team can be limited in number or very extensive (as was the case with your team). Again, the professionals who compose the team will depend on your baby's needs, which can begin even before birth.

As much as possible, you should plan before delivery for your baby's care. Obviously, you cannot provide for special care—that is the responsibility of the professionals. But you can arrange for well-baby care. Ask your doctor whom he or she recommends or, if you wish, get recommendations from family members or friends who have been pleased with the care their children are receiving from their family doctor or pediatrician. You can also obtain the names of several physicians from the local medical society.

We highly recommend that you and your partner meet with your baby's prospective doctor in the latter part of your pregnancy. In this way you can discuss with the doctor his or her philosophy of care, recommended schedule of office visits, well-baby care, newborn feeding, fees, etc. You can also find out which sub-specialists he or she would consult with if there were a problem with the baby. Some physicians charge a fee for this meeting, while others do not. You may wish to ask ahead of time.

If after the discussion with the doctor, you are satisfied that he or she and your family can work together in providing for your baby's health care needs, then ask the doctor how he or she wishes to be notified when your baby is born. If, on the other hand, you are not comfortable for some reason, then arrange to meet with another doctor(s) until you find the physician you feel can best meet your baby's needs and match your philosophy of care.

If you already have children, you may also already have a pediatrician or family doctor for them. Be sure to discuss your pregnancy with this doctor, and let him or her know when you expect to deliver. Be sure to tell him or her that you have been identified as high-risk, and where you will deliver, as well as who your doctor is. Your pediatrician may wish to discuss your risks with your own doctor before delivery, to try to determine any special needs your baby might have. Make sure you find out when and how the pediatrician or family doctor wishes to be notified when you are in labor or have delivered.

The following is a list of health professionals who may be members of your baby's health care team at some point:

Family physician: Many family doctors will care for both mother and baby (or just the baby) if the risk factors are low and there are no complications during labor, delivery or afterwards that require specialized care. If you already have a family doctor, it is best to discuss this to determine what role he or she would play in the care of your newborn.

Pediatrician: A pediatrician is a specialist in the care of infants, children and adolescents. To become a pediatrician, a doctor must complete a three-year residency in pediatrics, which includes in-depth training and experience in newborn care, including intensive care. After completing the residency, the pediatrician may become certified by the American Board of Pediatrics after passing an examination and completing other requirements. After becoming board-certified, the doctor can also become a *F*ellow in the *A*merican *A*cademy of *P*ediatrics and therefore can use the designation "FAAP" after his or her name. The pediatrician may be in attendance in the delivery room to care for your baby's needs at that time if difficulties are anticipated or be called in later, depending on the baby's problem(s).

Neonatologist: A neonatologist is a pediatrician who has completed two additional years of specialized fellowship training in neonatology (the care of newborns, especially those with known or potential problems). A qualified neonatologist can become board-certified in neonatology as well as in pediatrics. Most neonatologists practice in Level II or Level III nurseries (described in Chapters 18 and 19) and either provide direct care and management of high-risk newborns or work in consultation with your pediatrician or family doctor in the care of your baby if special care, evaluation or management are necessary.

If your baby is receiving care in a tertiary care center or regional perinatal center, you will meet doctors in various stages of specialty training.

Pediatric resident: A doctor in a three-year pediatric training program who cares for infants and children under the supervision of fellows, pediatricians and neonatologists. This kind of training most often takes place in a Level III facility, but some Level II infant care units may also train residents.

Neonatal fellow: A neonatal fellow is a fully trained pediatrician who is in a fellowship training program in the care of high-risk newborns (neonatology). The fellow works with and under the direction of a neonatologist, usually in a Level III (tertiary care or regional perinatal care center).

Pediatric and neonatal nurses: After your baby is born you will meet *registered nurses* or *vocational nurses* who have experience in caring for high-risk newborns if the baby needs special care. These nurses provide highly technical as well as loving care for infants. Some have additional training and experience as *clinical nurse specialists*, while others have completed special training programs in order to become *pediatric nurse practitioners*.

Other professionals: As is the case with your care, your baby may require the services of a variety of other professionals or paraprofessionals, all of whom have special training and experience in the care of sick or high-risk newborns.

Again, if at any time you do not understand the role of a professional in your care or that of your baby, make sure you ask. Although the various people and their roles on the health care team may often seem confusing to you, it is helpful to remember that each professional or paraprofessional plays a special part in your care or that of your baby, as his or her expertise or services are required.

EIGHTEEN

REGIONALIZED PERINATAL CARE: SPECIAL NETWORKS FOR MOTHERS AND NEWBORNS WITH SPECIAL NEEDS

As we have previously discussed, over the past 30 years alone, great strides have been made in all areas of medicine. In that time the most exciting, striking and impressive advances have taken place in perinatal care—the combined efforts of maternal-fetal medicine and neonatology. The statistics (as stated throughout this book) speak for themselves—statistics that translate into a saving of thousands of lives and an increase in the quality of life for countless others.

To put this into perspective, 20 years ago the concept of regionalized perinatal care was unheard of—because the technology and knowledge necessary were just starting to be developed. In fact, the term "perinatal" itself was not widely used by the public until the late 1970s. Today it is commonly used by professionals and laypersons alike to signify the *total care* of both mother and unborn/newborn infant.

For the past few decades obstetricians, pediatricians and other specialists have worked together for the betterment of both mother and baby. Whereas this interaction used to be more informal and less structured, in the last few years the cooperative efforts of these and other specialists have become progressively more structured and uniform, developing into a highly sophisticated network of care in many regions of the United States. Regionalized perinatal care was a logical extension of all those things we have discussed so far: the advent of sub-specialization in maternal-fetal medicine and neonatology; the tremendous growth in knowledge, skills and advanced diagnostic capabilities; and the importance of providing these specialized services to all those with potential or known high-risk problems (mothers and unborn/newborn babies alike).

Frankly, regionalization came about in part due to the enormous expense of providing the most sophisticated obstetrical and neonatal services available today. As you can imagine it would be virtually impossible for *all* hospitals in the United States to offer the most sophisticated level of care—considering the cost involved in having the most modern technical capabilities in all areas available, with specialists and sub-specialists working around the clock, and the backup services necessary to support the professionals.

For your safety and well-being and that of your baby, special guidelines have been prepared (and are revised as necessary) by a special "Committee on Perinatal Health"—a cooperative effort of the American College of Obstetricians and Gynecologists, the American Academy of Pediatrics, the American Academy of Family Physicians and the American Medical Association. These guidelines for regionalization of perinatal care and classification of hospitals based on the level of care they can safely provide—better ensure your safety and well-being and that of your unborn/newborn baby. (The guidelines have essentially established a coordinated system in many areas of the country.) The designation of a hospital—Level I, Level II and Level III—is determined by the level of care and services the hospital is able to provide based on stringent state licensing regulations and requirements.

These guidelines are not only useful to doctors and other health professionals but understanding the "why" and "how" hospitals are classified is quite advantageous to you as well. The fact is—the system can (at times) confuse, frustrate or make some women insecure—if they do not understand the basics about the different classifications and how certain professionals and the various levels of care interrelate (and cooperate) with one another. For example— if your doctor referred you to one hospital for tests—then the professionals there referred you to a maternal-fetal specialist (high-risk obstetrician/perinatologist) at another hospital—you might get the impression that you were being "bounced" from one place to another or (even worse) that no one knew what was going on, that no one cared or that something terrible was wrong! Not true. But these would be perfectly legitimate feelings if you did not understand the system of care.

Level III Hospital (The Highest Classification)

A regional perinatal center or a perinatal tertiary care center (if not in a regional network) has a Level III classification and was conceived and developed to provide you and your unborn/newborn baby with the most sophisticated care available today—if you need that level of care. If you are referred to a Level III facility for diagnostic tests, management or intervention, you can expect the state-of-the-art in maternal-fetal medicine and neonatology. These centers usually have a university affiliation—that is, medical students, residents and fellows are trained there. The regional perinatal center is also usually part of a major regional medical center and is capable of and responsible for managing the most complex medical problems as well. Essentially, the regional perinatal center acts as the hub of a network of hospitals that provide varying degrees of care and refer to the regional center as necessary.

What you will find at a Level III facility is a multidisciplinary approach to provide for your perinatal care needs. These professionals have the expertise and sophisticated equipment necessary to provide for your "total" care, including all the prenatal and perinatal methods of diagnosis, management, treatment and intervention we have discussed throughout this book:

- Amniocentesis
- Diagnostic ultrasound
- Genetic studies and counseling
- Specialized laboratory and pathology testing
- Management of the most complicated high-risk pregnancies
- Antepartum testing
- Antepartum transport (by land or air) of the expectant mother from hospitals in the network to other more specialized hospitals in the network or directly to the regional perinatal center
- Antepartum and intrapartum fetal monitoring
- Sophisticated surgical capabilities
- Transport of ill neonates or those requiring specialized care or evaluation
- A neonatal intensive care unit (discussed in detail in Chapter 19)
- Often, a neonatal followup program
- Sometimes, an alternative birthing center (within the regional perinatal center)
- Parent and community education
- Often, special programs for those identified as high-risk (such as programs for diabetic mothers and prepared childbirth classes)

The professionals at regional perinatal centers are also responsible for the continuing education of other professionals in the perinatal network and for providing consultation for the hospitals in the regional network. Close communications are constant between the professionals at the regional perinatal center and those at the hospitals in the regional network. (Often direct phone links are set up so the professionals at the regional center can be reached immediately.) Often, too, telemetry is utilized, so specialists at the perinatal center can help interpret oxytocin challenge tests (OCTs) or fetal heart rate monitoring data, for example, and offer recommendations. This kind of system allows for consultation to distant rural areas as well as to other hospitals in the regional network.

These close communications are important to you. If for some reason you need more specialized care (at any time) during your pregnancy—arrangements can be made for this care. The doctors caring for you will be in close contact with the perinatal center—as is necessary.

If at some point these recommendations include your immediate transport (before, during or after labor and delivery) or that of your newborn baby, a special transport team(s) will respond (by land or air). The team often includes a physician, nurse, respiratory therapist or other professional as is needed to provide safe transport (with management and/or intervention during transport, as is necessary) to the regional perinatal center. Those on the team will depend on the reason(s) for the transport, since continued stabilization and medical care are provided throughout the trip. If there is room, your husband or partner (or important other) may be able to go with you (however, policies differ from network to network).

If your newborn baby needs more specialized evaluation or management, a unique, mobile, battery-operated incubator is used for transport. This special unit, other portable equipment and the professionals in attendance allow for continual care of the baby during the trip. If you are well enough to travel (and there is room) you may be able to accompany your baby. However, if you are still recuperating from delivery and your baby must be transferred immediately, you will need to complete your recuperation period at the hospital where you delivered and see the baby as soon as you can be safely released from the hospital. Obviously, this situation is very difficult for new mothers. When at all possible, both mother and newborn are transported so they need not be separated. However, this is not always possible. It may be helpful to remember that your baby is being transferred for more specialized care for his or her safety and well-being. If you must be separated from your baby, keep in contact with the doctors and nurses in the special care nursery by telephone so you can know how your baby is doing and what treatment he or she is receiving.

While at the regional perinatal center, if you become confused about who your doctor is—simply ask which doctor is your "primary physician" or the physician in charge of your health care team. Often the physician "team leader" is obvious since he or she may be the maternal-fetal specialist whom you have been seeing throughout your pregnancy. In some situations, your obstetrician will be your "primary physician" or he or she may have identified a maternal-fetal specialist who will direct your total care. Things get confusing for most women when immediate transport to another hospital takes place and they come into contact with several doctors, none whom they know, in a short period of time. If you become confused or frustrated (or your husband or partner does), simply ask *who* your primary physician is, or who is the doctor directing your care.

Level II Classification

Those hospitals with a Level II classification should be able to provide care and services for normal pregnancy, some high-risk women and specific neonatal problems. Level II hospitals are usually found in suburban or urban areas and perform the majority of deliveries in this country. Generally, antepartum and intrapartum testing are available to some degree. If you are being seen at a Level II facility, you can be assured that consultation with the regional perinatal center occurs on a continuing basis, if necessary. If you or your baby need more sophisticated testing, management or intervention, then you and/or the baby would be referred to the regional perinatal center.

The fact is, many high-risk problems can be followed and managed at Level II hospitals. However, you should also realize that the Level II designation is (at times) a broad one, in that some of these hospitals have the facilities and expertise to handle many complications of pregnancy and of the newborn, while others are more limited. What this means is that experiences may vary from region to region, or Level II hospital to Level II hospital, or state to state. For example, if you were seen in one Level II hospital you might be evaluated and diagnosed as high-risk, then referred to the regional perinatal center for all further testing, management and intervention, depending on the reason for your high-risk status. However, if you were seen in another Level II hospital, even in the same network, for the same problem, you might be followed and cared for at that Level II facility, with consultation from the regional perinatal center as necessary.

In either situation the professionals at the Level II hospital (in concert with recommendations from the regional center) will refer you and/or your baby, or transport one or both (depending on the urgency of the situation) to the regional center when a greater degree of sophisticated care is needed. The perinatal network is a step-up approach, with each hospital in the network caring for you and your unborn/newborn baby up to a certain level, then referring to a higher level of care when it is appropriate to do so. It is important to remember that your experience may be different from that of someone else you know who is high risk. Your own experience will very much depend on the perinatal network, the hospital where your doctor has staff privileges and your needs and those of your baby.

Level I Classification

Low-risk pregnancies, uncomplicated deliveries and healthy newborns can be cared for by Level I hospitals. According to guidelines developed by the Committee on Perinatal Health, Level I hospitals should be those in which fewer deliveries are performed and should be located in primarily rural or semi-rural areas. These hospitals, whether rural, surburban or urban should be affiliated with a regional perinatal network which better ensures prompt consultation from and referral to the regional perinatal center or a Level II facility if an unexpected complication occurs for mother or unborn/newborn baby. Professionals at Level I hospitals in a regional network are trained to care for mother and/or neonate on a short-term basis when a situation warrants special management, until prompt transport to a Level II or III facility takes place.

The Effects of Regionalized Perinatal Networks

One of the first statewide programs to be developed for regionalization of perinatal care was in Wisconsin in 1967. All hospitals in the state with obstetrical services became involved in an ongoing education program, and Level II facilities were developed for all areas of the state, with a regional perinatal center at the University of Wisconsin, Madison. The overall neonatal mortality rate in the state declined by 49.7 percent from 1968 to 1977.

Iowa's regionalized perinatal system, which now includes all Iowa hospitals, has the University of Iowa Hospital as the system's only Level III center. Level II facilities throughout the state perform careful evaluation of patients and provide care at the level of their capabilities. They are prepared to transport high-risk women and/ or newborns to the nearest Level III center. (Patients closer to centers in Minnesota, Wisconsin or Nebraska are transported there.) Neonatal mortality declined by 44.4 percent in Iowa from 1968 to 1978.

There are many more examples, but what is important is the fact that the neonatal mortality rate has declined by 41.7 percent overall in the United States from 1968 to 1978. Although there is no way to prove cause and effect—it seems reasonable to deduce that the combination of great strides made in maternal-fetal medicine, advances in neonatal care and the development of regionalized perinatal networks (and their education programs) has had a major impact on infant mortality rates and ensured better outcomes for those at risk for problems.

The reduction of infant mortality has been complimented by a reduction in maternal mortality as well. In 1970 there were 21.5 maternal deaths per 100,000 births nationwide. In 1978 this nationwide figure had been reduced to 9.9 maternal deaths per 100,000 births. As we discussed in greater detail in Chapter 16, statistics on maternal mortality rates are somewhat misleading, in that the rate includes death from any cause while pregnant or within 90 days from the termination of the pregnancy, regardless of the pregnancy's duration. Therefore, the actual number of deaths due to pregnancy, labor or delivery may well be even much fewer than these statistics indicate.

When There Is No Regionalized Network

Some areas of the country have not as yet regionalized their perinatal care, and others are in the process of doing so now. If you live in an area where perinatal care has not been regionalized, you should remember that there is at least one tertiary care center (Level III equivalent) in virtually every major city in the United States, and that smaller cities usually have Level II facilities or their equivalent. If you are high risk, or your doctor believes you need more specialized care than can be obtained in your local hospital, you will usually be referred to one of these hospitals in a larger city. Your doctor will know where to refer you if this is necessary.

In some high-risk pregnancies, your own physician will follow you during pregnancy, even though not a specialist in high-risk obstetrics, and have specialists at the nearest center consult, make recommendations concerning your care or perform necessary tests when necessary. Other high-risk women will need to be followed by a maternal-fetal specialist (perinatologist) throughout the entire pregnancy, and their newborn baby will need to be evaluated and cared for by a neonatologist at birth. It will depend on the reason for your high risk status, as well as how your pregnancy progresses. If your personal physician is not a specialist in maternal-fetal medicine but a well-trained obstetrician who practices (has staff privileges at and delivers at) a Level III facility, is perfectly able to care for the great majority of high-risk problems.

A Word About Statistics

At times reports in the news media unintentionally mislead by misinterpreting data about infant or maternal mortality rates for a specific hospital or regional center. Sometimes it is reported that the rates are higher at the regional perinatal center or tertiary center, without any explanation of the reason(s) for the higher rates. All such statistics should be viewed in perspective. In general, mortality rates for mothers, babies or both will be higher at perinatal centers when compared to other hospitals (Level I or Level II and their equivalents). These major centers deal with the most complex and difficult situations, and higher rates do not necessarily mean that the quality of care should be in question. The point is, if a regional perinatal network is functioning efficiently and effectively, all Level I hospitals should have extremely low mortality rates, since they handle only uncomplicated pregnancies and provide care for normal newborns. Level II mortality rates should also be lower than those at the regional perinatal center, since they handle only certain maternal complications and provide care for only specific newborn problems.

Since each facility refers "up" as complications for mother and/or newborn increase, it is reasonable to expect that the institution handling the most serious problems would have the highest mortality rates, although those rates are significantly lower than ever before. In other words, comparing the mortality rates of hospitals with different designations is like comparing apples and oranges.

You should also realize that rates vary not only with level of care at a given center, but also are dependent on the population served by the center (or even by the perinatal regional network). Those factors that must be considered are: the health status (before pregnancy) of those in the population served, the compliance (or lack of compliance) with medical recommendations and even whether or not any prenatal care was obtained by the patients. The purpose of peer review boards (and some government agencies) is to objectively evaluate morbidity and mortality rates and to ascertain if these rates are too high or if the level of care is below what it should be in each hospital or region. Medical care given to mother and unborn/newborn baby is constantly evaluated in this way to better ensure appropriate care, timely referral and state-of-the-art intervention.

The Bottom Line

Not all high-risk women need the level of care provided by a regional perinatal center or its equivalent tertiary care center in a nonregionalized system. The ideal level of care in every case is dependent on the problem(s) or potential problem(s) that put you or your unborn/newborn infant at risk. A careful medical and maternal history by your personal doctor, routine prenatal visits, and indicated maternal and fetal screening tests can identify approximately 60 percent of all mothers and babies who will or may have problems and require special attention. Therefore, your obstetrician or family physician will be able to determine the need for specialized management and refer you to the appropriate specialist, sub-specialist or center that can meet the needs of your pregnancy.

If, however, you have questions at any time about the need for specialized care, be sure to ask your doctor. It is always better to know to whom you would be referred or to what hospital or center you or your infant might be sent if the need arose. In this way, you and your family will be less confused and bewildered if you, the baby or both are referred to specialists at a different hospital, or are transferred to a perinatal center. Everyone will be satisfied that this is being done for your safety and well-being and that of your baby.

NINETEEN

INFANT SPECIAL CARE UNITS: WHAT ARE THEY?

Infant special care (intensive care) units are an intrinsic component of quality perinatal care. In fact, as we discussed earlier in this section, the classification of a hospital in a regional perinatal network is based on many factors, including the level of care the hospital is able to provide for the mother—and the level of newborn intensive care available for the baby. The many advances in newborn care and the establishment of infant special care units (also called neonatal intensive care, newborn intensive care, infant intensive care) have had a major impact on saving lives and bettering the quality of life for countless numbers of babies in the United States.

The Establishment of Newborn Special Care

We know that perinatal care consists of the care of both the mother and her unborn/newborn baby. Newborn intensive care units are classified as Level I, Level II or Level III based on the type of care the units are able to provide. In almost all cases, the classification of the hospital matches the classification of the infant special care unit. Evaluation and classification of newborn units, as well as overall perinatal care available at hospitals was made possible in part by the National Foundation—March of Dimes which established the first committee on perinatal health care services in 1971. The Robert Wood Johnson Foundation also played a major role beginning in 1972 when it started supporting a national program to regionalize perinatal care. Because of this initial work, infant special care units were established nationwide.

Levels of Care

As was the case with your care, it is valuable for you and your partner to understand the various levels of care available to your baby. With this knowledge, you'll be less likely to become confused, frustrated or insecure about what is happening with your baby's care if he or she has a problem that requires transfer to another hospital, or if you're transferred to another hospital in order to have your baby where there is special care available for newborns.

Level III (tertiary care or regional perinatal care) centers would have the staff and specialized facilities to care for all perinatal needs, including all low- and high-risk mothers and newborns. Level III centers, then, offer the most sophisticated and intensive care available for you and your baby alike. In a regional perinatal center (Level III or tertiary center) the infant special care unit may be divided into several different nurseries (although this varies from center to center).

You can expect the *intensive care nursery* in an infant special care unit to provide specialized treatment and management by neonatologists in conjunction with pediatricians and other sub-specialists (such as pediatric surgeons, pediatric cardiologists, anesthesiologists and neurologists). Maximum and specialized nursing care is provided 24 hours a day for your baby (often there is one nurse for each one or two newborns). This nursery, which has the most sophisticated and abundant equipment for the stabilization and monitoring of ill newborns, is for those newborns in need of the most intensive medical supervision. The medical and nursing care in these units is very aggressive.

The unit may also have an *intermediate nursery* that generally serves several functions. If your baby has been in the intensive care nursery, but no longer needs that level of care, he or she may be moved to the intermediate nursery. Or, if your baby requires close observations or special treatment but not to the extent of that provided in the more intensive unit, he or she may be placed in the intermediate nursery right from the start. To put this into perspective, the intermediate nursery at a Level III center is the equivalent of the special care nursery at the Level II facility (which we will discuss in greater detail in this chapter).

In some facilities infants are discharged directly from the intermediate nursery, but in others there is another step before going home—the *growing nursery*. If your baby is very small or is still recovering from serious problems and needs nursing observation and care, he or she would be closely watched while gaining strength and weight. You and your partner would usually play an increasingly important role in this stage of your baby's care—feeding, bathing and caring for the baby's needs.

All regional perinatal centers or tertiary care centers (Level III) have *newborn nurseries* for healthy babies. If your baby was taken to a newborn nursery because there were no unusual problems, you should expect close observation by specially trained nurses of your baby for several hours to several days to detect any possible problems that might follow labor and delivery. Your baby's doctor would also perform a detailed examination on the day of his or her birth and would check on the baby's progress on a daily or twice-a-day basis until discharged from the hospital. The professionals in a newborn nursery also have the ability to intervene and stabilize infants who become ill and transport them to a more specialized nursery. They also have provisions for parent education and support in the initial care of the new baby. The newborn nurseries in a Level III center are basically the equivalent of the nursery in a Level I hospital.

Level II hospitals would have the staff and facilities to care for well newborns, as well as those with special needs transferred from Level I hospitals, and provide an intermediate level of special care for high-risk newborns appropriately delivered at these facilities. As we discussed earlier related to your care, a Level II classification is a very broad one and this holds true for Level II infant care as well. This means that if you had your baby in one Level II facility, they may be able to provide for all your baby's needs and consult with the specialists at the regional center as needed, or your baby may need to be transferred from another Level II facility to the regional perinatal center with the same problem. Each hospital recognizes the level of care it can best provide and (in concert with the sub-specialists at the Level III facility) decide when it is in the best interest and well-being of your baby to have more specialized, intensive care. So, if your experience is different from someone else you know, this should not concern you.

A *Level I hospital* would have the staff and facilities to care for well newborns until they are discharged, resuscitate newborns at the time of delivery or during the hospital stay, stabilize ill newborns for transfer to a Level II or III facility and continue care for those infants returned to the hospital after treatment and management at a Level II or III unit.

One note: The role of a children's hospital in a network of care often confuses people. A children's hospital itself can be a tertiary care center for infants and children. If it is not attached to or part of a major general medical center (or women's hospital) that provides the complimentary and necessary obstetrical care, however, it would not be a perinatal center—but could be a neonatal center. In other words, its neonatal classification could be Level II or III, and other hospitals in the area would transport ill newborns to its nurseries for the level of specialized care required, but babies would not be delivered there.

The Reasons Newborns Are Admitted for Special Care

The importance of an infant special care unit cannot be overstated. We know that approximately 3 percent of all infants will require intensive care because of life-threatening problems. Others will need observation and/or intervention as a protective measure, and still others may need to be transferred from a normal nursery (for newborns without problems) to some level of special care because of the development of an unexpected problem.

There are many and varied reasons for a newborn to be admitted to a special care unit:

- The need for careful observation for a suspected problem
- Known or suspected infection
- Severe jaundice
- Rh disease or other blood disorder
- Birth asphyxia
- Prematurity (gestational age of less than 36 weeks)
- Birth weight of less than 2,500 grams (5 pounds 8 ounces)
- Respiratory distress syndrome (hyaline membrane disease)
- Problems that require special surgical care
- Respiratory failure from any cause
- Life-threatening congenital abnormalities or those that require prompt intervention or management
- Suspected hereditary metabolic disease
- Any of a wide variety of other conditions that could potentially threaten a newborn infant's life and health

In some situations (for example, when the mother has a medical problem such as diabetes, heart disease or other chronic condition), the baby is placed in an intermediate care nursery for a few hours to a few days for close observation—although the baby seems to be doing well at birth.

Being Prepared for Infant Special Care

It is never easy for anyone to have a baby admitted to an intensive care unit. For most parents and family members, it is a very trying and stressful time—a time when concerns are magnified—often out of proportion to the actual seriousness of the baby's condition. Normally, anxiety about what is wrong with the baby and how serious it is, is enhanced by such factors as having to face much unfamiliar equipment, noise and confusion; not understanding the procedures performed and what they mean; and dealing with professionals who may be strangers. All contribute to the parents' confusion—and to their feelings of helplessness and loss of control. If your baby is placed in an infant special care unit and you experience these feelings, it is perfectly understandable—the rule rather than the exception.

Much of the time you and your partner will not know in advance that your newborn will need specialized care, while in other situations there is time to prepare for this necessary step. While there is really no way to totally prepare yourself for all of your concerns and feelings if your baby must be admitted to a special care unit, there are things that can be useful.

Talk to your doctor about the possibility of the baby's needing treatment in an intensive care unit. Learn all you can about the possible problems he or she might have, based on your risk status. Learn what you can about the equipment, so it does not frighten you—what it does, how it helps, even the noise it makes. Many women and their partners even visit the unit long before the delivery to see what it is like and to have the equipment and procedures explained to them.

Some perinatal centers give tours of the hospital and show expectant parents the neonatal intensive care areas, talk about the various professionals who work there and what they do, and discuss the unit's policies and procedures. If there is no special arrangement for such a "preview" of the unit, talk with your doctor in detail so your questions can be answered. It would also be helpful to meet with your unborn infant's doctor (pediatrician or even neonatologist) before delivery to discuss expected problems and ask questions.

Caring for the Basic Needs of Ill Newborns

All newborns must adapt to life outside the womb. They must learn to breathe air to obtain oxygen and eliminate carbon dioxide. Their heart and circulation must change to pump blood through the lungs rather than through the placenta. They must adjust to an environment that has changeable temperature—and must learn to stay warm. They must nurse or be bottle fed for their nutrition, instead of automatically receiving nutrients from the placenta.

The majority of babies—even those in high-risk pregnancies—have few problems adjusting to the outside world. They require careful observation for a few hours, are watched for up to several days and are then able to be discharged and sent home with their parents. If they have problems, these are temporary and require little if any intervention.

However, very small infants—and those who experience stress before birth (due to many reasons)—may have a difficult time adapting to life after birth. Some newborns need special, often heroic, assistance in order to survive. Such assistance involves the special expertise and capabilities found in infant special care units.

While each infant will receive individualized treatment based on his or her unique needs and specific situation, each ill newborn also has certain needs in common with all other ill infants. Therefore, much of what is done in a neonatal unit is devoted to the basics: keeping babies warm; assuring adequate oxygenation and proper elimination of carbon dioxide; providing optimal nutrition; preventing and treating infection; providing close, expert nursing observation and care to anticipate and detect as well as treat problems; and utilizing the latest in technology for diagnosis and treatment.

Nutrition and Feeding

Most very ill newborns have special nutritional needs and will require assistance in eating or total provision of their nutritional needs for some time.

The sick baby is almost always given fluids and nutrients intravenously (by IV) for the first day or so of life. A very small needle (called a "butterfly" or "scalp vein" needle) or a small plastic "catheter" is inserted into a vein of the scalp, hands, feet, arms or legs. Sometimes a small incision must be made in the skin in order to insert the catheter, a procedure called a "cutdown."

Some ill infants (those not able to tolerate breast milk or formula feedings for days to weeks) receive very special mixtures containing sugar, amino acids (the components of proteins) and fats, as well as vitamins and minerals. These mixtures supply all or nearly all the baby's needed calories and nutrients by vein. This technique of providing all necessary nutrients is called "total parenteral nutrition" or "hyperalimentation."

The amount of liquid given to the baby by IV must be regulated very carefully, so an "infusion pump" or "regulator" is used. One of the most common of these devices is called an "IVAC®," which regulates the IV flow and sounds an alarm when there is a problem with the flow. The alarm's sounding does not mean there is anything wrong with the baby, simply that the IV flow needs to be checked and adjusted.

When the baby is able to tolerate some feeding by mouth, he or she will begin to receive milk (pumped breast milk from the mother or special infant formula). If the baby is too weak to suck or would tire excessively, then "gavage feeding" is performed. A tiny plastic tube is inserted through the nose or mouth into the baby's stomach, and formula or breast milk is dripped in. The very small or ill baby may require this kind of nutritional therapy for days to weeks before he or she is capable of sucking on a special soft nipple. It may take much longer for the baby to be able to nurse from his or her mother's breast, because breast-feeding requires more effort on the baby's part. (Note: Breast milk has many advantages over formula for the small, sick infant and can be pumped with a breast pump or expressed by hand by the mother, stored in a freezer and fed to the baby by gavage or bottle until he or she is strong enough to nurse. Most doctors encourage breast milk feeding whenever possible.)

Prevention and Treatment of Infection

Careful *handwashing (scrubbing)* is a must in all special nurseries in order to help prevent the spread of infection to sick infants. All units have a required routine for handwashing, which is explained to parents at their first visit. Each time anyone goes into the nursery, he or she must scrub in a prescribed manner and wear a *protective gown* over his or her clothing. Both parents and professionals alike must follow this procedure.

Many babies in special care units receive *antibiotics* for known or suspected infection during their stay. Antibiotics are given by IV or injection into the muscle. (Because of the potention seriousness of most infections in newborns, antibiotics are rarely if ever given by mouth—because it is very difficult to adequately treat infections in newborns this way.)

Infection in the newborn can often be difficult to detect, and serious infections like "sepsis" (generalized blood infection) and "meningitis" (infection of the tissues around the brain) must be treated quickly. Therefore, if a problem is suspected, specimens of blood, urine, spinal fluid and other tissues are obtained and cultured in the laboratory. (A "culture" is a technique in which a specimen is specially treated in order to try to grow and identify bacteria.) Antibiotics are often started and continued for the one to three days it takes to get the results of the cultures from the laboratory. This allows doctors to get a "jump" on the infection, so it doesn't worsen during the time period in which they are waiting for the laboratory reports. If the cultures are negative (no bacteria can be grown), the antibiotics are often stopped.

Monitoring and Special Nursing Care

Sophisticated *electronic monitoring* is used to help doctors and nurses evaluate and care for very sick newborns. Through *special electrodes* that are attached to the baby's chest, his or her heart rate and breathing can be continuously monitored on a screen and recorded on paper for further evaluation, if necessary. If the baby's breathing stops (called "apnea") or slows down, or if the heart rate slows (called "bradycardia"), the sophisticated machine sounds a loud alarm. This is important because *apnea/bradycardia spells* are rather common in prematures and ill newborns, and this monitoring allows for prompt detection and intervention.

Special monitoring may also be used, when indicated, for continuous evaluation of blood pressure, oxygenation and intracranial (inside the head) pressure. All of these measurements assist the nurses and doctors in assessing the baby's status minute to minute and provide information that helps them determine the baby's needs and the best direction for care.

Specially trained, experienced neonatal nurses care for the very sick infants 24 hours a day and pay particular attention to any changes in the babies' general condition, breathing, color and activity. The nurses measure and record the babies' *vital signs* (temperature, heart rate, breathing rate, blood pressure), monitor fluids (IVs as well as urine and intestinal fluid), suction fluid and mucus from the mouth and lungs as needed, feed the babies and provide other necessary treatments.

The Environment and Noise in Intensive Care Units

The environment of an intensive care unit is very unfamiliar to parents. The abundance of machines and equipment, the tubes, lights, capsulelike isolettes—and in particular, the noise—can be a source of stress. Loud equipment can be anxiety provoking, with such sounds as the beeps of some monitors, the swooshing of respirators, the characteristic noise of suction apparatus, IVAC alarms that signal the need to adjust IV fluids, and loud alarms on respiratory or other equipment that at times signify the need for intervention but in other instances are only "false alarms."

When you put all these together and add the stress parents are experiencing from other causes, as well, you can see how a beep or an alarm can cause concern or fear. Parents usually over-react to the sounds until they get more familiar with the surroundings and can distinguish between noises that are normal for the equipment, those that alert a nurse or doctor to the need to make an adjustment or true alerts that require intervention. It helps to remember that skilled professionals are always right there, and they know what each alarm, beep and sound means and does not mean. They have been trained to respond when a response is required.

Try not to let all the noises and medical equipment overwhelm you. Most parents adjust well as soon as they understand the equipment and get used to the noises it makes, but it's normal to feel jumpy. It's also helpful to remember that this equipment is there to assist in the care of your baby—and that it is an invaluable resource for doctors, nurses and special technicians in following and directing the baby's care.

What Are They Talking About?

Medical terminology often confuses and concerns parents, because they are not sure what the doctor or nurse is really telling them. If at any time you don't understand what is being said, say so. Health professionals will try to explain a situation in non-medical terms as much as possible. At times, too, parents are so stressed that they forget what they were told or aren't really "hearing" what is said. Never feel embarrassed to ask again or to have something explained in more detail.

Medical terminology and jargon are used as a communications shorthand, and just as all people do not know shorthand or speak French, not all understand "medicalese." You may overhear discussions between professionals where medical terminology is used. This is particularly stressful for parents, because they may have heard some of the words before and have only an incomplete knowledge of this "foreign" language. If you are concerned, and the discussion involves your own baby—ask for a "translation" rather than worrying about "what" is being said.

Your Special Role on the Health Care Team

Many professionals work together as a team to care for the sick neonate (as was discussed in detail in Chapter 17.)

You, too, are an important member of your baby's health care team, as are all your family members. Unfortunately, parents of ill infants or those needing some type of intervention most often feel helpless and useless in caring for their new baby. While specialized medical care is needed, your role and your partner's in your new baby's care is very, very important. Today all parents are regarded as members of the health care team. Although nurses, doctors and other health professionals talk to and touch the baby, they understand the need for the baby to experience the special love and attention only you can give. Therefore, visiting the nursery—touching, caressing and talking to your baby and holding him or her when this is possible—is vitally important. Getting to know your baby better and showing love and affection do make a difference for your baby, your partner and yourself. This bonding of parents and infant plays an important role not only during the illness but also in laying the groundwork for future relationships.

It is also well documented that breast milk has distinct advantages over formula for sick and premature babies (as well as for well babies). Here is where you can make a difference as well. As previously noted even if the baby cannot yet nurse, you can successfully express or pump breastmilk for your baby. Many nurseries have special electrical breast pumps for mothers to use, so the baby can have a supply of milk available. Pumping or expressing milk also helps you to continue producing milk, so you can actually nurse your baby as soon as he or she is strong enough to do so.

Most intensive care nurseries have special educational programs for parents, in addition to the individualized instructions given by doctors and nurses about your baby. It is often helpful to know more about baby care, safety, first aid and how to perform CPR (cardiopulmonary resuscitation). Some classes also teach ways for you to help your baby reach his or her highest level of development over the years.

If the baby has a genetic (or other) abnormality that will require medical care throughout life or some special care at home, join a group (there are many) of parents with a child who has the same type of problem. Those in the intensive care nursery or the clinical social worker can direct you to the group or groups that can meet your needs. Not only are these groups very supportive to parents who have a child with a chronic problem, but they help with practical issues, as well—for example, the "tricks" to use for easier care and the like. Organizations for parents of children with Down's Syndrome, Muscular Dystrophy, Spina Bifida, Cystic Fibrosis and multiple handicaps are common. Your local National Foundation—March of Dimes office can also be a resource for finding such organizations.

The Bottom Line on Infant Special Care

Infant special care units, the many advances in neonatology and sophisticated perinatal care have resulted in better outcomes for many babies and saved the lives of so many others. This country has seen an overall decline of 41.7 percent in neonatal mortality from 1968 to 1978. As more areas of the United States become regionalized and as advances in neonatology and maternal-fetal medicine continue, we will see an even greater decline in neonatal death and an increase in the quality of life for countless other infants.

TWENTY

A GLIMPSE INTO THE FUTURE

They spoke of glimmering silver space suits, massive streamlined spaceships, space stations and humans walking on the moon. Some told of men and women who spoke with and saw one another over a small screen, although they were continents apart. Others described 200-yard-long vessels that traveled the ocean floor, powered only by special molecules.

There were those who told of doctors evaluating a pumping heart on a multicolored screen connected to a humming computer; hair-thin intensified light beams striking diseased tissue, destroying it and stopping blood loss; organs transplanted from one human donor to save the life of another; miraculous reattachment of hands, fingers, legs and arms; and babies conceived in test tubes with the embryos then implanted into their mothers to grow and thrive. The list of prophecies was seemingly endless.

Some called them fools, buffoons or daydreamers. But in reality they were science fiction writers—men and women with fantastic, futuristic dreams and visions of worlds to come. No one suspected they would be right. Even they never guessed that their prophecies were to come to pass long before they had ever imagined. The *Harvard Medical School Health Letter* (August 1981) noted that "Every time science fiction writers gather, they remove one or two items from their list of futuristic dreams—mostly because modern science has converted yet another fanciful idea into reality." The fact is, much of yesterday's science fiction has become today's reality, and more fantasy is turning into fact every year.

There are many technical advances that are now being applied experimentally in maternal-fetal medicine. Some others look very promising, and their application is just around the corner. Others are still only dreams, but ones that scientists say are reachable in the near future. Of course, time alone will tell what is possible, reasonable and acceptable.

Fetoscopy and Fetal Blood and Tissue Sampling

Fetoscopy is an experimental procedure performed in only a few major perinatal centers across the country. Because the technique needs to be refined further and there is presently a 3 percent to 10 percent risk of losing a fetus if fetoscopy is performed, it is used only when specific problems are suspected.

This procedure allows the doctor to look directly into the amniotic sac at the fetus and placenta. It is ideally performed between the 15th and 18th week of pregnancy if it is being done in order to look at the fetal anatomy. (At this point the amniotic fluid is clear, and the fetus is still small enough that it can be seen quite well with the tiny instrument.)

The procedure is done with the aid of ultrasound, which is used to determine the fetus's position, as well as the location of the umbilical cord and placenta. A local anesthetic is given by injection at a chosen point on the woman's abdomen, and a small incision is made. A special cannula (a small, hollow, tubelike instrument) is pushed down through the abdominal wall via the incision and passes through the uterus directly into the amniotic sac. The fetoscope (a very thin, telescopelike instrument) is inserted through the cannula so the physician can view the fetus by means of the "scope." In this way fetal malformations or serious structural problems may be identified by looking directly at the fetus.

Fetal blood sampling can be performed during fetoscopy by inserting a needle down alongside the fetoscope, which is still inside the cannula. A small needle puncture is made in a fetal blood vessel found on the surface of the placenta or, at times, in the umbilical cord near where it attaches to the placenta. Bleeding from the needle puncture stops within 10 to 30 seconds. Doctors prefer to wait until the 18th to 20th week of pregnancy to take fetal blood samples using fetoscopy, because the blood vessels are larger and the procedure is more likely to be successful.

Fetal blood samples can also be obtained without fetoscopy. Called "placental aspiration," this procedure is performed with the assistance of ultrasound and involves inserting a needle through the abdominal wall, the uterine wall and into the placenta. Considered

a more "blind approach," this technique sometimes needs to be
repeated several times in order to obtain fetal blood. The blood
sample removed must be tested immediately to determine whether
the blood is from the fetus or the mother. If the mother's blood
was accidentally obtained, the needle must be inserted again to try
to obtain a sample of the fetus's blood.

Besides fetal blood sampling, fetoscopy also allows for fetal tissue
sampling (biopsy), in which a small sample of skin tissue is taken
from the fetus's scalp, buttocks or trunk. This kind of biopsy heals
completely, and usually the scar is not noticeable when the baby
is born. This tiny sample of fetal tissue can be studied under a
microscope as well as through chemical analysis, and this sophisticated study can provide important information about the fetus's
cell makeup.

Fetoscopy and fetal blood and tissue sampling permit the identification of a number of potentially devastating fetal problems (such
as serious metabolic, brain, liver, skin and blood disorders) that
cannot be identified by analysis of amniotic fluid and the cells in
the fluid.

The most important use of this type of fetal blood sampling and
analysis is in the identification of certain important blood abnormalities. Such problems as sickle cell disease and thalassemia (very
serious abnormalities of the hemoglobin) and the bleeding disorders
(hemophilia and others in which blood clotting is abnormal) cannot
be detected by amniocentesis or other techniques. In addition, unusual conditions like chronic granulomatous disease (an unusual
disease thought to be caused by a disturbance in the body's immune
system, not yet fully understood) and some disorders of the blood
platelets, white blood cells and red blood cells, as well as alpha-
antitrypsin deficiency (a defect that results in serious liver and lung
problems) have been found. Muscular dystrophy has been detected
by measuring a muscle enzyme in blood samples obtained in this
way. However, this is not a reliable way to make that diagnosis.

Biopsy samples of fetal tissue (skin) have permitted the diagnosis
of several unusual hereditary skin diseases, such as some forms of
ichthyosis and other scaling or peeling diseases that can be life
threatening. Skin tissue can also be used in genetic diagnosis, because the skin fibroblasts (developing cells) multiply quickly. These
cells can be studied for chromosomal problems or metabolic diseases
if examination of amniotic fluid was not successful. It might also
become more and more possible to use this kind of tissue sampling
to measure the drug or chemical content of the fetus's cells.

While fetoscopy was developed at least in part in order to allow medical personnel to look directly at the fetus to diagnose malformations, this use is actually somewhat restricted now. Because of the small size of the instrument, only limited areas of the tiny fetus can be seen easily. Although neural tube defects as well as other major and minor abnormalities have been identified with this procedure, with the development of better ultrasound and other techniques, the use of diagnostic fetoscopy will probably always be rather restricted.

Although the diagnostic capabilities of fetoscopy may never be extensive, its most exciting potential use lies in the area of fetal therapy. The possibilities may be endless—the administration of vital medications directly into the fetus's blood, cell transplants that may induce the development of normal enzyme function, as well as the use of genetic material (involving a technique called "recombinant DNA technology") to treat and thereby potentially cure a wide spectrum of genetic or congenital diseases and disorders.

Imagine how fantastic it would be to actually be able to identify, then treat, a serious or life-threatening problem in the fetal stage and thereby improve the quality of the baby's life after birth!

Fetal Surgery

In April 1981 the first successful fetal surgery was reported by officials from the University of California. This surgery, performed through the university's Moffitt Hospital Prenatal Diagnosis Clinic, may well represent the beginnings of another milestone in maternal-fetal medicine. The fetus was suffering from a potentially life-threatening blockage of the urinary tract. This was complicated by the fact that he was a twin, and the well-being of his twin sister (who was without problems) could potentially have suffered from any procedure performed on him.

Using ultrasound, the physicians were able to identify the urinary blockage, which had caused severe pressure buildup. Kidney as well as lung damage would have continued to worsen unless the pressure was relieved. With the assistance of ultrasound to locate the fetus's bladder and to carefully determine the fetal position, a long, thin needle was inserted into the bladder, and the trapped fluid was removed. However, 10 days later another ultrasound told the team of doctors that a further step was necessary—the bladder had again become more distended. A one-inch long catheter (sometimes called a "shunt") was then inserted into the fetus's bladder, allowing the fetus's urine to drain directly into the amniotic fluid. Four days later ultrasound verified that the fluid from the bladder was draining properly. Although the pressure from the urinary blockage had caused abdominal wall stretching, after the baby's birth doctors removed the catheter, successfully corrected the urinary blockage problem and repaired the abdominal wall. His twin sister was not affected by the intervention, and both babies were reported to be doing well.

Within a few months two other babies on whom successful fetal surgery had been performed were born at the Medical College of Virginia Hospital. One had had a blocked kidney, resulting in a fluid-filled cyst. The cyst was larger than the fetus's head and was causing polyhydramnios (accumulation of excessive amniotic fluid), because the fetus was not swallowing the fluid, as he should have been. Ultrasound allowed doctors to identify the problem and permitted them to remove the excess fluid from the cyst. Once the fluid had been removed, the fetus's development could continue. This surgery was performed five months into the fetus's development and represented the procedure's first successful use.

Fetal surgery for hydrocephalus (abnormal accumulation of a large amount of fluid inside the fetus's head) is beginning to be reported. The *New England Journal of Medicine* has published a report of a fetus who was treated for this condition at 25 weeks of gestation. A long, thin needle was used to remove fluid from the fetus's head. The baby, whose fetal surgery was performed in Boston, was later born without evidence of the puncture marks but with some suggestion of mental retardation. (Retardation is a certainty with progressive untreated hydrocephalus, so it should not be assumed that this resulted from the surgery, which may well have reduced the degree of retardation experienced. In Colorado another type of fetal surgery for hydrocephalus has been successful. A small catheter was inserted into the fetus's head and left in place to allow the fluid to continue to drain.

Studies are being done with animals to develop techniques that may be able to be applied to humans. In addition to antenatal treatment of hydrocephalus, which is often associated with neural tube defects, attempts are being made to cover the spinal defects in some of these conditions with "bone paste" in the hopes that the graft will be successful. Still other investigators are studying limb defects—abnormalities that have many causes and result in deformities of arms, legs or digits. There has been some success in causing growth of a normal extremity following amputation of the deformed part, if the amputation is performed at the right time in the gestation of the animals being studied. Again these are *all only* studies in animals at the present time.

The point is—reports of fetal surgery are starting to come in, and the results look promising. Although fetal surgery is still in its infancy and current indications for it are rare, its potential is far-reaching in saving lives and improving the quality of life for many others. The day may come when it will be possible to perform extensive surgery on a fetus to correct or repair certain problems, so structural development or organ function may proceed normally. Such procedures may even include removing the fetus from the womb to surgically repair a problem, then returning it to the womb to permit normal prenatal growth and development to continue. This has been successfully performed in extensive animal studies.

In Vitro Fertilization (Test Tube Babies)

There are various reasons for infertility. Anovulation (lack of ovulation) results in infertility, because no ovum is released to be fertilized by the sperm. Fertility drugs developed in the last two decades have dramatically increased the number of women able to have children, but there are cases where the drugs simply do not work.

For other women (an estimated 500,000 in the United States), infertility results from Fallopian tube blockage or dysfunction, or because the Fallopian tube was removed as a treatment for ectopic pregnancy or other medical condition. These women are unable to conceive only because the ovum has no way of meeting the sperm. With normal Fallopian tubes conception occurs when the ovary releases an ovum that travels up into the Fallopian tube and is met by ejaculated sperm. The egg is fertilized when penetrated by a sperm. A woman with a problem in the Fallopian tubes, then, has a mechanical condition that interferes with fertilization, but it does not mean she (or the woman who does not ovulate) could not carry a pregnancy if there were a means to bring the sperm and ovum together. (With some Fallopian tube problems, microsurgery is recommended to see if the obstruction can be corrected. Although there have been some successes, many tubal problems cannot be corrected.)

For those women with blocked Fallopian tubes, a means to allow them to bear children needed to be developed. Although a very new and still unrefined procedure (in terms of its success rate), *in vitro* fertilization (coming from Latin, meaning "in glass"—in this case, in a test tube) holds great promise for the future.

The procedure involves aspiration (removal by a special needle) of an ovum from the ovary using a technique called "laparoscopy." A tiny incision is made just below the umbilicus (belly button), and a small, special telescopelike instrument—the laparoscope—is inserted so the reproductive organs can be viewed. This allows the doctor to see the ovary and remove an ovum.

In the meantime the woman's husband or partner deposits sperm into a special sterile container. The sperm are counted and evaluated then prepared for fertilization. The sperm may be frozen as part of this process if there will be any delay in the procedure. When the conditions are right, the ovum and sperm are placed in a special medium inside a test tube or petri dish (a flat glass dish).

A sperm must penetrate the ovum in order for fertilization to occur. Once meiosis (special cell division) takes place and the correct cell division continues, the embryonic stage of development is reached. If everything so far has been successful, the embryo is transferred through the cervix into the mother's uterus when conditions are favorable. The next step is for the embryo to implant into the endometrium (lining of the uterus) so further development can occur. The success of the procedure at this point can be determined by special analysis of the mother's blood or urine—if she begins to show signs of hormones that are produced by the placenta, the implantation has been successful.

Because of the newness of the entire procedure, there is much that still needs to be formalized to ensure optimal results, and many questions are still unanswered. Detailed recommendations about how the procedure should best be performed and when each of the various steps must be done will depend upon the results of further attempts at *in vitro* fertilization.

So far, successes with *in vitro* fertilization—successes that have produced healthy babies—have been well publicized. However, problems can occur at any of the various steps in the procedure: At times it is difficult or impossible to remove an ovum from the ovary; there may be a problem with sperm collection; the *in vitro* fertilization may not occur properly (no sperm or many sperm may penetrate the ovum); something may go wrong with cell division; embryo transfer may fail; implantation of the embryo may not occur, or for some reason it may come off the wall of the uterus;

and of course, there is always the problem of maintaining the pregnancy.

Although the steps of the procedure seem simple—none are. The success of *in vitro* fertilization is dependent on so many factors, and the overall success rate has been low. Part of the difficulty appears to be that the Fallopian tube's environment is presently impossible to match *in vitro*. New work in the field is now being done to find an answer to this problem. If it is somehow possible to either reproduce in the laboratory the environment of the Fallopian tubes or find a place in the body where fertilization and cell division can occur in a more natural environment before transfer to the uterus, the procedure will be more predictably successful.

Some experimentation is being done to determine the feasibility of placing egg-embryo chambers in the peritoneal cavity (inside the abdomen) of monkeys. Using this procedure, the ovum would be aspirated from the ovary, checked visually and placed in a small plastic chamber with the sperm collected from the father. This small plastic chamber is porous to allow the fertilized ovum to be surrounded by peritoneal fluid, which contains proteins, salts and other compounds that may make the environment more like that inside the Fallopian tube. After three to four days the embryo (if all is well) is then transferred to the uterus. According to Gary D. Hodgen, Ph.D. (chief of the Pregnancy Research Branch of the National Institute of Child Health and Human Development at the National Institutes of Health in Maryland, where the egg-embryo chambers were developed), results so far—although preliminary— have been promising.

With further investigation and refinement it may someday be possible to remove an ovum from a woman's ovary and allow it to be fertilized *in vitro*, then place the fertilized egg in he egg-embryo chamber inside her abdomen, just as is being studied in the monkeys. After the growing embryo underwent cell division in the chamber for several days, it would be transferred to the uterus, so it could implant and further embryological and fetal growth could continue. This kind of technique may someday provide a means for many or most women with an infertility problem to successfully have the children they and their husbands have so wanted. While all the answers are not yet known, much more research and experimentation will continue in the area of *in vitro* fertilization.

Genetic Engineering

The whole issue of genetic engineering and what it means is confusing to most people. Certainly it needs to be put into perspective and its potential advantages and the serious concerns regarding it explained. Genetic engineering is based on a technology called "recombinant DNA" (*deoxyribonucleic acid*). With this technique genetic material within a cell is essentially spliced and hereditary information rearranged.

To put this more simply, DNA is the basic blueprint for cell production and contains all the genetic information for the cell and the organism. Found in the center of the cell, the DNA directs all cellular activities. American scientists proved DNA's role in genetics in 1944. In 1953 the appearance of DNA—a tiny ladder-shaped molecule twisted like a corkscrew—was described. James Watson and Francis Crick called it a "double helix" and explained the zipperlike action of DNA. For the cell to divide and reproduce, the DNA unzips—splits down the center of its ladder—leaving the same genetic information on each half. Through a highly complex procedure, special enzymes attach to each half of the DNA by matching parts to each of the two equal half-ladders. These special enzymes rebuild the DNA to complete the new second half of each ladder. This splitting and rebuilding of DNA by the special enzymes results in two sets of DNA with the same genetic information. The cell then splits into two identical cells, each having one of the new strands of DNA. This process goes on endlessly, manufacturing cells with identical genetic information in each one.

Recombinant DNA, then, is the technique of rearranging—"recombining"—the genes found on the DNA ladder. Several important breakthroughs were necessary before this could occur. First, scientists had to purify the enzymes responsible for unzipping and rebuilding the DNA. With this information they had the ability to essentially cut pieces of genetic information out of one DNA molecule and insert these pieces into another DNA molecule. Scientists found that by using bacteria (the least complex form of life), they could get the bacteria to accept, then reproduce, the extracted segments of DNA—the genetic information.

As a result of this kind of research, human proteins could potentially be produced by inserting genes into bacterial DNA strands, with the help of special enzymes. In 1979 a human growth hormone was produced in bacteria. Other areas of research include the manufacturing of human insulin; a protein called Factor VIII, missing in hemophilia; interferon, which fights viral infections; and vaccines to provide immunity to viral diseases. The work performed so far has been directed toward manufacturing drugs and substances that could aid in the fight against disease.

However, there is hope that someday it will be possible to insert needed genes directly into those people who are missing them— for example, genes that govern the ability to produce growth hormone for dwarfs, Factor VIII for hemophiliacs or insulin for diabetics. Who knows? It may even be possible someday to remove or replace a faulty gene before or soon after conception, remove an extra chromosome or repair a faulty chromosome soon after conception. Obviously, all of these techniques—if they ever become possible—would be major breakthroughs and would allow each person the opportunity to reach his or her optimal potential and maintain a better quality of life without serious physical or mental abnormality. They would allow many who cannot survive today to live.

Although there is much good that might come from recombinant DNA/genetic engineering techniques, there are also some very legitimate concerns and fears. For one, some raise the possibility that "safe" bacteria used in recombinant DNA could accidentally be transformed into deadly bacteria, resulting in a devastating epidemic. Others fear that this technology could get into the wrong hands and be used in connection with bacteriological warfare. And of course, there is the fear that all of this intervention will lead to the manufacturing of a "super race"—little automatons looking, acting and thinking alike—totally lacking everything that makes each person a unique being.

Because of these concerns an international conference was held in 1975 to develop guidelines for safe experimentation. These guidelines are reviewed and revised periodically (the last revision was in 1980) by the National Institutes of Health in Maryland. One potentially major problem, however, lies in the fact that these very detailed guidelines only apply to research funded by the National Institutes of Health and other specific research funded by the federal government. This means that studies funded by and performed in the private industrial sector (and many companies perform such studies today) are not forced to conform to these or any other guidelines.

There are also those who fear that even if specific guidelines were put into law, an accident would occur, the guidelines would not be carefully enforced and followed, or some sort of sabotage would occur and endanger the lives and health of a substantial number of people. So far, no accidents are known to have occurred, and many scientists feel the dangers are merely hypothetical. Others feel that the technology is still very young, and there is no way to determine the possible long-range side effects and hazards. They primarily fear the lack of controls over private research and commercialization. (There does seem to be a great race to develop the technology to inexpensively mass-produce such drugs as interferon, Factor VIII and many, many others, because so much profit would be involved.) Obviously, with such a race it might be tempting to take shortcuts, and accidents could occur.

These various controversies will go on for some years to come. It is to be hoped that society will provide protection from potential (although hypothetical) accidents in all aspects of genetic engineering research and development—both federally funded and commercial endeavors. If the emphasis of research continues in the direction in which it is now going—to improve the health and well-being of all people—then the potential good and the number of lives that might possibly be saved would be phenomenal. With proper regulations and enforcement, as well as proper vision for its use, genetic engineering may well prove to be one of the most significant answers to many serious and life-threatening problems. Only the future will tell.

Fact or Fiction?

Science fiction writers have been correct in predicting many things. As the future turns fiction into fact, let us hope that the writers have been correct in envisioning developments that would make our world better and brighter and that they have been wrong in envisioning developments that would destroy, hurt or change the character and uniqueness of human life.

Since the time of Hippocrates, the basis for all medical work has been—above all, do no harm. All advances now being worked on must be judged by comparing their potential benefits to their potential risks. Those from which the greatest good can be attained are well worth pursuing.

Indeed, the future of perinatal care looks promising. All in all, we believe that each year will bring more advances to better ensure the health and well-being of mothers and unborn/newborn babies. New and exciting answers for many serious problems are just around the corner. Much has already been accomplished—and much more lies ahead. It is the responsibility of both professionals and the public alike to make sure no one strays from the intended goals—to make the world a better place to live—and to make life healthier and happier for those here today, as well as for our children, their children and all those who follow.

GLOSSARY

ABO INCOMPATIBILITY—Situation in which a mother and her infant have different blood types, and antibodies from the mother's blood destroy some of the baby's blood.

ABORTION—Expulsion of a fetus which is not able to survive; or termination of a pregnancy prior to the 20th week; can be spontaneous or induced. **THREATENED ABORTION**—bleeding experienced before 20 weeks gestation may be a sign of potential (threatened) abortion. **MISSED ABORTION**—bleeding took place, the conceptus stopped growing, did not survive, but did not pass spontaneously through the cervix and vagina; products of conception must be removed by "D & C" or suction extraction. **INCOMPLETE ABORTION**—some tissue has passed but some remain in the uterus; must be removed by "D & C" or suction. **INEVITABLE ABORTION**—bleeding and pain are occurring and spontaneous abortion cannot be avoided and will take place usually rather quickly.

ALPHA-FETOPROTEIN (AFP)—A protein produced by the fetus, found in the amniotic fluid and maternal blood in excessive amounts when a fetus has certain types of congenital malformations, especially neural tube defects.

AMNIOCENTESIS—A procedure in which a small amount of amniotic fluid is removed for analysis.

AMNIOTIC FLUID—Special fluid which surrounds the developing fetus within the uterus.

ANENCEPHALY—Serious congenital malformation in which the brain fails to develop.

ANESTHESIA—Complete absence of all sensation, including pain.

BETAMETHASONE—A cortisone-like hormone which, when given to a pregnant woman in premature labor, can induce fetal lung maturity.

BETASYMPATHOMIMETIC—Having actions or characteristics like those substances which stimulate beta receptors; among other actions, these agents relax the uterus and in pregnancy are used to slow or stop premature labor.

BRADYCARDIA—Slow heart beat.

BRAXTON-HICKS CONTRACTIONS—Intermittent tightening of the uterine muscles during pregnancy prior to active labor; sometimes called "false labor."

BREECH PRESENTATION—Condition in which the fetus positions itself buttocks and/or feet down prior to delivery, rather than the more common cephalic ("head down") position.

CEPHALIC PRESENTATION—Fetal "head down" position.

CEPHALOPELVIC DISPROPORTION (CPD)—The baby's head is too large in relationship to the mother's pelvis.

CESAREAN BIRTH (CESAREAN SECTION, C-SECTION)—Removal of the fetus through a surgical incision made in the mother's abdomen; surgical delivery.

CHROMOSOME—A structure which contains specific segments of DNA (genes) as part of the genetic material. AUTOSOME—One of 22 matching pairs of chromosomes (in the human). SEX CHROMOSOME—Pair of chromosomes (in the human) that determine the sex of the person.

CONTRACTION STRESS TEST (CST)—A means of measuring the placenta's function and the fetus's response to hypoxia by monitoring the fetal heart rate during uterine contractions.

DOWN'S SYNDROME—The common name for Trisomy 21, in which the affected person has an identifiable group of abnormalities. Often called mongolism.

DYSTOCIA—Abnormal labor.

ECLAMPSIA—Severe hypertension of pregnancy, with convulsions and possibly coma.

ENCEPHALOCELE—A neural tube defect in which a portion of the brain protrudes through an underdeveloped skull.

ENDOMETRITIS—Infection of the lining of the uterus, most commonly following a delivery in which the fetal membranes were ruptured for a prolonged period of time.

FETAL DISTRESS—A fetal condition in which the developing fetus shows one or more effects of sudden and/or chronic lack of oxygen.

FETOSCOPY—A technique in which the developing fetus can be seen through a special instrument inserted into the uterus through a tiny incision in the pregnant woman's abdomen.

GENE—The smallest unit of inheritance; a unit of DNA, located on a specific chromosome. DOMINANT GENE—A gene whose characteristic would always be expressed, or seen, in the offspring, whether one or two genes of a pair were present. RECESSIVE GENE—A gene whose characteristic would be seen only if two identical genes of a pair were inherited.

HIGH RISK PREGNANCY—Pregnancy in which there is a possibility or likelihood of a problem developing which might jeopardize the health or life of mother, baby or both.

HYALINE MEMBRANE DISEASE—See respiratory distress syndrome.

HYDROCEPHALUS—Brain abnormality in which there is too much spinal fluid ("water on the brain"), leading to an enlarged head.

INTRAUTERINE BLOOD TRANSFUSION—A procedure in which blood is introduced into the abdomen of a developing fetus; it is used with severe Rh disease.

INTRAUTERINE GROWTH RETARDATION—Reduction in fetal growth rate for any of a variety of reasons, such as uteroplacental insufficiency, infection, teratogens, etc.

LABOR—The process of giving birth, often referred to in stages. FIRST STAGE

OF LABOR—Extends from the start of labor until the time when the cervix is completely dilated. SECOND STAGE—Extends from the time of complete cervical dilatation until the baby has been delivered. THIRD STAGE—Extends from the delivery of the baby until the afterbirth has been expelled. FOURTH STAGE—newly recognized, the period of recovery during the first few hours after delivery.

L/S RATIO—A chemical test on the amniotic fluid that can predict fetal lung maturity; it reflects the relationship between two chemicals, lecithin and sphingomyelin.

MAGNESIUM SULFATE—A chemical compound with several actions useful in pregnancy: it is used to treat toxemia of pregnancy; may also be used to stop premature labor.

MISCARRIAGE—Spontaneous abortion; unexpected expulsion of an embryo from the uterus before 20 weeks of gestation.

MONGOLISM—See Down's syndrome.

NEONATOLOGY (NEONATOLOGIST)—A subspecialty of pediatrics involved with the care of the newborn infant; usually most concerned with the care of high risk newborns.

NEURAL TUBE DEFECTS—A group of congenital malformations caused by the failure of the embryo's primitive nervous system to develop normally.

OLIGOHYDRAMNIOS—Condition in which there is too little amniotic fluid around the fetus; associated with several types of congenital malformations.

OXYTOCIN—A hormone which stimulates contraction of the uterine muscles.

PERINATOLOGY (PERINATOLOGIST)—The field of specialized care of the expectant mother and her developing baby; usually involves care of high risk pregnancies—"high risk obstetrics."

PHOSPHATIDYL GLYCEROL (PG)—A compound which can be detected and measured in the amniotic fluid as a predictor of fetal lung maturity.

PLACENTA PREVIA—Condition in which the placenta is attached to the uterus in an abnormally low position, near or covering the cervix.

PLACENTAL ABRUPTION—Partial or complete detachment of the placenta from the uterine lining before the delivery of the baby.

PLACENTAL ASPIRATION—Technique by which a fetal blood sample can be obtained using a needle inserted through the mother's abdomen into the placenta.

POLYHYDRAMNIOS—Condition in which there is an excessive amount of amniotic fluid.

POST-DATE PREGNANCY—Pregnancy which goes more than two weeks beyond the expected delivery date.

POSTMATURITY SYNDROME—A group of problems in a fetus which result because of decreased placental function; may be the result of prolonged pregnancy.

POSTPARTUM—After delivery; refers to a period of six weeks after delivery.

PRE-ECLAMPSIA—A hypertensive disorder of pregnancy, not characterized by convulsions or coma.

PREMATURE—In pregnancy, labor and/or delivery which occurs after the 20th week but before the 36th week of gestation; also called *preterm*.

PROGESTERONE—A hormone normally produced in large amounts during pregnancy.

PROGESTIN—Progesterone-like compound.

PROLONGED PREGNANCY—Pregnancy which continues beyond 42 weeks.

PROSTAGLANDIN—Hormone which stimulates uterine muscle contractions as one of its actions. PROSTAGLANDIN INHIBITOR—Substance which prevents or slows the body's production of prostaglandins.

RESPIRATORY DISTRESS—Breathing difficulty. RESPIRATORY DISTRESS SYNDROME—A lung disorder of newborn infants, especially prematures, caused by a lack of surfactant; also called *hyaline membrane disease.* OTHER CAUSES of respiratory distress in the newborn include *transient tachypnea of the newborn, pneumonia* and *pneumothorax.*

RHOGAM®—Rh immune gamma globulin; a product which prevents the formation of Rh antibodies by an Rh negative person—that is, immunizes the person against Rh sensitization.

RUPTURE OF THE MEMBRANES—Breaking or leaking of the amniotic sac which surrounds the developing fetus; this allows the amniotic fluid to leak out into the vagina.

SEPSIS, SEPTICEMIA—Generalized infection of the body, in which the infection spreads in the body via the blood stream.

SPERM—Male germ cell, produced by the testicle.

SPINA BIFIDA—A neural tube defect in which the backbone fails to form normally, often allowing part of the spinal cord and its coverings to protrude.

SURFACTANT—A substance produced in the fetal lung which is associated with fetal lung maturity.

SYNDROME—A group of signs or symptoms that characteristically occur together in a specific disease.

TERATOGEN—Any substance able to induce malformation in the developing embryo.

TERM (PREGNANCY)—Pregnancy in which the fetus has developed fully; gestation of 37 weeks to 42 weeks.

THROMBOPHLEBITIS—Blood clot with inflammation.

TOCOLYTIC—That which stops labor; usually, tocolytic agents or drugs.

TOKODYNAMOMETER—Device which measures uterine contractions from the mother's abdominal wall.

TOXEMIA—Referring to the hypertensive diseases of pregnancy.

TRIMESTER—Three month period during pregnancy; as, the *first trimester*, which refers to the first three months, the *second trimester*, the middle three months, and the *third trimester* to the three months prior to delivery.

TRISOMY—Condition in which an offspring inherits an extra chromosome of a specific kind , so it has three rather than two of that type.

TUBAL PREGNANCY (ECTOPIC PREGNANCY)—Gestation in which the embryo implants in the Fallopian tube; as it grows the tube ruptures, causing bleeding and severe abdominal pain.

UTERINE CONSTRAINT—Crowding on the fetus or excessive pressure on it during intrauterine development; a cause of certain types of congenital malformations.

UTEROPLACENTAL INSUFFICIENCY (UPI)—Condition in which the placenta is not able to adequately meet the oxygen and/or nutritional needs of the developing fetus; can be either acute (sudden) or chronic (longstanding).

VENEREAL DISEASE—See Sexually Transmitted Disease.

VERSION—Procedure in which the fetus and uterus are manipulated to turn the fetus to the cephalic position.

BIBLIOGRAPHY

American Academy of Pediatrics Committee on Fetus and Newborn. Sixth Edition. Hospital Care of Newborn Infants, Evanston: American Academy of Pediatrics, 1977.

Committee on Perinatal Health, *Toward Improving the Outcome of Pregnancy*, White Plains: the Nahonar Foundation—March of Dimes, 1976.

Freeman, Roger K., M.D. and Garite, Thomas J., M.D. Fetal Heart Rate Monitoring, Baltimore: Williams & Wilkins, 1981.

Hayes, Arthur Hull, M.D., commissioner "Surgeon General's Advisory on Alcohol and Pregnancy." FDA Drug Bulletin 11 (1981): 1 & 10.

Hein, Herman A., M.D. "Evaluation of a Rural Perinatal Care System." Pediatrics 4 (1980): 540–546.

Hellman, Louis M.; Pritchard, Jack A.; and Wynn, Ralph M.: Williams Obstetrics. Fourteenth Edition. New York: Appleton—Century—Crofts, 1971.

James, Francis M., III, M.D. "A Guide to Anesthesia for Labor and Vaginal Delivery." Resident & Staff Physician April (1980): 89–98.

Johnson, John W. C., M.D. and Dubin, Norman H., Ph.D. "Prevention of Preterm Labor." Clinical Obstetrics and Gynecology 23 (1980): 51–73.

Kaback, Michael M., M.D. guest editor "Prenatal Diagnosis." Pediatric Annals 10 (1980): 13–65.

Merkatz, Trwin R., M.D.; Peter, John B., M.D.; and Barden, Tom R., M.D.: "Ritodrine Hydrochloride: A Betamimetic Agent for Use in Preterm Labor." Obstetrics & Gynecology 56 (1980): 7–12.

Queenan, John T., M.D., ed. A New Life. New York: Van Nostrand Reinhold Company, 1979.

Report of a Consensus Development Conference. Antenatal Diagnosis. Washington, D.C.: U.S. Department of Health, Education and Welfare (now Department of Health and Human Services), Public Health Services, National Institutes of Health, 1979.

Sinclair, John C., M.D. et al "Evaluation of Neonatal Intensive Care Programs." The New England Journal of Medicine 305 (1981): 489–494.

Smith, David W., M.D. and Wilson, Ann Asper The Child with Down's Syndrome (Mongolism), Philadelphia: W. B. Saunders Company, 1973.

Task Force on Cesarean Childbirth: Consensus Development Conference on Cesarean Childbirth (Draft Report), Washington, D.C.: U.S. Department of Health and Human Services, Public Health Service, National Institutes of Health, 1980.

INDEX

ABO Incompatibility
  (Blood)—30, 35–36
ACHONDROPLASIA
  —87, 88
AGE Risks
  (Maternal)—48–53,
  148
ALCOHOL—55–57
ALPHA-fetoprotein
  Levels—175–176
AMENORRHEA—64
AMNIOCENTESIS—
  163, 168–178, 241
AMNIOTIC Sac
  Rupture—206
ANALGESIA—213,
  217
ANEMIA—123
ANENCEPHALY—
  103
ANESTHESIA—
  215–217, 248–250,
  252
ANXIETY—150
APGAR Score—209
ASPHYXIA—108
ASTHMA—29
ANTICONVULSANT
  Medications—63
AUTOSOMAL
  Dominant
  Conditions—86–89

AUTOSOMAL
  Recessive
  Disorders—89–92

BANDING—96
BETAMETHASONE
  —233, 234
BETASYMPATHO-
  MIMETICS—
  228–231
BETA-
  THALASSEMIA—
  90, 91, 92
BIRTH Control Pill—
  64
BIRTH Defects—
  81–113; See also
  Congenital Defects
  and specific disorders
BIRTHS, Multiple—
  39–40; See also
  Delivery
BLEEDING,
  Vaginal—41–42,
  252
BLOOD
  Incompatibility—See
  RH Disease and
  ABO Incompatibility
  (Blood)
BLOOD Vessel
  Accidents—107–108

BRACHIAL Palsy—
  108–109
BRAXTON-HICKS
  Contractions—205,
  207
BREAST Enlargement
  and Tenderness—
  116–117
BREATHING
  Problems—117
BREECH Position—
  222
BRONCHIAL
  Asthma—See Asthma

CANCER
  (Childhood)—
  104–105
CARDIOMYOPATHY
  —22
CARPAL Tunnel
  Syndrome—115
CELLULAR
  Receptors—229
CEPHALOPELVIC
  Disproportion—239
CESAREAN Birth—
  235–260
CHLAMYDIA—79
CHROMOSOMAL
  Abnormalities—
  93–108

311

CHROMOSOME Breakage—99–100

CHROMOSOME Duplication (Trisomies)—96–99

CHROMOSOMES—82–85

CHROMOSOMES, Sex—100–102

CLEFT Lip (Harelip)—102

CLUBFOOT Deformities—102

CONGENITAL Defects—102–109, 243–244

CONGENITAL Hip Dislocation—102

CONGENITAL Infections—See Teratogens and specific types of infections

CONSTIPATION—119

CONTRACTION Stress Test (CST)—190–198

CORTICOSTEROIDS—198–199

CRAMPS, Leg—115

CROWNING—208

CYSTIC Fibrosis—90, 92

CYSTITIS—25

CYTOMEGALO-VIRUS Infection—70–71

DATING (pregnancy)—135–136

DDT (dichloro-diphenyl-trichloroethane)—67

DELIVERY—201–224; See also Breech Position and Cesarean Delivery

DENTAL Problems—118

DIABETES—16–20

DIET and Nutrition—127–132

DNA (Deoxyribonucleic Acid)—82–83, 302

DOWN'S Syndrome—97–99

DRUGS—58–63, 227–234

DYPLASIA—102

DYSTOCIA—218–219, 237–240

ECLAMPSIA—10–11, 14

EFFACEMENT—205

ENCEPHALOCELE—104

ENDOMETRITIS—252

ENVIRONMENTAL Hazards—67–68

EPISIOTOMY—208

ESTRIOL Testing—196–197

ETHANOL—227

EXERCISE—132–133

FACIAL Palsy—109

FAINTNESS—119-120

FAMILIAL Polydactyly—87, 88

FAMILIAL Polyposis—87, 88

FETAL Alcohol Syndrome—See Alcohol

FETAL Distress—112–114, 242–243

FETAL Fitness—190–198

FETAL hydantoin syndrome—63

FETAL Lung Maturity—173–174, 190–200, 232–234

FETAL Monitoring—179–189

FETAL Movement—140

FETAL Position—220–222; See also Breech Position

FETAL Surgery—297–299

FETAL trimethadione syndrome—63

FETOSCOPY—163, 295–297

FINANCIAL Considerations—448–149

FLUSHING—117

GALACTOSEMIA—90, 91

GAS—119

GENES—82–85, 89, 90, 92–93

GENETIC Counseling—109–112

GENETIC Engineering—302–304

GENETIC Defects—85–93; See also Autosomal Dominant Condition, Autosomal Recessive Disorders, and Congenital Abnormalities

GENETICS—82–85;
See also
Chromosomes,
Genes and specific
genetic defects
GENOTYPE—84
GERMAN Measles
(Rubella)—68–70
GLOMERULONEPH-
RITIS, Chronic—26
GONORRHEA—
74–75

HAIR Loss—117
HARELIP—*See* Cleft
Lip
HEARTBURN—
118–119
HEART Disease—
22–25
HEMOPHILIA—92,
93
HEREDITARY
Spherocytosis—87,
89
HERPES—75–77
HIGH Blood
Pressure—*See*
Hypertension
HUNTINGTON'S
Chorea—88
HYALINE Membrane
Disease—153
HYDROCEPHALUS
—104
HYPERTENSION—
10–16
HYPERTHERMIA—
66–67
HYPER-
THYROIDISM—
20–21, 91
HYPOXIA—108,
180–181

INCOMPETENT
Cervix—40–41
INFANT Special Care
Units—283,
284–285, 287
INFECTION—252
IN Vitro Fertilization—
See Test Tube Babies

KARYOTYPE—96
KIDNEY (Renal)
Disease—25–27
KLINEFELTER'S
Syndrome—101

LABOR—201–224
LAPAROSCOPY—300
LEG Cramps—*See*
Cramps, Leg
LIVER Disease—
27–28

MAGNESIUM
Sulfate—231
MEIOSIS—83
MENSTRUATION—
135, 136, 137
MENTAL
Retardation—90; *See
also* Down's
Syndrome
MISCARRIAGE—
45–46
MONOSOMY—101
MORNING Sickness—
121–123
MULTIFACTORIAL
Inheritance—102
MULTIPLE Births—
See Births, Multiple
MUSCULAR
Dystrophy
(Duchenne-type)—
92
MUSCLE Tone—116

NATURAL
Childbirth—213
NEONATOLOGIST
—272
NEURAL Tube
Defects—102,
103–104
NEUROFIBROMA-
TOSIS—87, 88
NON-Stress Test
(NST)—190–198
NURSES, Specialties—
270, 273
NUTRITION—*See*
Diet and Nutrition

OBSTETRICAL
Care—134–140, 166
OCCUPATIONAL
Hazards—67–68
OLIGOHYDRAM-
NIOS—162
OVER-the Counter
Drugs—*See* Drugs

PALMAR Erythema—
117
PCBs (Polychlorinated
Biphenyls)—67
PERINATAL Care—
261–293 passim
PHENOTYPE—84
PHENYLKETO-
NURIA (PKU)—90,
91
PHYSICIANS,
specialties—269, 272
PLACENTAL
Abruption—41–42,
240
PLACENTAL Previa—
42–43, 163, 240
PLACENTAL
Problems—41–43,
210, 223–224; *See*

also specific problems
POLYCYSTIC Kidney
  Disease (Adult-
  type)—87, 88
POLYGENIC
  Inheritence—102
POLYHYDRAMNIOS
  —162
POST-date
  Pregnancy—*See*
  Pregnancy, Post-date
PRE-Eclampsia—10–14
PRESCRIBED
  Drugs—*See* Drugs
PREGNANCY, Post-
  date—37–39
PREMATURITY—
  43–45, 225–232; *See
  also* Delivery
PROGESTINS—228
PROSTAGLANDIN—
  125
PROSTAGLANDIN
  Inhibitors—227–228
PTYALISM—117
PYLORIC Stenosis—
  103
PYELONEPHRITIS,
  Chronic—25

RADIATION—*See* X-
  RAY
Rh Disease—30–35
RUBELLA—*See*
  German Measles

SALIVA Increase—117
SEPSIS—252
SEX Chromosomes—
  See Chromosomes,
  Sex

SEX-Linked Recessive
  Defects—92–93
SEXUAL Intercourse—
  124–127
SICKLE Cell Anemia—
  91, 92
SMOKING—57–58
SONOGRAPHY—*See*
  Ultrasound
SPIDER Angiomas—
  117
SPINA Bifida—104
SPONTANEOUS
  Abortion—*See*
  Miscarriage
STILLBIRTH—46
STREET Drugs—*See*
  Drugs
STREPTOCOCCAL
  (Strep) Infections—
  78–79
STRESS—150
STRETCH Marks—
  115–116
STUFFY Nose—119
SYPHILIS—72–74

TAY-Sachs Disease—
  90, 91, 92
TERATOGENS—
  54–80
TEST Tube Babies—
  299–301
THROMBOPHLE-
  BITIS—253
THYROID Disease—
  20–22
TOXEMIA—10–11
TOXOPLASMOSIS—
  71–72
TRANSLOCATION
  (chromosomes)—99

TRISOMIES—*See*
  Chromosome
  Duplication
TUBEROUS
  Sclerosis—87, 88
TURNER'S
  Syndrome—
  101–102
TWINS—*See* Births,
  Multiple

ULTRASOUND—
  158–166
URINARY Tract
  Infections—25
UTERINE
  Constraint—
  105–107
UTERINE
  MALFORMATION
  —40–41
UTERINE Size—162
UTEROPLACENTAL
  Insufficiency
  (UPI)—190

VACUUM
  Extraction—
  212–213
VACTERL
  Syndrome—64
VAGINAL Bleeding—
  See Bleeding, Vaginal
VAGINAL
  Discharge—120–121
VENERAL Diseases—
  72–79
VERNIX—207
VISION—118
VITAMINS—130

X-RAY—64–66